J. Dissemond, K. Kröger
for Initiative Chronische Wunden (ICW) e.V. (Eds.)
CHRONIC WOUNDS

D1663756

Joachim Dissemond, Knut Kröger
for Initiative Chronische Wunden (ICW) e.V. (Eds.)

CHRONIC WOUNDS

Diagnostics – Therapy – Health Care

First edition

Edited by:
Prof. Dr. med. Joachim Dissemond
University of Essen
Department of Dermatology, Venerology and Allergology
Hufelandstraße 55
45147 Essen/Germany

Prof. Dr. med. Knut Kröger
Helios Hospital Krefeld
Clinic for Angiology
Lutherplatz 40
47805 Krefeld/Germany

Initiative Chronische Wunden e. V.
Wipertistr. 1a
06484 Quedlinburg/Germany

Contributors: Frank Assmus, Essen/Germany; Matthias Augustin, Hamburg/Germany; Christine Blome, Hamburg/Germany; Anke Bültemann, Hamburg/Germany; Adrien Daigeler, Tübingen/Germany; Joachim Dissemond, Essen/Germany; Richard Dodel, Essen/Germany; Sabine Eming, Cologne/Germany; Gerald Engels, Cologne/Germany; Peter Engels, Bergisch Gladbach/Germany; Cornelia Erfurt-Berge, Erlangen/Germany; Madeleine Gerber, Quedlinburg/Germany; Veronika Gerber, Spelle/Germany; André Glod, Löffingen/Germany; Wolfgang Hach, Frankfurt on the Main/Germany; Viola Hach-Wunderle, Frankfurt on the Main/Germany; Theresa Hauck, Erlangen/Germany; Katharina Herberger, Hamburg/Germany; Tobias Hirsch, Münster/Germany; Dirk Hochlenert, Cologne/Germany; Raymund E. Horch, Erlangen/Germany; Philipp Jansen, Essen/Germany; Anna Lena Kahl, Essen/Germany; Sigrid Karrer, Regensburg/Germany; Jonas Kolbenschlag, Tübingen/Germany; Jan Kottner, Berlin/Germany; Knut Kröger, Krefeld/Germany; Jan-Jakob Meyer, Leisnig/Germany; Anya Miller, Berlin/Germany; Stephan Morbach, Soest/Germany; Karl-Christian Münter, Hamburg/Germany; Kerstin Protz, Hamburg/Germany; Stephanie Reich-Schupke, Recklinghausen/Germany; Finja Reinboldt-Jockenhöfer, Essen/Germany; Gunnar Riepe, Boppard/Germany; Alexander Risse, Dortmund/Germany; Gerhard Rümenapf, Speyer/Germany; Manfred Schedlowski, Essen/Germany; Stephan Schreml, Regensburg/Germany; Andreas Schwarzkopf, Aura a. d. Saale/Germany; Rachel Sommer, Hamburg/Germany; Anja Stoffel, Karlstein on the Main/Germany; Ingo Stoffels, Essen/Germany; Markus Stücker, Bochum/Germany; Eike-Phillip Tigges, Hamburg/Germany; Wolfgang Paul Tigges, Hamburg/Germany; Christian Willy, Berlin/Germany; Johannes Wohlrab, Halle/Saale/Germany; Gernold Wozniak, Bottrop/Germany
Translated by: Bonke Tim Funke, Hamburg/Germany; Diane Eng Li Kheng, Singapore; Marieke O'Connor, Oxford/Great Britain and Joachim Dissemond, Essen/Germany

ELSEVIER

Elsevier GmbH, Hackerbrücke 6, 80335 Munich, Germany
Please send your feedback and your suggestions to kundendienst@elsevier.com

Chronische Wunden, Diagnostik – Therapie – Versorgung
© Elsevier GmbH, Germany, 2019. All rights reserved.
ISBN: 978-3-437-25641-7

This translation of Chronische Wunden, Diagnostik – Therapie – Versorgung, first edition, by Joachim Dissemond, Knut Kröger and Initiative Chronische Wunden (ICW e.V.) was undertaken by Elsevier GmbH.

ISBN   978-0-7020-6762-4
eISBN   978-7020-6763-1

Disclaimer
The translation has been undertaken by Elsevier GmbH at its sole responsibility. Practitioners and researchers must always rely on their own experience and knowledge in evaluating and using any information, methods, compounds or experiments described herein. Because of rapid advances in the medical sciences, in particular, independent verification of diagnoses and drug dosages should be made. To the fullest extent of the law, no responsibility is assumed by Elsevier, authors, editors or contributors in relation to the translation or for any injury and/or damage to persons or property as a matter of products liability, negligence or otherwise, or from any use or operation of any methods, products, instructions, or ideas contained in the material herein.
Although all advertising material is expected to conform to ethical (medical) standards, inclusion in this publication does not constitute a guarantee or endorsement of the quality or the value of such product or the claims made of it by its manufacturer.

The publisher accepts no liability for the completeness and choice of drugs listed
Protected brand names (registered trademarks) are usually specially indicated (®). The lack of references to such trademarks is not meant to imply that a name or trademark is free of third party rights.
When required, in the case of translations: Information on diagnosis and therapy may differ from standards which are generally accepted in Germany.
Caution: The dosages and instructions for use given for the pharmaceutical products mentioned may deviate from those approved by the local medical regulatory authority.

Bibliographic information of the German National Library
The German National Library catalogues this publication in the German National Bibliography; detailed bibliographic data can be accessed on the Internet via www.dnb.de

22   23   24   25   26   5 4 3 2 1

Please refer to the list of illustrations for copyright details relating to the photographic material used.

When referring to patients and professional titles, the gender-neutral form has been used for the sake of improving the text's readability. All references in the text always refer to **all genders** equally.

Content Strategist: Dr. Bernhard Gall, Munich/Germany
Content Project Management and Production: Julia Stängle, Munich/Germany
Copy Editing: Dr. Antje Kronenberg†, Gronau/Germany
Typesetting: Thomson Digital, Noida/India
Printing and binding: Drukarnia Dimograf Sp. z o. o., Bielsko-Biała/Poland
Cover Design: SpieszDesign, Neu-Ulm/Germany
Cover photo: © stock.adobe.com – swisshippo

Current information is available on the Internet **www.elsevier.com**

Foreword

At a time when we are facing a global crisis caused by the emergence of a new disease why is a book on chronic wounds of interest and relevance to us all?

There is no question that wounds are a common, expensive and often poorly managed aspect of clinical care that is delivered to patients in 2021. Data is emerging from a number of countries to suggest that in Western Countries around 10% of health care expenditure is used to treat patients with wounds. In a paper published at the end of 2020 it was shown that in the United Kingdom there had been a 70% increase in the number of patients and a 45% in the cost of treating patients a year over a 5 year period.

This alone is sufficient reason for good quality educational resources on wound healing to be produced. The need for education is apparent very quickly if you visit clinical areas or if you ask a clinical colleague for help and advice. In addition the research and evidence base on wound healing, although still weak, has increased in recent years. A wound journal which I act as the Editor in Chief has seen an increase in submissions of papers from 40 to 750 a year over the past 15 years.

This book is written and edited by a plethora of Nationally and Internationally known individuals and without doubt provides a huge amount of up to date and relevant information. It provides sufficient detail on the science underpinning clinical practice but remains focused on a wide range of clinically relevant diagnostic and therapeutic interventions. It is well illustrated and includes a large number of clinical images that are extremely helpful. The skill of the authors and editors allow this book to be both comprehensive and concise at the same time.

This book is a valuable resource for clinicians working in this area and with its link to an educational module provides the reader with a large amount of information and as such I would commend the book to you all without reservation as it will assist all in our daily clinical work.

The patients we all look after, the clinical colleagues we work with and the Health Care system we are part of need educational resources of this quality to ensure this subject is given the profile and support that is commensurate with the challenges we all face in 2021.

Cardiff/Great Britain, January 2021
Keith Harding CBE, FRCGP, FRCP, FRCS, FLSW
Professor of Wound Healing Research

Preface

The Initiative Chronische Wunden (ICW) e.V. is the largest professional society in the field of wound healing in the German-speaking countries. It was founded by nurses, doctors and others committed individuals interested in wound care in 1995. ICW works to improve the prophylaxis, diagnosis and therapy of people with chronic wounds.

A guiding principle of the ICW is: 'If all the knowledge and experience in the prevention and treatment of chronic wounds already available were used consistently and everywhere – a lot of suffering and also costs could be avoided'.

To ensure that this knowledge and experience in the prevention, diagnosis and therapy of patients with chronic wounds reaches nurses, doctors, and other committed individuals, ICW offers a wide range of education courses since many years. In recent years, these courses have been held worldwide. Therefore, it has seemed useful to translate teaching materials into English. Thus, it is a special pleasure to present the book '**Chronic Wounds – Diagnostics, Therapy, Care**', a further part of this advanced training programme.

In a compact form, it bundles medical and nursing knowledge that corresponds to the current state of the art and underlying science. Wherever there is relevant evidence, it is presented. In the many areas of prevention and therapy of chronic wounds for which there is no study-based evidence, it reflects the current state of clinical knowledge. It was our aim to create a common platform for doctors and nurses with this book. Therefore, we have been able to enlist the most renowned experts from the German-speaking countries as authors. We would like to take this opportunity to thank the authors who have worked for the ICW without honorarium!

Many good books that present partial aspects of chronic wounds are currently available. However, up to now there is hardly any up-to-date-book that present the diagnostic and therapeutic aspects in such a comprehensive and interdisciplinary way.

Therefore, we hope that this comprehensively written book will convey the important concerns of patients with chronic wounds very well to all interested parties, so that together we can improve the care of people with chronic wounds and their quality of life.

January 2021
For the ICW
Veronika Gerber, Anke Bültemann, Martin Motzkus, Christian Münter, Knut Kröger und Joachim Dissemond

Editors

Prof. Dr. med. Joachim Dissemond
University of Essen
Department of Dermatology, Venerology and
Allergology
Hufelandstraße 55
45147 Essen
Germany

Prof. Dr. med. Knut Kröger
Helios Hospital Krefeld
Clinic for Angiology
Lutherplatz 40
47805 Krefeld
Germany

Initiative Chronische Wunden e. V.
Wipertistr. 1a
06484 Quedlinburg
Germany

Authors

Frank Assmus
Nordlandaue 9
45357 Essen
Germany

Prof. Dr. med. Matthias Augustin
Universitätsklinikum Hamburg-Eppendorf
Institut für Versorgungsforschung in der Dermatolo-
gie und Pflegeberufen
Martinistraße 52
20251 Hamburg
Germany

Priv.-Doz. Dr. phil. Christine Blome
Universitätsklinikum Hamburg-Eppendorf
Institut für Versorgungsforschung in der Dermatolo-
gie und Pflegeberufen
Martinistraße 52
20251 Hamburg
Germany

Anke Bültemann
ASKLEPIOS Klinikum Hamburg-Harburg
Wundcentrum/Gefäßchirurgie
Eißendorfer Pferdeweg 52
21075 Hamburg
Germany

Univ.-Prof. Dr. Adrien Daigeler
BG Klinik Tübingen
Klinik für Hand-, Plastische, Rekonstruktive und
Verbrennungschirurgie
Schnarrenbergstraße 95
72076 Tübingen
Germany

Prof. Dr. med. Joachim Dissemond
University of Essen
Department of Dermatology, Venerology and
Allergology
Hufelandstraße 55
45147 Essen
Germany

Prof. Dr. med. Richard Dodel
Universität Duisburg-Essen
Geriatriezentrum Haus Berge, Contilia GmbH
Germaniastraße 1–3
45356 Essen
Germany

Prof. Dr. med. Sabine Eming
Universitätsklinik Köln, Klinik und Poliklinik für
Dermatologie, Venerologie und Allergologie
Kerpener Straße 62
50937 Cologne
Germany

Dr. med. Gerald Engels
MVZ St. Marien GmbH
Bayenthalgürtel 45
50968 Cologne
Germany

Dr. rer. nat. Peter Engels
EngelsConsult
Gartenstraße 25
51429 Bergisch Gladbach
Germany

Dr. med. Cornelia Erfurt-Berge
Hautklinik, Universitätsklinikum Erlangen
Ulmenweg 18
91054 Erlangen
Germany

Madeleine Gerber
Leitungsteam Qualitätsmanagement (QM)
Geschäftsstelle der Initiative
Chronische Wunden
Pölle 27/28
06484 Quedlinburg
Germany

Veronika Gerber
Schulung und Beratung im Wundmanagement
Anne-Frank-Straße 10
48480 Spelle
Germany

Dr. med. univ. André Glod
Untere Dorfstraße 19
79843 Löffingen
Germany

Prof. Dr. med. Wolfgang Hach
Gemeinschaftspraxis für Innere Medizin
Fahrgasse 89
60311 Frankfurt on the Main
Germany

Prof. Dr. med. Viola Hach-Wunderle
Gemeinschaftspraxis für Innere Medizin
Fahrgasse 89
60311 Frankfurt on the Main
Germany

Dr. med. sci. Theresa Hauck
Plastisch- und Handchirurgische Klinik
Krankenhausstraße 12
91054 Erlangen
Germany

Priv.-Doz. Dr. med. Katharina Herberger D.A.L.M.
Institut für Versorgungsforschung in der Dermato-
logie und bei Pflegeberufen
CeDeF – Dermatologische Forschung und
Ambulanzen
Universitätsklinikum Hamburg-Eppendorf
Martinistraße 52
20246 Hamburg
Germany

Univ.-Prof. Dr. med. Tobias Hirsch
Plastische, Rekonstruktive und Ästhetische
Chirurgie, Handchirurgie
Fachklinik Hornheide
Dorbaumstraße 300
48157 Münster
Germany

Dr. Dirk Hochlenert
Praxis für Diabetologie, Endoskopie und
Wundheilung
Merheimer Straße 217
50939 Cologne
Germany

Prof. Dr. med. Dr. h. c. Raymund E. Horch
Plastisch- und Handchirurgische Klinik
Krankenhausstraße 12
91054 Erlangen
Germany

Dr. med. Philipp Jansen
Klinik und Poliklinik für Dermatologie, Venerologie
und Allergologie
Universitätsklinikum Essen
Hufelandstraße 55
45147 Essen
Germany

Anna Lena Kahl
Institut für Medizinische Psychologie und
Verhaltensimmunbiologie
Universitätsklinikum Essen (AöR)
Hufelandstraße 55
45147 Essen
Germany

Prof. Dr. med. Sigrid Karrer
Dermatologische Klinik und Poliklinik
Universitätsklinikum Regensburg
93042 Regensburg
Germany

Dr. med. Jonas Kolbenschlag
Klinik für Hand-, Plastische-, Rekonstruktive und
Verbrennungschirurgie an der
Eberhard Karls Universität Tübingen
BG Klinik Tübingen
Schnarrenbergstraße 95
72076 Tübingen
Germany

Prof. Dr. rer. cur. Jan Kottner
Einheit Klinische Pflegewissenschaft
CharitéCentrum 1 für Human- und Gesundheits-
wissenschaften
Charité – Universitätsmedizin Berlin Charitéplatz 1
10117 Berlin
Germany

Prof. Dr. med. Knut Kröger
Helios Hospital Krefeld
Clinic for Angiology
Lutherplatz 40
47805 Krefeld
Germany

Dr. med. Jan-Jakob Meyer
Helios Klinik Leisnig
Colditzer Straße 48
04703 Leisnig
Germany

Dr. med. Anya Miller
Präsidentin der Deutschen Gesellschaft für
Lymphologie
Wilmersdorfer Straße 62
10627 Berlin
Germany

Dr. med. Stephan Morbach
Diabetes-Fußzentrum Westfalen
Marienkrankenhaus Soest
Widumgasse 5
59494 Soest
Germany

Dr. med. Karl-Christian Münter
Wundzentrum Hamburg
Heilholtkamp 54
22297 Hamburg
Germany

Kerstin Protz
Wundforschung am Universitätsklinikum Hamburg-
Eppendorf
Bachstraße 75
22083 Hamburg
Germany

Prof. Dr. med. Stephanie Reich-Schupke
Privatpraxis für Haut- und Gefäßmedizin
Hertener Straße 27
45657 Recklinghausen
Germany

Dr. med. Finja Reinboldt-Jockenhöfer
Klinik und Poliklinik für Dermatologie, Venerologie
und Allergologie
Universitätsklinikum Essen
Hufelandstraße 55
45147 Essen
Germany

Priv.-Doz. Dr. med. Gunnar Riepe
Gemeinschaftsklinikum Mittelrhein
Krankenhaus Heilig Geist
Hospitalgasse 2
56154 Boppard
Germany

Dr. med. Alexander Risse
Klinikum Dortmund, Diabeteszentrum
Münsterstraße 240
44145 Dortmund
Germany

Prof. Dr. med. Gerhard Rümenapf
Diakonissen Speyer-Mannheim
Diakonissen-Stiftungs-Krankenhaus Speyer
Paul-Egell-Straße 33
67346 Speyer
Germany

Prof. Dr. rer. biol. hum. Dipl.-Psych.
Manfred Schedlowski
Institut für Medizinische Psychologie und
Verhaltensimmunbiologie
Universitätsklinikum Essen (AöR)
Hufelandstraße 55
45147 Essen
Germany

Priv.-Doz. Dr. med. Stephan Schreml
Dermatologische Klinik und Poliklinik
Universitätsklinikum Regensburg
93042 Regensburg
Germany

Priv.-Doz. Dr. med. Andreas Schwarzkopf
Institut Schwarzkopf
Otto-von-Bamberg-Straße 10
97717 Aura a. d. Saale
Germany

Dr. med. Rachel Sommer
Zentrum für Psychosoziale Medizin
Institut für Versorgungsforschung in der Dermato-
logie und bei Pflegeberufen (IVDP)
Bethanien-Höfe Eppendorf
Martinistr. 41
20251 Hamburg
Germany

Anja Stoffel
Im Sandfeld 13
63791 Karlstein on the Main
Germany

Prof. Dr. med. Ingo Stoffels
Klinik und Poliklinik für Dermatologie, Venerologie
und Allergologie
Universitätsklinikum Essen
Hufelandstraße 55
45147 Essen
Germany

Prof. Dr. med. Markus Stücker
Klinik für Dermatologie, Venerologie und
Allergologie
Venenzentrum der Dermatologischen und Gefäß-
chirurgischen Kliniken
Kliniken der Ruhr-Universität Bochum
im St. Maria-Hilf-Krankenhaus
Hiltroper Landwehr 11–13
44805 Bochum
Germany

Dr. med. Eike-Phillip Tigges
Heinrich-Kock-Weg 18
22529 Hamburg
Germany

Dr. med. Wolfgang Paul Tigges
Ansorgestraße 26
22605 Hamburg
Germany

Prof. Dr. med. Christian Willy
Abteilung Unfallchirurgie, Orthopädie und septisch
rekonstruktive Chirurgie
Bundeswehrkrankenhaus Berlin
Scharnhorststraße 13
10115 Berlin
Germany

Prof. Dr. apl. Johannes Wohlrab
Universitätsklinik und Poliklinik für Dermatologie
und Venerologie
Martin-Luther-Universität Halle-Wittenberg
Ernst-Grube-Straße 40
06120 Halle/Saale
Germany

Prof. Dr. med. Gernold Wozniak
Klinik für Gefäßchirurgie
Knappschaftskrankenhaus Bottrop
Osterfelder Straße 157
46242 Bottrop
Germany

Abbreviations

A.	arteria
ABI	ankle-brachial index
AC	alternating current
ACE	angiotensin-converting enzyme
ADSC	adipose-derived stromal cells
AGAST	Arbeitsgruppe Geriatrisches Assessment
AHA	American Heart Association
AHCPR	Agency for Healthcare Research and Quality
ALA	δ aminolevulinic acid
ASA	acetylsalicylic acid
ASIC	acid-sensing ion channel
ATA	absolute atmosphere
AU	arterial ulcers
bFGF	basal fibroblast growth factor
BID	body integrity disorder
BMI	body mass index
BMR	basal metabolic rate
BP	bullous pemphigoid
BRT	bio-resonance therapy
BW	body weight
CAP	cold atmospheric plasma
CCL	compression class(es)
CDT	complex/complete decongestive therapy
CEA	cultured epidermal autografts
CEAP	Clinical-Etiology-Anatomy-Pathophysiology
CERAD	Consortium to Establish a Registry for Alzheimer's Disease
CFU	colony-forming unit
C-GAG	collagen-glycosaminoglycan
CHD	coronary heart disease
CI	confidence intervall
CLCI	cumulative life course impairment
CLI	critical limb ischaemia
CML	chronic myelogenous leukaemia
CN	Charcot neuropathy
CNS	central nervous system
CPG	clinical practice guidelines
CRP	C-reactive protein
CT	compression therapy
CT	computertomography
cUCA	cis-urocanic acid
CVC	central venous catheter
CVI	chronic venous insufficiency
CWIS	Cardiff Wound Impact Schedule
DACC	dialkylcarbamoyl chloride
DBD	Dielectric Barrier Discharge
DC	direct current

DFS	diabetic foot syndrome
DFS-SF	Diabetic Foot Ulcer Scale – Short Form
DFU	diabetic foot ulcers
DGE	German Nutrition Society
DGEM	German Society for Nutritional Medicine
DIF	direct immunofluorescence
DIP	distal interphalangeal joint
DLQI	Dermatology Life Quality Index
DMSO	dimethyl sulfoxide
DNOAP	diabetic neuro-osteoarthropathy
DOAK	direct oral anticoagulation
DRG	diagnosis-related group
DSA	digital subtraction angiography
DVT	deep vein thrombosis
EBM	evidence-based medicine
ECM	extracellular matrix
ECPA	Echelle comportementale de la douleur pour personnes âgées non communicantes
EDP	electronic data processing
EGF	epidermal growth factor
EHEC	enterohaemorrhagic *Escherichia coli*
ELISA	enzyme-linked immunosorbent assay
EMA	European Medicines Agency
eNOS	endothelial NO-synthase
ENT	ear, nose, throat
EPUAP	European Pressure Ulcer Advisory Panel
Er:YAG laser	erbium-yttrium-aluminium-garnet laser
ESDP	endoscopic subfascial dissection of perforator veins
ESR	erythrocyte sedimentation rate
EST	electrostimulation
ESWL	extracorporeal shockwave lithotripsy
ESWT	extracorporeal shock wave therapy
EWMA	European Wound Management Association
FAST	Functional Assessment Staging Test
FGF	fibroblast growth factor
FLQA-w	Freiburg Quality of Life Assessment for Wounds
FSH	follicle-stimulating hormone
GDS	Geriatric Depression Scale
GDS	Geriatric Disability Scale
GLOBIAD	Ghent Global IAD Categorisation Instrument
GPCR	G-protein-coupled receptors
H_2O_2	hydrogen peroxide
HBOT	hyperbaric oxygen therapy
HDL	high-density lipoprotein
HiTop	high tone therapy

HMG-CoA	3-hydroxy-3-methylglutaryl coenzyme A	OECD	Organisation for Economic Cooperation and Development
HP	hydropolymer	OM	osteomyelitis
HRWD	hydro-responsive wound dressing	OR	odds ratio
HSAN	hereditary sensory and autonomic neuropathy	PAD	peripheral artery disease
ICD	International Classification of Diseases	PAINAD	Pain assessment in advanced dementia
ICW	Initiative Chronische Wunden e. V.	PAL	Physical Activity Level
IDSA	Infectious Diseases Society of America	PAMP	pathogen-associated molecular pattern
IEG	immediate early genes	PBI	Patient Benefit Index
IIF	indirect immunofluorescence	PBS	phosphate-buffered saline
IL	interleukin	PCNA	proliferating cell nuclear antigen
IP	interphalangeal joint	PCRA	patient controlled regional anaesthesia
IPC	intermittent pneumatic compression	PDGF	platelet-derived growth factor
IU	international unit	PDT	photodynamic therapy
IWGDF	International Working Group on the Diabetic Foot	PEG	percutaneous endoscopic gastrostomy
KGF	keratinocyte growth factor	PET	positron emission tomography
LDL	low-density lipoprotein	Ph. Eur.	European Pharmacopoeia
LILT	low intensity laser therapy	PHI	polyhydrogenated ionogens
LLLT	low-level laser therapy	PHMB	polihexamethylene biguanide = polihexanide
LOPS	loss of protective sensation	PIP	proximal interphalangeal joint
MAO	monoamine oxidase	PM	polymeric membrane
MAS	medical adaptive systems	PPPIA	Pan Pacific Pressure Injury Alliance
MCP1	monocyte chemotactic protein 1	PTF	paratibial fasciotomy
MCS	medical compression stockings	PTS	post-thrombotic syndrome
MCT	monocarboxylate transporters	PU	polyurethane
MDCTA	multidetector computed tomographic angiography	PU	pressure ulcers
MLD	manual lymphatic drainage	PU-QOL	Pressure Ulcer Quality of Life Questionnaire
MMP	matrix metalloproteinase	PV	pemphigus vulgaris
MMST	Mini Mental Status Test	PVA	polyvinyl alcohol
MNA	Mini Nutritional Assessment	PVP	povidone-iodine
MoCA	Montreal Cognitive Assessment Test	RCT	randomised controlled trial
MPG	Medizinproduktegesetz	ROS	reactive oxygen species
MRA	magnetic resonance angiography	RTC	randomised controlled trial
MRI	magnetic resonance imaging	SAg	silver sulfadiazine
MRO	multiresistant organisms	SA-β-Gal	senescence-associated β-glucocerebrosidase
MRSA	methicillin-resistant Staphylococcus aureus	SCC	spinocellular carcinoma
MTH	metatarsal head	SCT	stem cell transplantation
MTP	metatarsophalangeal joint	SHI	statutory health insurance
MTPS	medical thrombosis prophylaxis stockings	SIRS	systemic inflammatory response syndrome
MUST	Malnutrition Universal Screening Tool	SNRI	serotonin-norepinephrine reuptake inhibitor
NO	nitric oxide	SSD	silver sulfadiazine
NOS	nitrogen species	SSRI	selective serotonin reuptake inhibitor
NOSF	nano-oligo-saccharide factor	TBI	toe-brachial index
NPUAP	National Pressure Ulcer Advisory Panel	TCA	tricyclic antidepressant
NPWT	negative pressure wound therapy	TCC	total contact cast
NPWTi	NPWT instillation therapy	tcPO$_2$	transcutaneous partial pressure of oxygen
NRS	numerical rating scale	TEP	transepithelial potential
NRS	Nutritional Risk Screening	TFDD	Test for the Early Diagnosis of Dementia with Differentiation from Depression
NSAID	non-steroidal anti-inflammatory drug		
NTM	non-tuberculous mycobacteria	TGF	transforming growth factor
O$_2$	oxygen	TIMP	tissue inhibitor of metalloproteinases

TLC	thin-layer chromatography		**VLU**	venous leg ulcers
TNF	tumour necrosis factor		**VRE**	vancomycin-resistant enterococci
TRPV	transient receptor potential channel vanilloid		**VRS**	verbal rating scale
			VSS	Vancouver Scar Scale
TUG	timed up and go test		**VW-TCC**	Ventral Windowed Total Contact Cast
UCS	ulcer compression stocking system		**WDR**	wide-dynamic-range
UV	ultraviolet		**WHO**	World Health Organisation
V.	vena		**WHR**	waist-to-hip ratio
VAS	visual analogue scale		**wIRA**	water-filtered infrared A
VEGF	vascular endothelial growth factor		**WWS**	Würzburg Wound Score

Illustration credits

Reference to the relevant source of all the illustrations in this work can be found at the end of the legend title in square brackets. Any other graphics and illustrations not explicitly marked © are protected by copyright of Elsevier GmbH, Munich, Germany.

E645   Telser. Elsevier's Integrated Histology, 2007, Elsevier Mosby

F210-025   Buggy D. Can Anaesthetic management influence surgical-wound healing? The Lancet 2000; 35 (9227): 355–357

F1023-001 Voisin T, Vellas B. Diagnosis and Treatment of Patients with Severe Alzheimer's Disease. Drugs & Aging 2009; 2: 135–44

F1024-001 Mostafalu P, et al. Smart bandage for monitoring and treatment of chronic wounds. Small 2018; 6: e1703509

F1025-001 Blome C., Baade K., Debus ES., Price P. and Augustin M. The „Wound-Qol": A short questionnaire measuring quality of life in patients with chronic wounds based on three established diseasespecifi c instruments. Wound Repair Regen 22: 504-14

F1026-001 Korn P, et al. Why insurers should reimburse for compression stocking in patients with chronic venous stasis. J Vasc Surg 2002; 35 (5): 950–7

F1032-001 Friedel G. Operative Behandlung der Varicen, Elephantiasis und Ulcus cruris. Arch Klin Chir 1908; 86:143–59

F1033-001 Madelung O. Ueber die Ausschälung circoider Varicen an der unteren Extremität. Verh Dtsch Ges Chir 1884; 13:114–7

F1034-001 Hemmati, A. A./Mojiri Forushani, H./Mohammad Asgari, H.: Wound healing potential of topical amlodipine in full thickness wound of rabbit. In: Jundishapur Journal of Natural Pharmaceutical Products. 2014;9(3):e15638. Published 2014 Jun 16.

F1035-001 Serra R, et al. Doxycycline speeds up healing of chronic venous ulcers. Int Wound J 2015; 12: 179–184

G840   Schörcher F. Kosmetische Operationen. Lehmann. Munich/Germany 1955

L190   Gerda Raichle, Ulm/Germany

L231   Stefan Dangl, Munich/Germany

M291   Kerstin Protz, Hamburg/Germany

O1014   Bernd von Hallern, WOUND ADVERTISING Foto & Video-produktionen, Stade/Germany

O1089   Prof. Dr. Knut Kröger, Krefeld/Germany

P573   Prof. Dr. med. Wolfgang Hach, Frankfurt on the Main /Germany

P574   Prof. Dr. jur. Volker Großkopf, Cologne/Germany

P575   Dr. med. Stephan Morbach, Soest/Germany

P576   Prof. Dr. rer. cur. Jan Kottner, Berlin/Germany

P577   Dr. med. Jonas Kolbenschlag, Tübingen/Germany

P578   Klinik für HPRV, vertreten durch: Univ.- Prof. Dr. Adrien Daigeler, Tübingen/Germany

P579   Dr. med. Anya Miller, Berlin/Germany

P580   Prof. Dr. med. Joachim Dissemond, Essen/Germany

P581   Dr. Wolfgang Paul Tigges, Hamburg/Germany

P583   PD Dr. med. Andreas Schwarzkopf, Aura a. d. Saale/Germany

P584   Prof. Dr. med. Ingo Stoffels, Essen/Germany

P585   Prof. Dr. med. Christian Willy, Berlin/Germany

P586   Prof. Dr. med. Stephanie Reich-Schupke, Bochum/Germany

P587	Dr. med. Dirk Hochlenert, Cologne/Germany	**T1060**	Uniklinik Essen, Abteilung für Dermatologie, Wundambulanz
P588	Dr. med. André Glod, Löffingen/Germany	**U349**	Mölnlycke Health Care GmbH, Erkrath/Germany
P589	Frank Assmus, Essen/Germany	**V481**	medi GmbH & Co. KG, Bayreuth/Germany
P590	Dr. med. Finja Jockenhöfer, Essen/Germany	**V600**	Julius Zorn GmbH, Aichach/Germany
P591	Prof. Dr. med. Sabine Eming, Cologne/Germany	**V858**	Bösl Medizintechnik GmbH, Aachen/Germany
P592	Veronika Gerber, Spelle/Germany	**V859**	Adtec Europe Limited, Hounslow/UK
P593	Prof. Dr. med. Matthias Augustin, Hamburg/Germany	**V860**	Medline International Germany GmbH, Kleve/Germany
P607	Prof. Dr. med. Dr. h. c. Raymund E. Horch, Erlangen/Germany	**V861**	LEVABO®, Skanderborg/Denmark
P608	Dr. med. Karl-Christian Münter, Hamburg/Germany	**V862**	Mit freundlicher Genemigung der Firma SastoMed GmbH, Georgsmarienhütte/Germany
P609	Anja Stoffel, Karlstein on the Main/Germany	**V863**	LINET spol. s r.o., Slaný/Czech Republic
P610	Dr. med. Gerald Engels, Cologne/Germany	**V864**	Brümmer Orthopädie GmbH, Cologne/Germany
P611	Prof. Dr. med. Markus Stücker, Bochum/Germany	**W1012-01**	THE NATIONAL PRESSURE ULCER ADVISORY PANEL, Westford, MA/USA
T1012	CWC Comprehensive Wound Center Universitätsklinikum Hamburg-Eppendorf/Germany	**W1083**	Deutsches Historisches Museum Berlin/Germany
T1051	Prof. Amit Gefen, Department of Biomedical Engineering, Faculty of Engineering, Tel Aviv University/Israel	**W1084**	Wund-DACH Deutsch-Österreichisch-Schweizerische Wundheilungsorganisation, Wien/Austria
T1052	University Centre for Nursing and Midwifery, Ghent University Hospital, Ghent/Belgium	**W1085**	Initiative Chronische Wunden (ICW) e.V., Quedlinburg/Germany
T1054	Földiklinik Hinterzarten, Fachklinik für Lymphologie, Hinterzarten/Germany	**W1093**	Dr. Gunnar Riepe, Boppard/Germany
		W1094	Anke Bültemann, Hamburg/Germany

Contents

I

The basics

Wolfgang Hach, Viola Hach-Wunderle

History of the treatment of chronic wounds

1.1 Introduction

Dealing with an acute wound is as much a part of our lives as eating and drinking. It is vital that an organism which has been injured by external influences is healed quickly with a programmed repair. Otherwise, life could be in danger. In human history, acute wounds such as those caused by hunting, fighting in a war, or using tools have played the most crucial role. They occurred in all areas of the body.

A chronic wound used to be referred to as 'old damage' or 'old ulcer' and could last for years or decades. Poor people were most affected.

One aspect has special significance for chronic wounds: the relationship to the venous system of the lower extremity or in other words to the hydrodynamics of the circulatory system. Thinking in this way leads us to human anthropology. With the appropriation of the upright gait as a characteristic of *Homo sapiens,* unique adaptations of the circulatory system were required to overcome the hydrostatic pressure. In evolution, these 'auxiliary organs', such as the venous valves, immediately turned out to be significant risk factors for the chronification of a corresponding wound. The connection between heavy physical work while standing and a chronic venous leg ulcer would probably have been obvious.

Today, of course, the pathophysiology of chronic wounds lists other causes in addition to venous circulation disorders, e. g. chronic infections or metabolic disorders. These were also known and feared in the history of medicine just think of leprosy or St. Antonius fever (ergot) but at that time, the causal connections were obscure. We would like to discuss here chronic ulcer diseases of the lower leg and its history over the last two millennia, along with the physicians and their suffering patients.

1.2 Venous leg ulcers

In human phylogeny, as a result of the upright gait, the circulatory system required special anatomical and physiological conditions from the peripheral veins due to the increased hydrostatic pressure. Dysfunction of these mechanisms due to poor functioning and overloading leads to the pathophysiological situation of venous hypertension, i. e. the peripheral venous pressure does not drop physiologically by using the muscles and the effect of suction-pumping of the legs during physical work. As a result of this venous hypertension, chronic venous ulcer disease develops over the years.

The most common cause of venous hypertension is secondary venous insufficiency due to trunk varicose veins. Accordingly, both internal pathophysiological and external environmental or social influences are involved in the development of chronic venous ulcer disease. These facts have remained unchanged over thousands of years.

1.2.1 Varicose veins and chronic venous ulcers throughout history

The smaller size of the human body in ancient times may have been advantageous for venous haemodynamics, as well as lessening the frequency of diseases with venous hypertension. *Homo sapiens neanderthalensis* had an average height of 1.60 m and a weight of 60–80 kg. Acceleration in growth only began 100 years ago, at least in the white-skinned population. However, it has not been proven that chronic ulcer disease has become more common since then.

Most frequently, in the entire history of medicine, chronic venous leg ulcers were caused by trunk and perforator varicose veins. During the last 200 years, postthrombotic syndrome caused by leg and pelvic vein thrombosis has additionally been described.

Sporadic congenital malformations such as aplasia of the venous valves or Klippel-Trenauney syndrome played a lesser role.

The severe varicose vein disease with its pronounced varicose veins and tissue swelling, ending up with an open wound, was recognisable at first sight. The 'old ulcer' or longlasting sore used to be a painful condition for many patients, severely affecting their lives. Due to their inability to work, these people fell into deep social misery. Thromboembolism or bacterial infections such as erysipelas could also lead to death which is why we speak of venous leg ulcers as a *Morbus ulceris cruris venosi chronici*.

In the drafting of this chapter, a new medical-historical approach towards older accounts is emerging. Today we distinguish between uncomplicated (reticular) varicose veins without serious health significance and so-called *Morbus ulceris cruris venosi chronici*, the chronic venous ulcer disease with severe complications which was not clinically relevant in former times against the background of severe diseases such as plague, cholera and a generally short life expectancy. Both venous diseases have absolutely nothing to do with each other.

Physical strain on the patient played a decisive role in the development of chronic venous ulcer disease. They reflected the different circumstances of the personal individual, as well as the social environment as a whole, and it could not have been better described by Adolf von Bardeleben (see below). Little has changed over the millennia since Wolfgang Hach coined the term 'Berlin triad' for the old Berlin of Heinrich Zille (1858–1929): social misery, hunger and chronic leg ulcers (➤ Fig. 1.1).

Before the invention of anaesthesia and antisepsis in the 19th century, all so-called 'varicose vein surgeries' were performed not because of the varicose veins themselves, but due to chronic venous leg ulcers, because up till then even the smallest operation was associated with severe pain and various dangers.

Varicose veins and chronic venous ulcers in ancient Greece and Rome

Our modern medicine has its roots in the advanced cultures of ancient Greece and Rome. In particular, two medical personalities have shaped the image

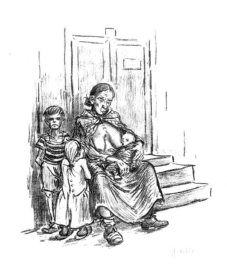

Fig. 1.1 Heinrich Zille 'Hunger'; Hach's Old-Berlin triad: social misery, hunger and chronic leg ulcers. [W1083]

of medical art and science over thousands of years: Hippocrates (460–375 BC) and Galen (130–200 AD).

De vulneribus et ulceribus from/according to Hippocrates in the 4th century BC

Hippocrates was born in 460 BC on the Greek island of Kos to a family of doctors. For 12 years he travelled the country as a doctor to learn and teach. Then he settled on the island of Kos and founded the Koan school (➤ Fig. 1.2). His doctrine of diseases was based on the theory of the four primary elements of fire, water, air and earth, the qualities of which had to be *warm, humid, cold and dry*, relative to each other.

The teaching of the elements is documented in the *Corpus hippocraticum*, a collection of more than 60 original writings. It contains the treatise Περι ελκων (on wounds and ulcers) with various recipes for the conservative treatment of old ulcers on the shins.

In the translation of Grimm and Lilienhain in 1838, it says: *'Dryness of the wound approaches the healthy, dampness is closer to the sick.'* Cleaning old wounds with a sponge is beneficial. The Caric ointment appeared to be particularly suitable for various external

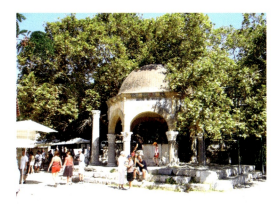

Fig. 1.2 The (alleged) plane tree of Hippocrates on the island of Kos. [P573]

applications. Caria was a country in Asia Minor with the capital Heraclea.

Caric ointment according to Hippocrates

- Helleborus niger ~ black hellebore
  dissolves tataric moisture
- Sandaracha Graecorum ~ rother arsenic
  sharp corrosive salt
- Cuprum ~ copper shavings
  cleans and is used for ointments
- Roasted lead with a lot of sulphur
  it dries, halts infection and heals in an ointment
- Arsenicum album ~ arsenic
  externally, to 'etch away' the flesh
- Spanish fly ~ Cantharides
  base for blister plasters
- Compounding with cedar oil

The later translation by Robert Fuchs from 1895 deals in particular with the surgical therapy of chronic leg ulcers.

Surgical therapy by Hippocrates

'If an ulcer develops as a result of the blood flow (varicose veins) mediated by the blood vessels, the blood must be drawn from these vessels. If this is not the case, the swellings (varicose veins) must be treated with quite deep and frequent bleeding using the sharpest and thinnest iron instruments possible. Rinse off with vinegar, cover with adipose, carded, soft wool which has been soaked in wine and olive oil, and keep the body part in such a position that the blood flows upwards, not downwards (elevation)'.

Grimm, Lilienhain 1838

Old ulcers at Cornelius Celsus in ancient Rome around the turn of the millennium

Celsus (30 BC 45 AD) is considered to be the most significant medical writer in ancient Rome. He reported on the sciences which every educated Roman had to master. He also found the causal relationship between varicosis and chronic leg ulcers in the writings of Hippocrates.

Celsus writes: *'However, if an old ulcer is ongoing, cut around it with a knife, cut out its margins and make incisions into the surrounding bluish areas. If there is a small varicose vein in the ulcer preventing healing, cut it out as well ("si varicula intus est, quae id sanari prohibet, ea quoque excidenda")'.*

Note   Similar operations were later reported by Adolf von Bardeleben and Nußbaum (see below).

Claudius Galenus after the turn of the millennium in Rome

Galen (131–200 AD) was one of the greatest doctors of all time. With his theory of the four bodily humours he created an ordering system of medicine based on the elementary theory of Hippocrates as well as the anatomical and physiological bases of the Alexandrian school. According to Galen's humoral theory, the bodily fluids *blood, yellow and black bile, and mucous* are generally in a healthy relationship with each other; dyscrasia causes illness.

Galen was born in Pergamon but mainly lived in Rome. Most of his writings were lost in the great fire of the Temple of Peace in 191, but 83 genuine and 19 ambiguous documents have survived; they were published in Latin or Greek editions, such as the famous Aldina of Venice in 1525.

Galen was a doctor and a pharmacist. His pharmacy was next to the Peace Temple and burned down with it. But Galen's recipes carried on being followed for centuries. The prescription for cabbage for 'old damage' can be read in the Lorcher Kräuterbuch (book of herbs) from 1731:

'Galenus writes/cabbage clamps the wounds together: Experience shows/that cooking the leaves in red wine/ and covering the wound/often heals large/deep/hollow wounds. The urine from someone/who has eaten

cabbage leaves for a number of consecutive days/is supposed to heal boils and cavities/cancer and similar skin impurities. Cabbage herb taken late in the 'Hew' month/with the middle ribs removed/the leaves cooked in a white wine/the limbs washed with the broth/then covered with the warm leaves/extracts the pain and heals all the old damage and festering gently.'

Galen was an advocate of using dressings as therapy, as was Hippocrates. He used various techniques. He also described the varicose vein operation on the lower leg, but without emphasing the relationship to 'old ulcers'; he was not a surgeon himself.

Varicose veins and chronic venous ulcers in the Middle Ages and before the introduction of anaesthesia and asepsis in the 19th century

The Middle Ages are the period from the 6th to the 15th century. Arabic-Islamic medicine, monastic medicine and also the western medicine schools had written down their teachings in a number of famous manuscripts. The first universities were founded.

From the 15th century onwards, the modern era brought great scientific discoveries and the rapid development of all sciences. The invention of letterpress printing around 1450 proved to be an absolute prerequisite for the preservation and dissemination of knowledge. New developments in medicine could now be followed well. However, in the beginning everything continued as it always had. The decisive turning point in medicine did not come until the 19th century with the invention of anaesthesia in 1844 and asepsis in 1865. Several impressive forms of treatment came up thereafter.

The *Hauß-Apotheck* of Joannis Gufer in 1689

The widespread disease of chronic venous leg ulcers had always been dependent on folk medicine among ordinary people in rural and urban areas, but hardly anyone had written about it. A little book by Joannis Gufer introduces the reader to the life of the poor people at that time. Not much is known about the author except that he was a practising doctor (*Arztney*

Doktorn) in Memmingen. He wrote prescriptions 'of minimal things/that should only be thrown away or not cared for/or of otherwise traditional means/which I either tried and experienced myself/or heard about from others. The catalogue has been brought together/so that a medic/can treat a sick person/who has no money/rurally where there are no pharmacies.' Even old shoes held a healing power for Gufer in treating a chronic ulcer.

Gufers recipe using old shoes

'To dry and heal old ulcers on shins/take eggshells and soles of shoes/burn them to make a powder/add cattle excrement which has been collected in the stomach and then dried/sprinkle it over the ulcer several times. One can also distil a delicate oil from collected shoes/which eradicates all sorts of tumours.'

The art of Doctor Weinhold for the healing of old skin ulcers in 1810

Using bandages as therapy, also with compression, has been a tradition since ancient times. Again and again, healers have invented new materials and techniques, with a great deal of success when used by experienced practitioners. An example of this is known from the early 19th century.

Dr. Karl August Weinhold (1782–1829) had studied philosophy, physics and other subjects in addition to medicine. After extensive travel, even to America, he was appointed professor of surgery at the University of Halle-Wittenberg in Germany. His books dealt among other things with historical and philosophical topics.

According to Weinhold, the previous therapies for treating chronic varicose veins had often shown no satisfactory effect. *'Annoyance with unsuccessful treatments finally prompts the surgeon to abandon such patients and to leave them to their fate.'* Weinhold invented an elaborate adhesive bandage for the treatment of ulcerations lasting many years.

Weinhold's adhesive bandage

The localised treatment starts with a series of four different mercury preparations used up to the granulation tissue, which is followed by the application of the 'Circulair plaster':

'The first patch is placed in the middle of the ulcer. It now divides the ulcer into two halves, which are covered each time so that one plaster overlaps the other, like the turns of the woodchip bandages. Then a light compress is placed on top so that the excreted serum is absorbed and the afflicted part is not contaminated. I let common and poor people carry on doing their housework during the cure, otherwise they would not bother getting treatment. Rich people with foot ulcers needed to rest and keep their legs raised. The poor were rebandaged once every 24 hours, the rich two and three times, depending on the flow of the serum.

This treatment must continue until the epidermis has finally healed: then the healed wound is exposed to the open air as much as possible to get it used to this beneficial stimulation again. Whoever has felt the uplifting experience of having removed a twenty-, even thirty-year-old evil so quickly, so safely and so pleasantly will not begrudge the time and effort it takes to teach poor sick people how to use compression plasters, if he can carry that sweet feeling in his heart as a reward.'

Bernstein's saphaena surgery for ulcer disease in 1820

Even the operation described by the surgeon Bernstein at the beginning of the 19th century, long before anaesthesia and asepsis, corresponds entirely to the spirit of the ancient world. Johann Gottlieb Bernstein (1747–1835) initially travelled through Austria and Germany as a journeyman barber. He then settled in Ilmenau as barber and wound care doctor. In 1896 he went to Jena University with the title of court surgeon, later to Halle and finally in 1810 as a professor to the new Friedrich University in Berlin. He wrote many articles and books, including a *Praktisches Handbuch für Wundärzte* ('Practical manual for wound care doctors') in four volumes in 1794.

Bernstein distinguished different forms of ulcers according to the secretion of *'bad pus or gauche. Ulcers which are surrounded by varicose veins derive great benefit from wrapping and a horizontal position. However, if there is a considerable dilatation of the blood vessels, the most straightforward cure is surgery.'*

Bernstein's operation

'Around the saphaena, where it crosses the knee joint, a ligature is applied. Since the veins are only full to bulging when the patient is standing, the operation must also be performed standing. The patient is placed next to a chair, holding onto the back. The affected limb must be turned to the light. In this position, the patient's skin is lifted into a transverse fold and is held on one side by the wound doctor and on the other by an assistant. Through this fold, the wound doctor stabs a sharp knife. A curved silver needle with a rounded tip can then pierce the cell tissue connected to the vein without risk of damaging the blood vessel, and a ligature thread can be guided around. The patient is then made to lie down, and the ligature threads are tied together over the vein. The edges of the skin around the wound are now pulled together by adhesive plasters, and a compress and bandage are applied so that the vein is gently compressed both above and below the site of the injury. The ligature falls off on about the ninth day, after which the parts usually heal.'

Note   The procedure was certainly rarely performed before applying anaesthesia. It is based on the idea that the V. saphena magna has a causal implication in the course of the disease.

Von Bardeleben's electropuncture of varices and ulcer excision in chronic venous ulcer disease in 1852

Adolf von Bardeleben (1819–1895) was one of the great surgeons of the 19th century. He received his surgical training in Heidelberg under Franz Carl Naegele (1778–1851) and was appointed professor at the University of Greifswald in 1868. Here he gained a reputation as a brilliant surgeon. In 1852 he published a three-volume *Lehrbuch der Chirurgie und Operationslehre* ('Textbook of surgery and surgical theory'). In 1868 he succeeded Johann Christian Juengken (1793–1875) at the Berlin Charité.

Adolf von Bardeleben impressively described the devastating situation of patients with chronic venous leg ulcers during his time at the 19th Congress of the German Society of Surgery in Berlin in 1891:

'On the ward, which I have the honour to preside over, there are often 80 to 100 patients with lower leg ulcers and varicose veins known to be a real nuisance for a surgical ward. In Greifswald, too, I had already had to suffer from the onslaught of tramps with varicose ulcers, migrating from one hospital to the next and who, since the new hospital opened in Greifswald, preferred to settle down there. A special ward was even constructed for them, in the warehouse, and even occasionally, if there were too many of them, bedding was laid down to accommodate them.'

We merit von Bardeleben with distinguishing the varicose ulcer from various other ulcers as a disease entity: *'In the case of the oedematous ulcer, the therapy is to be directed essentially against the oedema and the varicosities of the veins in the lower leg, where ulcers occur very frequently, which is why treatment of the ulcers is often combined with that of the varicosities.'* Palliative or 'radical' remedies were available (see box). Von Bardeleben surgically recommended *'electropuncture with multiple needle punctures in the varices'*. The undermined callous edges were removed from the ulcer, and pressure dressings with adhesive plaster strips (so-called Baynton's dressings) made it possible to achieve *'the transformation of the secretion into benign pus of relative quantity'*. Thus the ulcer was transformed into a festering surface, which then scarred in a familiar manner. However, *'every operation had to be regarded as a life-threatening intervention'*.

Von Bardeleben's palliative measures for venous leg ulcers in 1859

- Compression dressings with bandages, rubber strips,
- Bayton wraps/bindings with adhesive plaster,
- Lace-up leather stockings,
- Elastic compression stockings made of rubber fabric,
- Staying still and elevation,
- Cold compresses.

Von Bardeleben's radical measures to treat venous leg ulcers in 1859

- French methods according to Delpech, Velpeau, Sanson and others,
- Implementation of the tangential wound,
- Prevention, cutting out, peeling out,
- Viennese etching paste according to Marchal,
- Electropuncture.

Note   Celsus in ancient Rome had already described the surgical method of circumcising the ulcer.

The Von Nußbaum dissection in venous leg ulcers in 1873

With Johann Nepomuk Ritter von Nußbaum (1829–1890), the era of modern development in surgery was about to start with the invention of antisepsis, around 1864. Von Nußbaum was already appointed at the age of 31 as a full professor of surgery at the University Hospital of Munich. He became highly distinguished, and became Privy Councillor and the consultant General Staff Doctor for the Army. Many of his scientific works dealt with war surgery. He was active on the battlefields in 1859 and 1866 (Austria/Italy) as well as 1870/71 (Germany/France). He was the first German to visit Joseph Lister in England to learn about antisepsis. The procedure was first used by him in emergency operations on the battlefield, but from 1874/75 it was also used consistently in his Munich clinic.

From a scientific point of view, Von Nußbaum was particularly interested in orthopaedic operations. For severe pain, he introduced the nerve stretching method (see below). In the course of his life, he is said to have performed a total of 204,441 operations, of which most were big. His ulcer dissection was performed worldwide (➤ Fig. 1.3).

Von Nußbaum's operation

'Since 1857 I have even attempted operating on ulcers which are very difficult to cure, which soak five and six towels daily with their muck and which are an indescribable burden for patients and those around them, especially in summer, and which produce such an enormous and rapid change in such callous ulcers that I repeat it on the hour, and have already healed more than 60 cases with it. I narcotise such a sick person and make an incision around his foot ulcer, one finger wide from the edge, an incision going down to the fascia, cutting through a large mass of vessels which would result in severe bleeding if I did not immediately stuff a small strip of fine lint into the incision and compress the whole ulcer firmly. The insertion of the lint is also necessary so that the incision does not heal up before tomorrow [Note: in the time before asepsis]. What happens now? The ulcer, which yesterday was nourished

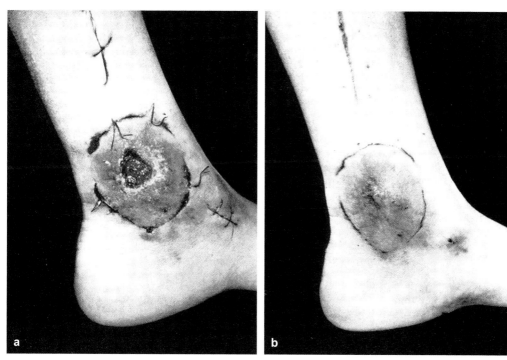

Fig. 1.3 a, b Circular dissection of the leg ulcer according to Von Nußbaum in 1873. Picture from Schörcher, here with direct suture of the cut. Before adoption of asepsis, Von Nußbaum left the wound wide open for the development of 'good pus'. [P573-1]

by a vast quantity of vessels, an abnormally large blood supply and produced large quantities of liquid muck so that one lot of exudate washed away the other, is today cut off from every blood supply surrounding it. For this reason, instead of 3 and 4 quarters of serous secretion, we have today a tablespoonful of thick, white, creamy pus. But where there is thicker, nicer pus, there is also regeneration, the forming of new connective tissue and vessels. Once the cavity has been filled up to the level of the skin, the popular Baynton plaster bandage, which always remains in place for 48 to 60 hours, is the most suitable bandage, or skin formation can be accelerated by the Reverdin pinch grafting method.'

Note The procedure is still performed today.

Varicose veins and chronic venous ulcer disease after the invention of anaesthesia and antisepsis in the 19th century

After the breakthrough of modern surgery in the middle of the 19th century, new treatment methods also emerged for the chronic venous leg ulcer. Extended pathophysiological knowledge and increasing understanding of the disease played a leading role.

First of all, the partial removal of the V. saphena magna quickly set a precedent. In most cases, however, this was not sufficient to heal the deep chronic ulcer. Therefore, the surgeons devised various additional procedures, which sound astonishing today even though they may have been useful in their time.

Bardescu's nerve extension operation in 1899

The operation was based on the theoretical assumption that in a chronic varicose lower leg ulcer, there are trophic innervation disorders as well as haemodynamic impairments. Bardescu's first publication was in a Bucharest journal in 1897. Manipulations were performed on the saphenous nerve and the superficial peroneal nerve, depending on the location of the leg ulcer.

Bardescu's case report

The procedure was performed on a 45-year-old farmer with a chronic leg ulcer for eight years.

'On the 28th of September, the resection of the V. saphena magna in the middle third of the lower leg was performed under local anaesthesia with cocaine. On the 8th of October, the stretching of the common peroneal nerve behind the fibular head, just above its end branches, was performed under chloroform anaesthesia. After stretching, the nerve was frayed out, and its fasciae separated with the tip of the scalpel so that the varicose vessels of the nerve would be destroyed as much as possible. The nerve was then moved to its former location. After the operation, we noticed temporary anaesthesia of the superficial peroneal nerve. The patient was released on November the 27th as healed.'

Note   The method was used in many clinics at that time, also for other indications.

Circular incisions in chronic venous ulcers at the end of the 19th century

Circular and spiral incisions were introduced by several authors to completely interrupt venous blood backflow in patients with chronic varicose veins. Dissections of all subcutaneous varicose veins were performed beyond the truncal vein. At its peak, dissections were performed worldwide.

Moreschi (1893) and von Schede (1897) performed the circular incisions above and below the leg ulcer (➤ Fig. 1.4). Mariani (1903) conducted the incision only above the ulcer. Petersen (1896) recommended circumcision below the knee and Wenzel (1902) at the lower third of the thigh.

From Buenos Aires, Wenzel reported on 26 cases where he had operated with the best results. The patients remained in bed without moving for 12 days after the operation in the Trendelenburg position and were then discharged with a compression bandage up to the groin.

Schede's case report

'A 47-year-old washerwoman, mother of six children, lean, haggard, bronchiectasis. Palm-sized, greasy, extremely painful ulcer for five years. She is now very ill, plagued by the ulcer which robs her of sleep. When she decides to go to bed, desperately tired, her rest is short-lived, because the father is a stupid drunkard, and if the mother doesn't work, the children have nothing to eat.' After the operation, the ulcer healed over for 2½ years. The scar appeared to be sunken like a gutter. The patient explained: 'Yes, you know, doctor, I always tie my garter there, it holds so beautifully.'

Spiral incisions in chronic venous ulcers of Rindfleisch and Friedel in 1908

In principle, Rindfleisch and Friedel wanted to completely remove all varicose veins in patients with varicose ulcers. However, this was not possible in scarred and ulcerous or oedematous tissues. Thus they arrived at their unusual method via a horseshoe-shaped incision of the leg ulcer and small circular incisions. The operation consisted of a long incision in five to six spiral incisions from the lower leg to the thigh and right down to the fascia (➤ Fig. 1.5). The wounds remained open. During postoperative treatment, fresh granulations were repeatedly removed or etched away with a Höllenstein (silver nitrate etching pen) so that the wound margins were as far apart as possible. After 14 days, the patients could leave their beds. Rindfleisch worked as a surgeon at the Johanniter Hospital in Stendal. The method was published by his assistant Friedel.

Rindfleisch's case report

'O. H., farm labourer, 56 years old, has been on the local surgical ward for about four months due to varicose veins on his left leg. The Vena saphena magna descends from the thigh as a two-finger width cord and then disappears into the oedematous tissue of the lower leg. Since the fistula did not close, the V. saphena was cut out on the thigh to a width of 10 cm on 05.04.1907. At a handwidth below the knee, starting from the medial side, a spiral incision is then made five times around the lower leg, ending before the outer ankle joint. In the

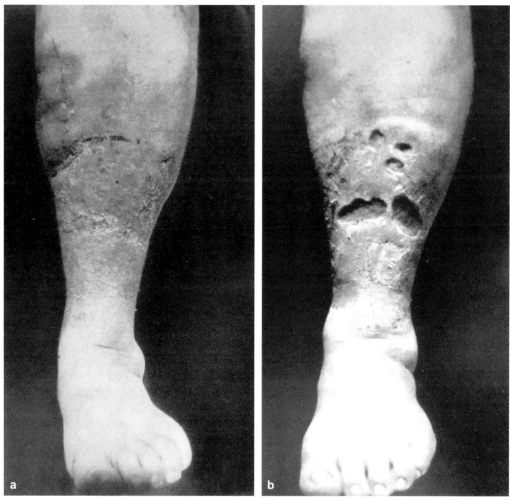

Fig. 1.4 a, b Circular incision of the lower leg above the chronic leg ulcers according to Moreschi in 1893; Figure from Schörcher: Anamnesis of the ulcers for seven years. [G840]

process, varices lying below the muscle fascia are also severed. The spiral heals within approx. eight weeks, abscesses and fistulas have disappeared; the oedema has considerably decreased.'

The surgeon Kayser (1910), senior physician at the Kümmell University Clinic in Hamburg-Eppendorf in Germany, later made up to 12 incisions during this 'garter operation' or 'peritomy', plus three long skin incisions on the instep from the outer to the inner side. The ulcer came to lie between two turns and additional longitudinal incisions as if on an island. Due to the tendency to bleed, the edges of the incision had to be sutured extensively. In most cases, the ulcer had

already closed up after four weeks, before the surgical wound healed.

Today, the Rindfleisch-Friedel operations may appear as an extreme form of venous and ulcer surgery. At that time, however, the method had become established at all significant clinics in Germany and Austria. It was later discredited because of the high blood loss, postoperative sensitivity disorders, severe stasis with limited use of the extremity as well as a long inpatient treatment period of up to 20 weeks. Even so, the length of the surgical wound reached 156 cm. Only one death was recorded in the literature, even though the patient population consisted of older patients, often well over 70 years of age. A critical

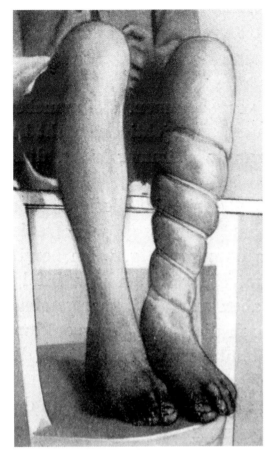

Fig. 1.5 Scar after spiral incision of the leg according to Rindfleisch and Linton, 1908; five circles; healing of the surgical wound after eight weeks. [F1032-001]

follow-up examination was carried out by Friedrich Bode, chief physician of the Surgical Clinic in Bad Homburg, in 1919.

Bodes' report of the follow-up examination

'Disappointed and disheartened, the sick left the institution unhealed, and the doctor, too, soon lost the courage and desire for further activity of this kind during these experiences.'

By chance, one of the most dissatisfied patients was admitted to the Bad Homburg hospital later because of another illness. Bode was surprised at the good late result. He then requested a follow-up examination with all 18 patients who had undergone the operation

and, apart from sensitivity disorders, found excellent new results.

Total removal of the V. saphena magna according to Madelung in 1884

For the first time in medical history, the removal of the V. saphena magna proved to be a causal treatment concept for severe truncal varicosis with leg ulcers, which led to reproducibly good results. The first report about such an operation using Esmarch's tourniquet comes from the London surgeon John Marshall in 1875. Since then, the operation has been modified in various ways. Initially, the Madelung operation was considered an extreme variant (➤ Fig. 1.6).

Otto Madelung (1846–1926) was full professor for surgery in Rostock, Göttingen and Strasbourg. Many vital findings in surgery such as the Madelung's disease or lipomatose can be traced back to him.

Madelung removed the whole V. saphena magna, including the lateral branches, using long skin incisions, and also performed extensive subfascial

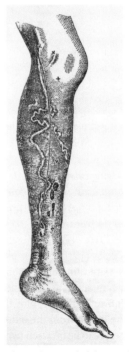

Fig. 1.6 Incision for total removal of the V. saphena magna according to Madelung 1884 with extensive resection of the lateral branches and the perforated vein. [F1033-001]

perforator dissections. In his publication in 1884, he reported on eleven operations. In many cases, major surgery was associated with complications.

Madelung's operation

'I have performed the radical peeling of the venous plexus degenerated by cirsoid varicose veins. The skin of the lower leg has to be prepared over more than the length of the foot and more than the width of the hand. A sleeve loosely wrapped around the thigh makes the peripheral veins bulge. A great number of subbindings are particularly necessary to close the small vessels penetrating the fascia of the lower leg muscles. I have earned more thanks with this operation, which is so easy to perform, than with many difficult operations.'

1.2.2 Summary

The chronification of a wound is today traced back to various causes in pathophysiological terms. In most cases, it is a chronic leg ulcer. At its time of origination, the failure of circulation to adapt to the conditions of the upright gait played a decisive role in human history.

On the one hand, there are endogenous factors and on the other hand external influences, such as hard physical work, which potentiate each other and can cause the patient many years of suffering, even death. The term **Morbus ulceris cruris venosi chronici** or **chronic venous leg ulcer disease** comprehensively defines the course of the disease.

Wound doctors have had to deal with chronic venous ulcers throughout the history of humanity. In ancient times, various ointments and dressings were available, including minor surgeries on varicose veins. But it was not possible to help them effectively. It is therefore not surprising if magic and superstition interfered with the therapy.

The decisive breakthrough in treating the disease was only achieved with modern surgery after the introduction of anaesthesia and asepsis in the middle of the 19th century. Although connections between ulcer disease and varicose veins were suspected for a long time, they could only now be specifically addressed. Sclerotherapy, Babcock surgery, Hach's partial saphenous resection and modern endovas-

cular procedures were important milestones. Nevertheless, chronic venous leg ulcers are still present today. The solution to this particular condition, the pathophysiology of venous hypertension, has not yet been found, even after 2.6 million years of human history since the Palaeolithic Age.

REFERENCES

Bardeleben A von. Lehrbuch der Chirurgie und Operationslehre. 2. Band. 3. A. Berlin: Reimer 1860, 253–291.

Bardeleben A von. Diskussionsbemerkung. Verh Dt Ges Chir 1891; 20: 163.

Bardescu N. Eine neue operative Behandlung der varikösen Unterschenkelgeschwüre. Centralbl Chir 1899; 26: 769–771.

Bernstein JG. Praktisches Handbuch für Wundärzte, nach alphabetischer Ordnung in vier Bänden. 5. Ausg. 4. Band. Leipzig: Schwickertsche Verlage 1820, 480.

Bode F. Grundlagen und Erfolge der Rindfleisch'schen Varicenoperation. Arch Klein Chir 1919; 112: 592–606.

Bopp C. Alfred Schönwerth (1865–1941) – Ein Münchner Chirurg in der Nachfolge von Johann Nepomuk von Nußbaum. Dissertation an der Technischen Universität München, 2005.

Eckart WU. Geschichte der Medizin. Berlin, Heidelberg, New York: Springer, 1990.

Friedel G. Operative Behandlung der Varicen, Elephantiasis und Ulcus cruris. Arch Klin Chir 1908; 86: 143–159.

Fuchs R. Hippokrates, Sämmtliche Werke. 3. Band. München: Lüneburg 1900, 294.

Grimm JFG, Grimm JJC, Lilienhain L. Hippocrates Werke. 2. Band. Glogau: Praußnitz 1838, 454.

Gufer J. Tabulae medicae sive Medicina domestica. Das ist kleine Hauß-Apotheck. Augsburg: Kronigers und Gobels seel. Erben 1689, 130.

Gurlt E . Geschichte der Chirurgie und ihrer Ausübung. 1. Band. Berlion: Hirschwald, 1898.

Hach W. Die merkwürdigen Therapien des Ulcus cruris – Medizinhistorische Betrachtungen über Jahrhunderte hinweg. Vasomed 2005; 17: 6–11.

Hach W. Die Kunst des Dr. Weinhold zur Heilung veralteter Hautgeschwüre. Phlebologie 2013; 42: 252–256.

Hach W, Hach-Wunderle V. Die Wandlung der theoretischen Konzepte in der Chirurgie der Stammvarikose vom 19. Jahrhundert bis in die Gegenwart. Gefäßchirurgie 2001; 6: 111–118.

Hach W, Mumme A, Hach-Wunderle V. Venen-Chirurgie. 3. A. Stuttgart: Schattauer, 2013.

Hirsch A. Biographische Lexikon der hervorragenden Aerzte aller Zeiten und Völker. Wien, Leipzig: Urban und Schwarzenberg, 1886.

Kayser P. Zur Behandlung des varikösen Symptomenkomplexes mit dem Spiralschnitt (nach Rindfleisch-Friedel). Beitr Klin Chir 1910; 68: 802–810.

Laqua K. Die Behandlung der Varizen. Bruns' Beiträge Klin Chir 1930; 150: 215–251.

Lovejoy CO. The origin of man. Science 1981; 211: 341–350.

Madelung O. Ueber die Ausschälung circoider Varicen an der unteren Extremität. Verh Dtsch Ges Chir 1884; 13:114–117.

Marshall J. A new method of treating bad cases of varicose veins of the leg. Brit Med J 1875 (no journal volume known).

Nußbaum, N von. Neue Heilmethoden bei Geschwüren. Aerztliches Intelligenz-Blatt 1873; 20: 205–211.

Plinius Secundus G. Naturgeschichte. 36. Band. Übersetzung Ph. H. Külb. Stuttgart: Metzler 1864, 4528.

Richtern CF. Vollständiges Materialien-Lexikon. Leipzig: Braun, 1721.

Schede M. Ueber die operative Behandlung der Unterschenkelvaricen. Berliner Klin Wochenschr 1877; 14: 85–89.

Scheller E. Aulus Cornelius Celsus. Über die Arzneiwissenschaft in 8 Büchern. Hildesheim: Olms 1967, 276.

Schörcher F. Kosmetische Operationen. München: Lehmann, 1955.

Tabernaemontanus DJT. Kräuterbuch (Lorcher Kräuterbuch). Reprint. Offenbach am Main: Königs 1731, 788.

Weinhold KA. Die Kunst, veraltete Hautgeschüre besonders die sogenannten Salzflüsse nach einer neuen Methode sicher und schnell zu heilen. Dresden: Arnold, 1810.

Wenzel C. Der Circulärschnitt am Oberschenkel bei der operativen Behandlung der Varicen und des Ulcus cruris. Berliner Klin Wochenschr 1902; 39: 122–127.

Joachim Dissemond, Knut Kröger

2
Current definitions and spellings for the treatment of chronic wounds

---

Key notes

- Various medical professions with varying backgrounds of training are involved in wound therapy.
- A necessary prerequisite for communication and documentation is a standard nomenclature.

- By using standard definitions, diagnostic and treatment strategies are optimised and easier to understand.
- In consultation with the Scientific Advisory Board, the board of the ICW has outlined various definitions, spellings and terms as the basis for a uniform standard.

2.1 Introduction

Experts from various professional groups with very different training are involved in the very complex processes of wound treatment. It is necessary to use uniform terminology to ensure proper communication and joint documentation. Therefore, in consultation with its scientific advisory board, the board of the European Wound Management Association (EWMA) has begun to publish definitions, spellings and the clarification of terms in recent years. By using standard terms, diagnostics and treatment strategies are to be optimised and made more comprehensible.

2.2 Definitions

Wound   A wound is defined as the loss of the barrier between the body and the environment due to the destruction of tissue on external or internal body surfaces.

Chronic wound   A wound that has not healed after eight weeks is called chronic. Irrespective of this time-oriented definition, some wounds must be considered as chronic from their very beginning since their care requires the treatment of their underlying cause. For example, these include the diabetic foot ulcer, wounds

in peripheral artery disease (PAD), venous leg ulcers or pressure sores.

Acute wound   Each wound that is not chronic is considered to be acute.

Erosion   An erosion is a superficial wound that exclusively affects the epidermis of the skin.

Ulcer   An ulcer is a deep wound that extends at least into the dermis of the skin.

Wound edge   The wound edge is the border between the wound and the intact epithelium.

Periwound tissue   The periwound skin is the area that starts at the wound edge and surrounds the wound.

Necrosis   A necrosis is a non-vital tissue that was previously vital.

Gangrene   The term gangrene defines obsolete body parts. Thus, when describing non-vital tissue in wounds, we use the term necrosis and not gangrene.

Wound exudate   The expression wound exudate refers to all fluids which are released by a wound. Depending on the wound status, the exudate can include lymph, blood, proteins, pathogens, cells and cell remnants.

Relapse   Recurrence after treatment distinguishes between disease and symptom relapse.
- **Relapse of a disease:** relapse of disease describes the recurrence of this disease after temporarily successful treatment or after spontaneous healing. Example: tumour relapse.
  Comment: in chronic diseases such as diabetes mellitus or chronic venous insufficiency (CVI), healing is not possible. There is therefore no relapse in these cases.
- **Relapse of a symptom:** relapse of a symptom describes the recurrence of this symptom after temporarily successful treatment or after spontaneous healing.

A distinction is made between the following:
- Local relapse: relapse reoccurring at the same anatomical location.
- Symptom relapse: relapse reoccurring at a different anatomical site.

Example: A venous leg ulcer is the symptom of the underlying disease, CVI. During the disease, an ulcer may be found at different locations.

Compliance   The patient closely follows the instructions given by the healthcare professional. Comment: the patient doesn't have to understand the instructions.

Adherence   Based on the understanding of the disease, the patient and the healthcare provider together choose a therapy which the patient can integrate into his everyday life. Comment: The patient should actively participate in the decision-making process. To this purpose, individualised education of the patient must be performed based on the patient's prior knowledge.

Maceration   Maceration refers to the swelling or softening of tissues as a result of prolonged contact with the fluid. In wound care, maceration of the epidermis at the wound edge and the periwound skin is often a sign of inadequate exudate management.

Capillaritis alba vs. atrophie blanche   Preliminary remarks: In patients with chronic venous insufficiency, livedoid vasculopathy or chronic vascular damage – for example due to taking hydroxyurea – white skin alterations often develop in the progressing disease due to vasculopathy of the capillaries. During the further course of the disease, very painful ulcerations may form. In this case, the terms capillaritis alba and atrophie blanche are mostly used as synonyms. However, since the painfulness and especially the therapeutic consequences vary, it makes sense to differentiate the inflammatory earlier form as capillaritis alba from the less inflammatory atrophie blanche derived during the disease.
- **Capillaritis alba:** very painful vasculopathy of the skin capillaries.
  Comment: treatment consists of short-term, topical use of high-potency glucocorticoids.
- **Atrophie blanche:** less painful chronic status of capillaritis alba.
  Comment: important is the treatment of the underlying disease, e.g. compression therapy in case of CVI.
- **Pseudoatrophie blanche:** scar after an ulcer has healed.
  Comment: In CVI this corresponds to stage IIIa according to Widmer, or respectively stage C5 of the CEAP classification. No specific therapy is necessary.

Erythema   Redness of the skin.

Eczema   Non-infectious inflammatory reaction of the skin. Eczema is clinically characterised by the following typical symptoms:
- **Acute eczema:** redness, desquamation, pruritus, vesicles, erosions, discharge.
- **Chronic eczema:** redness, lichenification (thickened and leathery skin structure), desquamation, pruritus.

Comment: Eczema only describes a symptom. A distinction must be made concerning the aetiology, e.g., allergic contact eczema, toxic contact eczema, stasis dermatitis, or atopic dermatitis.

2.3 Conclusion

Currently, many terms are used very differently by the different health care professionals. Thus it comes again and again to misunderstandings and inconsistent documentation. By describing definitions, spellings and terms, the EWMA has now attempted to develop a uniform standard that should be the basis for documentation and also for clinical studies.

REFERENCES

Dissemond J, Bültemann A, Gerber V, Jäger B, Münter C, Kröger K. Diagnosis and treatment of chronic wounds: Current standards of the Initiative for Chronic Wounds (ICW) e.V. from Germany. J Wound Care 2017; 26: 727–732.

3

Knut Kröger, Joachim Dissemond

Epidemiology

Key notes

- There is no global population-based study that describes the incidence and prevalence of chronic wounds worldwide.
- There is no accepted definition of the term chronic wound that is generally used in the few existing epidemiologic studies.

- The interpretation of all published data must take into account the specific population being analysed, the underlying definitions and the type of data collection.

3.1 Introduction

A chronic wound can be defined in various ways. The ICW has published a definition (➤ Chap. 2), but there are very different points of view worldwide. The terminology therefore does not conform to any standard. Also, there are other terms, such as 'therapy refractory', 'complicated' or 'hard-to-heal'. The healing period seems to vary between four weeks and three months.

Based on the causal etiologies, the most common types of chronic wounds are divided into four categories: pressure ulcers, diabetic foot ulcers, venous leg ulcers and ulcers in peripheral artery disease.

Although epidemiological and clinical data on chronic wounds, including prevalence and incidence, infection rates, hospital stays, amputations, healing and recurrence are available, these data are very heterogeneous. They have never been systematically summarised. Therefore, there is no valid or reliable data basis to describe the epidemiology of chronic wounds.

3.2 Prevalence estimation

The interpretation of all published data must take into account the specific population being analysed, the underlying definitions of the wound and the type of data collection.

Point prevalence is the prevalence of a particular day and period prevalence is of days, weeks or years. Since people with specific diseases are more likely to be in medical facilities, the prevalence rates are systematically higher than the period prevalence rates. Data sources collecting statutory health insurance billing data are collected by health insurance funds to provide services such as reimbursement and health care. They comply with legal requirements and usually contain information on benefits, regulations and details of their reimbursement. However, there is often a lack of relevant information about the services and treatments provided that are not covered by health insurance, as well as information about medical issues such as complications, laboratory tests, out-of-hospital mortality, etc. Patient registries are organised database systems with a specific scientific, clinical or health purpose. The data is collected prospectively to examine a group of patients with specific characteristics, such as a particular disease or treatment. These are cohort studies developed with a predefined health-related objective.

A recent publication by McKosker et al. (2018) has attempted to describe the prevalence of chronic wounds in Australia. Some representative results are summarised in ➤ Table 3.1. The results show that an accurate estimate is not possible. For each type of chronic wound, the prevalence rates show a significant variation depending on the attitude on which they are based.

Table 3.1 Prevalence of various chronic wounds in various settings in Australia

Chronic wounds	Prevalence and setting
Arterial ulcers (AU)	Prevalence in people with lower-extremity ulcers: prevalence of AU as a primary cause of ulceration in this population ranged from 3.0%–19.0%.
	Prevalence in people with all types of wounds (including chronic, surgical and traumatic wounds): prevalence of AU as a primary cause of ulceration in this population ranged from 1.0%–10.9%.
Diabetic foot ulcers (DFU)	Prevalence in people with lower-extremity ulcers: prevalence of DFU as a primary cause of ulceration in this population ranged from 2.5%–12.0%.
	Prevalence of DFU in people with all types of wounds (including chronic, surgical, and traumatic wounds): prevalence was 2.6%.
	Prevalence of DFU in all people with diabetes: prevalence ranged from 1.2%–2.5%; prevalence of DFU in the first year of diabetes diagnosis was reported to be 1.0%.
Venous leg ulcers (VLU)	Prevalence in people with lower-extremity ulcers: prevalence of VLU as a primary cause of ulceration in this population ranged from 1.0%–70.5%.
	Prevalence in people with all types of wounds (including chronic, surgical, and traumatic wounds): prevalence of VLU as a primary cause of ulceration in this population was reported to be between 3.1% and 53.1%.
Pressure ulcers (PU)	Prevalence of PU in acute health care facilities (e.g., hospitals): prevalence ranged from 0.2%–29.6% in hospital settings.
	Prevalence of PU in non-acute health care facilities (e.g., residential aged care settings): prevalence ranged from 0.03%–25.9%.
	Prevalence of PU in the community (involving general practitioners or community nursing services): prevalence of PU – as a percentage of total presentations – ranged from 7.7%–42.3%.
Leg ulcers	Prevalence in people presenting to community health care services: prevalence was reported at 1.1–7.0 per 1000 patient encounters and 0.1% and 0.3% of all patient encounters.
	Prevalence among people presenting to a community healthcare service with a wound (including chronic, surgical, and traumatic wounds): prevalence was 48.2%. Prevalence in hospitalised patients: prevalence ranged from 2.3%–2.8%.

3.3 Costs and outlook

On the one hand, the treatment of patients with chronic wounds represents a high-quality medical challenge. On the other hand, it is an economic challenge against the background of rising costs in the healthcare system. Exact figures on the number of patients with chronic wounds are not available. Thus, the statistics for the direct and indirect costs caused by patients with chronic wounds are still based on estimates. The costs are composed of, among other things:

- Inpatient hospital stays
- Outpatient hospital stays
- Home care
- Care period
- Number of dressing changes
- Dressing material costs
- Personnel costs

The average direct costs of wound care for a patient with lower leg ulcers from the statutory health insurance (SHI) were calculated between 8,000 and 10,000 € per patient and year. This cost is mainly due to the long duration of treatment, the lack of patient adherence, incorrect use of materials, inadequate diagnostics, inpatient accommodation, wound infection coupled with a high tendency to relapse after healing, and the co-morbidity of the patients. The consequences of the disease led to further indirect costs of economic importance, which are difficult to measure. In addition to lost working days, patients can become unemployed in the long term, suffer a social decline and thus burden the social security funds.

Demographic change and the associated problems in the cost sector are presenting the healthcare system with new challenges in dealing with people with chronic wounds. It can be assumed that the steady increase in average life expectancy and the associated increase in the number of risk diseases such as diabetes, peripheral artery disease (PAD), etc. This assumption of growth will considerably increase the number of patients with chronic wounds and will increase the associated direct and indirect costs significantly. In this respect, solving the problem of healing chronic wounds is one of today's most critical medical topics.

3.4 Conclusion

Even though the exact numbers on incidence and prevalence of people with chronic wounds in the different countries are unknown, the available data show that this is a common problem. A systemic assessment of people with chronic wounds would be an essential prerequisite for assessing the influence of the ageing of society and the increase in immobility, obesity and diabetes mellitus on the incidence of chronic wounds and the effectiveness of modern prevention and treatment strategies.

REFERENCES

Augustin M, Brocatti LK, Rustenbach SJ, Schäfer I, Herberger K. Cost-of-illness of leg ulcers in the community. Int Wound J 2014; 11: 283–292.

Heyer K, Herberger K, Protz K, Glaeske G, Augustin M. Epidemiology of chronic wounds in Germany: Analysis of statutory health insurance data. Wound Repair Regen 2016; 24: 434–442.

Järbrink K, Ni G, Sönnergren H, et al. The humanistic and economic burden of chronic wounds: a protocol for a systematic review. Syst Rev 2017; 6: 15.

McCosker L, Tulleners R, Cheng Q, et al. Chronic wounds in Australia: A systematic review of key epidemiological and clinical parameters. Int Wound J 2019; 16: 84–95.

Pannier-Fischer F, Rabe E. [Epidemiology of chronic venous diseases]. Hautarzt 2003; 54: 1037–1044.

Purwins S, Herberger K, Debus ES, et al. Cost-of-illness of chronic leg ulcers in Germany. Int Wound J 2010; 7: 97–102.

4

Knut Kröger, Joachim Dissemond

Evidence and guidelines

Key notes

- Evidence-based medicine (EBM) is a more recent development in medicine, which explicitly claims that patient-oriented decisions should be made in medical treatments based on empirically proven efficacy wherever possible.
- With the advent of EBM, there has been a shift in emphasis towards randomised controlled trials (RCTs) and a hierarchisation of the value of study types. Thus, meta-analyses based on RCTs are particularly valued in EBM.
- Good evidence in wound medicine is often problematic as wounds are a symptom and not a

circumscribed disease, passing through various stages, and various therapeutic approaches build on each other.
- Generally accepted guidelines regarding prevention, diagnosis and treatment of chronic wounds published as a uniform standard by one of the significant wound associations are not available. For each type of chronic wound, there are many guidelines from the different countries and different societies focusing on various aspects of the diseases. Recent publications tried to compare these guidelines and to summarise the joint statements.

4.1 Introduction

Evidence-based medicine (EBM) means 'medicine based on evidence'. EBM is a more recent development in medicine that expressly demands that patient-oriented decisions should be made in medical treatment based on empirically proven efficacy wherever possible. EBM, if understood correctly, thus describes something that goes without saying, namely the consideration of scientific principles in diagnostics and therapy. The term was proposed in the early 1990s by Gordon Guyatt of the Department of Clinical Epidemiology and Biostatistics at McMaster University in Hamilton, Canada.

Originally, EBM was conceived as a learning concept for physicians to bring clarity and transparency into the daily growing data jungle, to critically evaluate new scientific findings and, if necessary, to put them into practice quickly. What was new with the emergence of EBM, however, was a shift in emphasis towards randomised controlled trials (RCTs) and a hierarchisation of the significance of study types (➤ Table 4.1, ➤ Table 4.2). Thus, meta-analyses based on RCTs are particularly valued in EBM.

Table 4.1 Following the recommendations of the Agency for Healthcare Research and Quality (AHCPR), the evidence is divided into different classes

Meta-analyses describe a statistical procedure in which the results of scientific studies on the same or very similar questions are systematically summarised quantitatively.
Randomised controlled studies (RCTs) are usually the best possible study design for medical, experimental questions.
When a study is performed in a controlled manner, the results of the study group can be objectively compared with the results of a control group. This control can be achieved with placebo or standard therapy, for example.

In contrast to the original approach of the learning concept for physicians, EBM is used today in many cases as an instrument for the central control and rationalisation of medicine with the consequence of increasing legalisation.

Central aspects of EBM:

- To find answers to medical questions in a structured and systematic way. For example, it

Table 4.2 Classification of the evidence

Class Ia	Evidence through meta-analyses of multiple RCTs
Class Ib	Evidence based on at least one RCT
Class IIa	Evidence from at least one high-quality, but non-randomised and controlled study
Class IIb	Evidence based on at least one high-quality quasi-experimental study
Class III	Evidence from well-designed, non-experimental descriptive studies such as comparative studies, correlation studies or case-control studies
Class IV	Evidence based on reports from expert committees or expert opinions, or clinical experience of recognised authorities
Class V	Case series or expert opinion

should be clarified whether one treatment is more beneficial than another.

- It offers a high degree of certainty in decision-making. A standard element of EBM is the systematic identification and compilation of all qualitatively appropriate studies on a question, summarising the current state of knowledge.
- EBM serves as a protection against incorrect decisions and the wrong expectations. For example, useful treatments not being included in the care should be avoided, as well as ineffective treatments which can harm patients.

Although many decision-makers in the various health policy structures refer to EBM, the criticism of EBM as the only actual point of view goes on and on. This criticism is based, among other things, on the fact that studies with large numbers provide a statistically exact result, but it is unknown, however, to whom it applies. Studies with small numbers provide a statistically useless result, but one knows better who it affects. The more data collected in extensive studies, the more difficult it is to compare the average patient in the study with a specific case. Thus, reviews with a large number of patients are not readily applicable to a specific individual case.

4.2 Guidelines

Generally, accepted guidelines based on sound evidence for the prevention, diagnosis and treatment of patients with chronic wounds are insufficiently available internationally. For each type of chronic wound, there are several guidelines from different countries and professional societies focusing on various aspects of the disease. Recent publications have attempted to compare this guideline and summarise the joint statements.

Sun et al. from China analysed a total of 22 clinical practice guidelines (CPG) on diabetes foot syndrome. They assessed the consistency of the recommendations, the quality of the CPGs and presented an evidence map to explain research trends and gaps in 2019. The authors looked for recommendations for diabetic foot complications with diabetic foot ulcers (DFUs), Charcot neuropathy (CN) and osteomyelitis (OM). They concluded that the recommendations in some CPGs were not very specific, explicit and even inconsistent. They recommend the use of evidence mapping to facilitate the process of knowledge transfer and reduce research effort. In 2019, Tan et al. from the UK evaluated the quality of 14 CPG to venous leg ulcers (VLUs) published between 1999 and 2016. The majority of the recommendations come from Europe or North America. Overall, there was excellent reliability of results between the evaluators with an intra-class correlation coefficient of 0.986 (95% confidence interval 0.979–0.991). No single CPG achieved the highest score in all six areas.

Significant methodological heterogeneity was observed in VLU CPGs. Only four CPGs were considered qualitatively sufficient for clinical use. Consolidation of efforts to promote high-quality, comprehensive VLU CPGs is necessary to reduce the number and heterogeneity of currently published guidelines. The European Pressure Ulcer Advisory Panel (EPUAP), the Pan Pacific Pressure Injury Alliance (PPPIA) and the National Pressure Ulcer Advisory Panel (NPUAP) have updated the CPG on pressure ulcer prevention and treatment and published their protocol 2019. A Guideline Governance Group will define and monitor all steps of CPG development. An international consumer survey will be conducted to identify consumer needs and interests. Systematic evidence searches in relevant electronic databases will cover the period from July 2013 to August 2018. The risk of distortion of the included studies will be assessed by two evaluators using established checklists and overall strength of evidence associated with the cumulative body of evidence. Small working groups review the evidence available for each topic, review or draft the guidance chapters and recommendations, or best practice statements. Finally, the strengths of the levels of recommendation are assigned. Recommendations are evaluated against their significance and potential to improve individual patient outcomes in an international formal consensus process.

In summary, it can be said that much is currently being done internationally to improve better and more meaningful guidelines as an aid to clinical activity.

4.3 Evidence in wound medicine

As a term, evidence in wound medicine is associated with many problems, as wounds are a symptom and not a circumscribed disease, they go through different stages, and different therapeutic approaches can build upon each other. Also, alternative therapy approaches are possible, which in turn are convenient, effective and economical. Most products used in wound therapy are medical devices. Medical devices are objects or substances that are used for medical-therapeutic or diagnostic purposes for humans. In contrast to drugs, the intended main effect is not primarily pharmacological, metabolic or immunological, but usually physical or physicochemical. Medical devices are divided into different classes (➤ Table 4.3). Wound products are generally approved by the European Medicines Agency (EMA), which defines the scope of application, requires a biological safety test and checks compliance with the general regulations for carrying out conformity assessment. In this way, the EMA guarantees that the product does not cause any biological damage and comes onto the market to a defined quality standard. Also, § 19 of the EMA requires proof of the suitability of medical devices for the intended use, utilising a corresponding clinical evaluation. The clinical evaluation is based on clinical

Table 4.3 In the European Union, medical devices are classified by Annex IX of Directive 93/42/EEC

Class I	
Features and benefits	Low application risks, low degree of invasiveness, no or non-critical skin contact
Dressing materials	Mechanical barrier, compression, absorption of exudate Use for superficial wounds (erosions)
Examples	Cotton woll gauze, compression stockings
Class IIa	
Features and benefits	Medium application risk, a moderate degree of invasiveness
Dressing materials	Influencing the microenvironment of a wound Use for superficial wounds (erosions)
Examples	Disposable syringes, polyurethane film dressings
Class IIb	
Features and benefits	Increased risk of application, systemic effect
Dressing materials	Use in wounds where the dermis is severed (ulcer), secondary wound-healing
Examples	Alginates, hydrogels
Class III	
Features and benefits	High risk of application, implantable or highly invasive
Dressing materials	Medical devices with supportive, active pharmaceutical components or animal components Use, e.g. for wounds at risk of infection/infected wounds
Examples	Silver bandages, bandages with collagen/hyaluronic acid

data which contain both safety and performance data resulting from the use of the medical device. Clinical data originate from the following sources (§ 3 No. 25 MPG):
• a clinical trial of the medical device in question, or
• clinical trials or other studies reproduced in scientific literature relating to a similar device, the identity of which can be demonstrated with the medical device concerned, or
• published or unpublished reports on other clinical experience, either with the medical device concerned or with a similar device, the identity

of which can be shown with the medical device concerned.

Irrespective of this approval, product properties ('claims'), identified as advantageous by the manufacturers based on product development, are advertised in wound medicine. The clinical user must be able to weigh up these different product advantages and justify the costs incurred if necessary. This pressure to evaluate leads to a call for evidence based on studies (➤ Table 4.2).

4.4 Randomised controlled trials in wound-healing

Although the call for RCTs is urgent in relation to the treatment of patients with chronic wounds, the usefulness of the findings of such studies should be queried, including aspects of patient selection, blinding, standardisation and endpoints. In the following, therefore, some of the points of criticism under discussion in the wound-healing sector will be presented.

- Blinding is easily possible in pharmacological studies by taking similar drugs without active ingredients (placebos). Blinding to wound products presupposes that these cannot be differentiated visually, but this is only really the case in rare cases. With physical methods such as vacuum therapy, blinding is virtually impossible.
- Even when talking generally of wound-healing, there are wounds of different genesis. For example, a venous leg ulcer cannot be compared exactly with arterial wounds or pressure ulcers. The type of wound and the extent of the underlying disease have a significant influence on the chances of recovery. RCTs should, therefore, only include a distinct entity of chronic wounds. The results of studies of this entity cannot be easily transferred to other entities.
- To generate as homogeneous a population of volunteers as possible for RCTs, inclusion and exclusion criteria are described in advance. Patients with specific comorbidities or a long duration of ulcer, for example, can often not be included in studies. Thus, RCTs usually represent a kind of 'positive selection' of patients and not reality.

- The optimal endpoint of a study for the benefit of a wound product is usually complete healing. Similar to pharmacological studies in which endpoints such as mortality or heart attack are defined as endpoints, complete healing would be a hard endpoint. Wound-healing takes time, and not all wounds can ultimately be healed. Endpoints such as quality of life, debridement, painlessness or reduction of antibiotic consumption play a subordinate role in the current approach. Also, various wound-healing products are usually used in phase-adapted wound treatment, so that it is often difficult to assess a component of the complex therapy.
- Unlike in pharmacological studies, solely taking the trial drug is not viable as a wound treatment. Treatment by a wound expert following a standard of care is necessary and requires a close regional connection.

All these aspects make it difficult to carry out RCTs on the various approaches to wound-healing and require a rethink to create the conditions for practice-relevant assessments. A standard definition of health policy endpoints is currently lacking.

4.5 Conclusion

If current guidelines or expert standards exist for the topic in question, taking into account existing good evidence, these should always be made known and, if necessary, included in the decision-making process. In the field of wound treatment, however, there are currently several limitations in this regard, so that many procedures in daily practice must continue to be based on individual empirical values. It is desirable that in future, there will be more high-quality evidence from scientific studies, for example from registry studies, which form a reasonable basis for the implementation of EBM in the field of wound-healing.

REFERENCES

Kottner J, Cuddigan J, Carville K, et al. Prevention and treatment of pressure ulcers/injuries: The protocol for the second update of the international Clinical Practice Guideline 2019. J Tissue Viability 2019; 28: 51–58.

Scott IA, Guyatt GH. Suggestions for improving guideline utility and trustworthiness. Evid Based Med 2014; 19: 41–46.

Sun Y, Gao Y, Chen J, et al. Evidence mapping of recommendations on diagnosis and therapeutic strategies for diabetes foot: an international review of 22 guidelines. Metabolism 2019; 100: 153956.

Tan MKH, Luo R, Onida S, Maccatrozzo S, Davies AH. Venous leg ulcer clinical practice guidelines: What is AGREEd? Eur J Vasc Endovasc Surg 2019; 57: 121–129.

5

Gernold Wozniak, Alexander Risse

Ethical aspects

Key notes

- Basic ethical attitudes have a significant influence on medical practice and are therefore ahead of technical expertise.
- People have a fundamental right to self-damaging behaviour.
- Patient management is not the task of doctors.

- *Nihil nocere* (first do no harm) and pain control are the highest ethical maxims in medical treatment.
- Ethical action is threatened by economic constraints.

Healthcare is not just a business. Patients are not only customers, and doctors are by no means medical engineers.

O'Donovan 2003

5.1 Introduction ethics

Immanuel Kant's definition of philosophy according to the cosmic concept encompasses the questions:
What can I know? (metaphysics)

So we have to deal with the question, what is behind it? Today, scientific metaphysics is decisive, creating the corresponding pathophysiological constructs behind the phenomena, e.g. patient complaints. Large parts of this book deal with this. It should not be forgotten that the decisive factor for the patient is not the organic correlation, but the complaint. The term 'merely subjective' is misleading. The complaint leads the patient to the doctor, the 'subjective fact', not the 'objective', quantifiable disorder: The patient does not come and complain: 'Doctor, please help me, my nerve conduction velocity has decreased'. Likewise, pain is not 'merely subjective', but painful for the patient. The prescribing of saline tablets or solutions is, therefore, immoral (although placebo effects have been proven to be highly effective).
What can I hope for?

These are questions for religion, i.e. questions about a personified God or a world spirit; not topics of this book.

What is a human? (anthropology)

The preoccupation with the nature of man. In the old European, post-aristotelian world of objectification, man is usually viewed as a construction of the body (machine) and the soul (modern: consciousness) ('anthropological dualism', 'psychosomatic medicine'). This concept has led to groundbreaking insights and treatment methods, but for people with a diabetic foot syndrome (DFS), it doesn't deliver as expected.
What do you want me to do? (subject area of ethics and morals)

Morality describes the ethics and morals of human action. The judgemental assessment of actions and their relationship to norms is a result of ethics. Norms are programmes for possible obedience: the validity of imperativist standards are based on an order (law, scientific guidelines within certain limits); non-imperativist standards are valid without needing an order, e.g. social tact or conventions of dealing with patients. In addition to non-binding norms (recipes, rules of the game), there are also binding norms that are equipped with either automatic or exigent coercion. They are based on the authority of feelings (anger and shame) and are at the same time the foundations of every legal system and legal consciousness.

Ethics does not depend on absolute values or of the need for standards applying to everybody.

The validity of any norm is relative in two ways:
1. To the audience of whom the norm is required
2. To the supporter for whom it is bindingly or non-bindingly valid

A norm can only be binding from the perspective of a person who is subject to its relative existential coercion (as an individual or as integrated into society).

For the validity of ethical standards, for ethically correct action, the audience (here: wound therapists) must be possible to embarrass the public. Moreover, lack of shame only results when a certain way of thinking in a community (e.g. wound therapists) is regarded as moral. Lack of shame reflects (unethical) behaviour when integrated into a community's way of thinking (medicine). For example, the use of military expressions against patients ('the patient denied …') or reducing patients to categories is common in all medical hierarchies and is regarded as unobjectionable. Morally acceptable language is also strongly fixed in time. As an example, in the 1990s, diabetologists of the German Diabetes Society viewed the term 'diabetics' as devaluating and replaced it with the phrase 'people with diabetes'. Twenty years later, the term 'diabetic' is back – unquestioned – with specialist staff as well as with the patients themselves; accompanied by the 'asthmatics' or the 'gallbladder in room 17', etc.

5.2 Medical ethics

Four principles of ethical action in medicine are repeatedly quoted and also called the 'Georgetown mantra':

1. The patient's right to self-determination (patient autonomy/respect for autonomy)
   Everyone has the right to his or her views, to make his or her decisions and to act according to his or her lifestyle and values. This applies in particular to peculiarities which run counter to the old habits of traditional European medicine and care: fast driving and skiing, smoking, regular alcohol consumption, a sedentary lifestyle accompanied by a rich, high-calorific diet. To act ethically means to not interfere with the patient's lifestyle, or to try to correct it, but to limit oneself to the somatological necessities (e.g. appropriate compression therapy). Commenting on body weight or the harmfulness of smoking are not only unethical but also redundant in terms of content and therefore superfluous.
   Informed consent means that practitioner and patient agree on a standard procedure, i.e. that the patient has understood the suggestions first and foremost and that these suggestions can also be implemented in the context of his/her life.

2. Principle of damage prevention (nihil nocere/nonmaleficence)
   Avoidance of harm means an obligation to train up to the limits of physical endurance, and lifelong training and practice for the practitioners. It presupposes knowledge of the medical bases for treatment (the guidelines should be read and understood), including the critical position on recommendations: following therapy 'in the house style' ('We have always done it this way', 'It has proved its worth with us …') is immoral. Unfortunately, this rarely induces a feeling of shame on the part of the practitioners.
   Damage avoidance also means abstaining from unethical medical curiosity, and especially avoidance of financially lucrative but medically uncovered treatment options: 'Hippocrates knew nothing about individual health insurance.' A Swiss working group led by the philosopher Jean-Pierre Wils has therefore drawn up a new oath for medicine (Working Group 2015). It says, among other things: 'I am a medical practitioner with good judgement and do not recommend or take any measures that are not medically indicated.' However, the number of financially very lucrative hip and knee joint operations is increasing inexorably. For every 100,000 people in Germany, for example, there are 624 cardiac catheter interventions, while the OECD (Organisation for Economic Co-operation and Development) average is 177 less than a third.

3. Principle of care (beneficence)
   Informed consent and patient autonomy apply when the patient can make decisions. This changes when patients need external help due to dementia or loss of corporeal islands (see below). Creeping transitions at the onset of dementia are challenging to diagnose and require at least a basic psychopathological knowledge from the

therapist. Equivalents to directive psychotherapy also lead to the regression of the patient and must be considered carefully.

In the social context, while the principle of care in individual contact with patients requires active intervention by the therapist – ideally without interfering or abuse, it also refers to preventive measures. Holding back on certain behaviour, but even more so, on the development of inappropriate relationships, often leads to delusions of grandeur on the part of the protagonists and cannot be discussed further at this point.

4. Social equity (justice)

The original Hippocratic oath refers to the 'usefulness and piety of the sick', and thereby certainly implies the equal treatment of all regardless of their social position. Recent developments in economisation, mercantilisation and the transition of decision-making powers from doctors to managers and stockholders are forcing us to discuss the equitable distribution of increasingly scarce resources to patients, as well as the consequences for health care professionals. In Germany, the introduction of per capita flat rates for patients (DRGs or diagnosis-related groups) led to a drastic reduction in hospital stays and the so-called 'English' hospital discharge: transferred to unmanaged outpatient care before sufficient recovery, possibly for billing reasons, then reinstated with a different diagnosis. The simultaneous market-driven recruitment of patients, partly for unnecessary medical interventions, all leads to an untenable situation.

The shortened cycle of care in the outpatient sector, especially in wound care, as well as care and custody in old age homes, sometimes with fatal consequences, is – measured against the economic possibilities of the industrialised countries – scandalous. Medical ethicists and historians are increasingly referring to this deconstruction of the medical and nursing sector. Efforts to modify the Hippocratic oath and at least ethically counterbalance the health care system are well-intentioned but precarious given the sliding power of the economy.

5.3 Practical ethics for the treatment of people with chronic wounds

If morality describes the entirety of ethical and moral norms, principles and values which regulate the interpersonal behaviour of a society and are accepted as binding by it, and if it can further be determined that in the medical field, the four principles of the Georgetown Mantra naturally determine the conduct of our medical actions, then these cannot be considered separate from the principle of morality. They are contained by it and also born out of it.

These four principles are by no means unconflicting, although this is not a claim that is made. Moreover, none of the principles lose in significance if one leads in the realisation, but hinders another; if, for example, the respect of the practitioner for patient autonomy makes the principle of avoidance of harm only conditional or even impossible to implement. Thus, not every treatment scenario allows for the equal consideration of the four principles of the Georgetown mantra.

The question of the 'right or wrong' treatment can usually be checked by medical experts and evaluated, based on guidelines, recommendations for action or simple evidence.

The question of 'good or bad' in a treatment evaluates medical objectivity against the background of the ethics of the medical profession, which in turn is, however, part of the social image of morality.

It is precisely here that various areas of tension arise for those who (must) initiate, carry out or terminate treatment.

1. At best, the ethics of the healing profession are passed on and not taught.
2. The parameters for our medical actions are politically or socially initiated. They are created under the precondition of an underlying morality of the health profession, but without due consideration of this morality.
3. A change in the social structure concerning age, incidences of disease, etc., or a change in the social, moral image, may mean that the morals of the health profession may no longer have an appropriate place.

The prospect of fundamental change in our increasingly enforced economisation is slight. Therefore, it does not make much sense to remind other supposedly 'responsible people' (political or professional representatives) of this change, supposedly necessary, because minor corrections are continuously made, but never any fundamental differences. The apparently new 'responsible people' (shareholders, business economists, health insurance companies …), are however probably divesting themselves of this responsibility by introducing a new market-oriented regulator of supply and demand via economisation.

The fact that the 'new responsible people' can wash their hands of this so easily will not be stopped by our profound misery and exhortations, despite other aspects – suddenly of unforeseen importance – questioning the regulation of supply and demand.

One of the main problems of the present situation, with its current and impending shortage of skilled workers, presents a new aspect – suddenly we are a scarce commodity and we have become important. This situation allows us to disect the conflict between economisation and the ethics of the health profession.

Neither of the concepts present a contradiction in terms or even an exclusion. But for conflicts to become 'solvable', we must be and remain authentic.

At a time when the market situation is causing us significant problems, we cannot refer to the ethical conflict of the health profession and argue against it, to then behave like an army of mercenaries in a changed market situation – because now we are in short supply.

'Ethics and equity and the principles of justice do not change with the calendar.'

D. H. Lawrence

REFERENCES

Arbeitsgruppe der „Stiftung Dialog Ethik". Schweiz Ärztebl 2015; 25: 930–934.

Beauchamp T, Childress J. Principles of biomedical ethics. 6th ed. Oxford: University Press, 2008.

Gallagher SM. The ethics of compassion. Ostomy Wound Manage 1999; 45: 14–16.

Wils JP. Ärztlicher Ethos, Zeit für einen neuen Eid. Dtsch Arztebl 2017; 114: A-358.

Schmitz H. Der unerschöpfliche Gegenstand. Bonn: Bouvier, 1990.

Strech D, Börchers K, Freyer D, Neumann A, Wasem J, Marckmann G. Ärztliches Handeln bei Mittelknappheit. Ergebnisse einer qualitativen Interviewstudie. Ethik Med 2008; 20: 94–109.

Unschuld PU. Das System droht zu entgleisen. Dtsch Ärztebl 2017; 114: 2264–2266.

Wehkamp KH, Naegler H. Ökonomisierung patientenbezogener Entscheidungen im Krankenhaus. Dtsch Ärztebl 2017; 114: 797–804.

6

Andreas Schwarzkopf

Hygiene

Key notes

- Wounds are not sterile. However, cleanliness is essential for wound-healing. The healing process is a complex biochemical reaction and should not be impeded by a mass of bacteria, medical products with uncertain status and non-disinfected hands. Besides legal aspects there are good reasons to take hygienic precautions.
- Standard hygiene means hygienic measures need to be followed by everybody at all times. Extended hygiene measures are important if

further risks (e. g. infection with MRSA) are identified. Hygiene management is based on three mainstays: personal hygiene measures, hygiene measures in the environment (like surface disinfection) and the correct use and disposal of medical products, drugs and waste.
- Self-protection is also an essential part of hygiene in wound management. Therefore, gloves are essential, and the waste should be disposed of in durable and sealable bags or containers made of a stable material.

6.1 Introduction

Wound care is carried out by doctors, nurses and careworkers in various ward or ambulant environments. The degree of hygiene needed in wound care comes up repeatedly. Often there are disputes between those offering ward and outpatient care, especially ambulant care. As an example, we take a quick look at the situation in Germany. The German Society for Hospital Hygiene has not published any general recommendations for hygiene in wound care. However, in 2008, the board of the ICW presented the first version of a publication giving hygiene guidelines, prepared by Vice President Schwarzkopf and handed over to practitioners and interdisciplinary experts for consensus. Elements of these guidelines were updated and form the basis for this chapter.

Each wound is contaminated by microorganisms immediately after damage to the skin barrier. However, this does not mean that asepsis does not play an important role in wound care. Besides legal aspects there are good reasons to take hygiene precautions.

Complications and infections, especially surgical infections, depend not only on the pathogenic profile of the microorganisms but also on the general condition of the patients. Customised treatment therefore needs

to run alongside medical measures such as disinfection and dressings, as in the case of comorbidities such as diabetes mellitus. These measures are part of active infection prevention, treating the patient and not just the disease.

6.2 Infection of wounds

Pathogenesis and virulence of infecting microorganisms

Bacteria may cause (limited) harm to wound healing mechanisms due to the metabolism. For nourishment, enzymes such as proteases, lipases and DNases, as well as other specialised enzymes, such as iron, are released. Some of them have capsules with immune cells within which they can hide, with a greater risk to patients with splenectomies. The ability to increase intracellularly does not prevent neutrophile granulocytes and macrophagy, and even allows an increase. As they can survive and reproduce, they have an advantage over the cellular body defence mechanism, if the quantum of oxygen in tissue is low. Special enzymes, e. g. hyaluronidase, may allow bacteria to spread outwards from a wound – examples are *Streptococcus pyogenes* and *Staphylococcus aureus*.

In many species, some strains may be extremely virulent, meaning they are the cause of hazardous infections. An example is necrotising fasciitis by the highly virulent *Streptococcus pyogenes*. *Staphylococcus aureus* strains may harbour Panton-Valentine-Leucocidin (PVL+) and cause abscesses with a high rate of relapse.

Fungi may infect wounds as well. Especially yeast fungi of the genus *Candida* are found in and around wounds, and also the more rare mould fungi. According to data of the Hospital Infection Surveillance System, *Candida*-species were found, for example, to play a role as the sole infectious agent in 0.1–1.4% of postoperative surgical site infections.

Viruses do not have an own metabolism and need to annex the host cells to multiply. They play no role as infectious agents in a hygienic context, but they may be present in exudate and blood, and personal protection care needs to be taken, therefore, with hepatitis viruses and HIV infections.

Parasites do not play a significant role in wound infections. A significant exception is leishmaniosis of the 'old world'. These protozoans are transmitted through being bitten by the sandfly *Phlebotomos*, causing chronic infection, partly through chronic wounds.

In Germany, common ectoparasites such as *Sarcoptes scabiei hominis* cause itchy areas, with scratching leading quickly to bacterial or secondary infections.

6.3 Hygiene in wound care

Hygiene measures should be chosen based on a risk assessment needing professional knowledge with planning and putting into practice. Not following regulations is contraproductive. Using the standards of experts and other sources, every institution should develop procedural instructions. Usually, everyone involved should follow these regulations. In certain cases a deviation can be allowed but should be documented. Hygiene law offers valuable advice in this case. In criminal and civil proceedings, documentation will be the primary basis for a legal review.

Table 6.1 Possible relevant legal aspects

Topic	Possible regulations
Infection prevention	General aspects of hospital hygiene like infection control teams, the role of federal departments and institutes
Medical products	Different aspects of medical products Buying, engaging, cleaning, disinfecting, sterilisation and storage of medicinal products Single-use of medical products
Security of employees	Use of secure needles and scalpels, correct disposal of waste Personal protective equipment (gloves, masks etc.) Immunisation (hepatitis B, influenza, etc.)
Drugs	Definition, use, storage
Social laws and acts	Payment, insurances
Drinking water protection act	Quality of drinking water, engagement of filters, whether tap water is used for wound rinsing

6.3.1 Legal aspects of wound care

Different aspects to look at

Wound care can be complicated, and local laws may regulate some of the processes. ➤ Table 6.1 shows some examples.

Standards (ISO, EN) and recommendations

Standards

Standards are consensual decisions of interprofessional circles, generally with a significant part played by industrial lobbyists. These standards represent the 'actual state-of-the-art'. Nonetheless, rules are not laws and there is constant room for deviation. In case of harm befalling patients, one should demonstrate that one's own solution will have the same effect as the standardised process.

Recommendations

Recommendations may be published by expert panels, interprofessional groups or even single experts. Using different evidence levels, they may reflect actual medical knowledge. Nonetheless, publications of state departments usually have a greater legal impact. These publications then have to be integrated into the process for management and quality.

Above and beyond this advice, recommendations from certain experts should be adhered to if they are coherent, consistent and appropriate.

6.3.2 Practical hygiene: basic hygiene and extended hygiene measures

Basic hygiene needs to be followed by all employees; for example, hand hygiene, surface disinfection and use of sterile medical products. Extended measures mean the use of protective suits which is indicated in cases of contaminated patients. The personal protective equipment depend on the microorganisms or virus. The appropriate protective measures need to be taken for corresponding infections or microorganisms. Hygiene management is based on three aspects: personal hygiene measures, environmental hygiene measures (such as surface disinfection) and the correct use of medical products, medicines and the disposal of waste.

Measures for personnel Basic measures for personnel are hand hygiene and disposal of accidentally contaminated workclothes. Extended measures mean protective material, such as gowns, gloves, masks and goggles. 'Personal hygiene' in hygiene management includes the points given previously and is based on a risk assessment providing for the virulence of possible pathogens, transmission pathways and manifestation index (how many infections occur in correlation to infection). In some countries, legal aspects have to be obeyed.

Workclothing

Generally, there are no special requirements for workclothing. Nonetheless, they should be of a light colour and washable at 60 °C, although reasonable disinfection takes place at a temperature of 40 °C. Contaminated working clothes must not be washed at the home of the employees. Most institutions have standard workclothing or a uniform (corporate identity), which are removed and disinfected in laundromats with a certificate.

Accessories like ties should not form part of the workclothing. When changing a dressing, doctors' scrubs should be taken off. Short-sleeved tops and trousers are optimal. Religious headgear is usually no problem. One has to make sure that nothing will drop onto the wound during treatment.

Protective equipment

Protective clothing (single-use gowns, aprons) and protective equipment (gloves, masks, goggles and face shields) are provided by institutions. In the case of reusable protective clothing, the institutions have to use a certified laundry service. Protective clothing must not be washed at the home of personnel.

Hand hygiene

Hand hygiene includes washing, disinfection, skincare and the use of gloves. The World Health Organisation (WHO) has initiated a 'clean hands'-program including advice for compliance checks and motivation of personnel, patients and patients' relatives. Hand hygiene results have shown that hands are not disinfected nearly enough. However, hand disinfection is still the cheapest and most effective preventative method to avoid transmission.

Handwashing is performed at the beginning and end of a working day, before and after breaks and before leaving the institution. In cases of higher contamination, once thorough removal of the object has taken place, a single-use cloth or wipe soaked in disinfectant can be used after washing the hands. To protect the skin, washing should take place as little as possible. To dry hands thoroughly, single-use towels from a dispenser should be used.

A **hygienic disinfection of the hands** should now take place. A handful of disinfectant should now be rubbed into clean and dry hands for 30 seconds. Spe-

cial attention should be paid to the tips of the fingers and the thumbs:
- **Before** and **after** contact with patients,
- **Before** aseptic work (like preparing injections or wound dressings),
- **After** contact with contaminated materials (used wound dressings, toilet use) and contact with the area around a patient,
- **Before** taking gloves out of the box and immediately **after** taking off gloves.

Surgical disinfection of the hands includes hands and forearms, at least 10 minutes after washing! – taking 1.5–3 minutes. Handbrushes are now only used for cleaning fingernails. Hands should be dry before putting on gloves, to avoid skin irritation.

Gloves are always indicated if contact with body fluids like blood or wound exudate is expected, as in wound care. Hygiene gloves (out of a box containing 100) are adequate for self-protection. If direct contact with the wound site is necessary, sterile gloves are mandatory. Disinfection of gloves is not recommended and one pair should not be worn longer than 15 minutes. However, even new gloves have micro-perforations, and hand disinfection after taking off gloves is obligatory.

Use of **medical skin protection lotions and hand cream** is an integral part of hand hygiene. People with allergies may use disinfection based on pure alcohol, which necessitates intensive skincare.

Hygiene measures for patient's environment

Hygiene measures for the patient's environment includes surface disinfection, use and preparation of medical products, use and application of drugs, use and cleaning of eating utensils and laundry as well as correct disposal of waste.

Cleaning and disinfection of surfaces

Each change of the wound dressing may spread bacteria from a wound to the surrounding surfaces, such as with bacteria carried by dust particles or tiny splashes when rinsing a wound. Therefore, disinfection of surfaces after the end of a dressing change makes sense. Useful are medical wipes which allow quick disinfection.

Use of medical products

All reusable medical products need a carefully managed process within the institution, including transport, cleaning, disinfection, sterilisation, quality management and storage. It is recommended to make a risk assessment like this:
- Non-critical medical products: regular contact with intact skin only (blood pressure unit, stethoscope, etc.),
- Semi-critical medical products: regular contact with intact mucosa only,
- Critical medical products: regular contact with open skin or mucosa.

Single-use (sterile) medical products have to be stored and protected from dust and ultraviolet radiation due to changes in the package stability.

Use of drugs and multidose units

Storage according to the manufacturers' recommendations. Medical fridges do not need regular disinfecting.

Drug dispensers should be washed; disinfection is not necessary.

Multidose units should be marked with the date and time of first use. The use-by date, which depends on the expiration time of the unit, needs to be noted and adjusted accordingly.

Infusions without an expiration date, such as physiologic sodium chloride solution, are for a single-time use only.

Waste

Sharps – even those with security mechanisms – should be collected in safe, unbreakable and non-penetrable containers. Wound dressings can be disposed of in sacks in regular waste.

6.4 Basic hygiene during patient treatment

These include injections and wound debridement. **Injections** should be prepared under aseptic conditions. Skin disinfection should be performed by spraying with a disinfectant and wiping, or using a medical wipe.

Subcutaneous injections only need simple disinfection by spraying. After 30 seconds, residues can be wiped off with **sterilised** swabs (sterilised by manufacturer, stored in sterile conditions by the institution). Intramuscular injections in the gluteal area need to be sprayed with disinfectant, then wiped using sterile swabs and then sprayed again and left to dry for the disinfectant to be effective.

Injections should be prepared in an aseptic environment. In ambulant care, this should be performed with a disinfected tray, e. g. wiped with a sterile wipe.

If available, **secure sharps** should be used and collected in safe containers, for needle disposal. If empty boxes of labelled products are used, signs of the former content should be eliminated and replaced with the word 'waste'. As these types of containers have no mechanism for the cleaning of cannulas, it is recommended to dispose of the whole syringe (including the cannula) inside. If containers with a wipe-off mechanism for cannulas are used, cannulas may be separated, and syringes can be disposed of in regular waste.

Once set in place, **infusion pumps** can be used for a maximum of 72–96 hours (without physiologic sodium chloride or Ringer's solution). If solutions with amino acids or lipids are used, this time decreases to 24 hours and 12 hours, respectively. If possible, avoid disconnections.

Puncturing of medical ports can be performed after antisepsis with a remanent antiseptic (alcohol + octenidine or alcohol + chlorhexidine, mixed and ready to use). One should wear sterile gloves and use special cannulas. Transparent dressings are recommended.

6.5 Risk assessment as basis for hygiene measures

Hygiene instructions should be based on certain measures. Important questions are:
- Which pathogens may occur in the relevant situation?
- Which patients are at risk and which areas in greater institutions?
- What special risks for infection does the identified group of patients have?
- Which measures can I take to break transmission pathways?

6.6 Hygienic surgical debridement

Surgical interventions for wound cleaning can be performed in an operating theatre (including airlocks for patients and personnel, and air conditioning preventing bacteria) or in smaller spaces without special technical equipment. Appropriate protective scrubs should be chosen to prevent possible risk of contamination and to protect the patient (e. g. sterile gloves instead of medical gloves).

More significant surgical sites require sterile protection suits and use of a fully equipped operation theatre.

Whichever theatre or space, the cleansing of aseptic wounds should be performed before those of septic ones. Biosurgical interventions using maggots need the same risk assessment.

Smaller or less invasive debridements can be treated in doctors' surgeries or even at the patient's home. Minimal requirements for hygiene in these situations are:
- An aseptic or sterile absorbent surface for the preparation of the required instruments and dressings; each item to be sterile,
- Use of medical gloves in the case of performing non-touch technique, sterile gloves in the case of direct wound contact,
- Protective apron (waterproof) in case of wound rinsing.

Biosurgical debridement with maggots will need a change of dressing from a hygienic point of view; methodologically, reference is made to the relevant literature and the EWMA handbook. In general, sterile instruments and compresses or swabs should be used.

Waste should be collected in waterproof, opaque, closed containers. Other methods of collecting waste depend on local legal regulations.

6.7 Hygienic requirements for the changing of wound dressings

6.7.1 Rooms

It should be possible to clean and disinfect rooms for changing wound dressings quickly; this includes all working surfaces, interior and the floor. Furthermore, the following is important:

1. Generally, when changing wound dressings, bacteria including multiresistant variants will be transmitted from wound environment to its surroundings. Therefore, sheets and beds or other places to lie on should be covered with a single-use protective cloth. If smooth surfaces are easy to disinfect, regular disinfection is adequate.
2. Sterile medical products have to be kept free from dust or ultraviolet light.
3. An antiseptic work surface is required.

6.7.2 Procedure

Preparation

Preparation requires:
- All the necessary instruments and dressings
- Opaque waste container
- Secure container for sharps disposal (see 'waste')
- Protective suits or aprons, if required, possibly a mask
- Removed dressings to be disposed of in appropriate containers

Cleaning and rinsing of the wound are now performed, followed by antiseptic treatment if necessary.

Mechanical cleansing of wounds is always performed from the centre of the wound to its periphery, from the inside to the outside.

Single-use instruments are disposed of in a safe container. Re-usable instruments have to be transported safely to be processed.

Gloves are removed, and after disinfection of hands, documentation such as photos or measurement of a wound size can be performed. After disinfecting hands once more, new medical gloves, and in the case of direct wound contact, sterile gloves, are put on.

Performance and finishing

New wound dressings are unwrapped while avoiding contamination. Cutting dressings to size (following manufacturers' instructions) can also lead to contamination. Application of new dressings, including tamponades, must be performed with the non-touch technique or otherwise sterile gloves.

After the new dressing is in place, waste is disposed of in a container and surfaces are disinfected. Disposing of gloves and disinfecting the hands completes this process.

6.8 Wound care in the case of infected patients

Multi-resistant organisms

All well-known variants of multi-resistant organisms (MRO) may infect wounds. These are:
- MRSA (methicillin-resistant *Staphylococcus aureus*)
- Acylureidopenicillin-, cephalosporin- and ciprofloxacin-resistant enterobacteriaceae
- Acylureidopenicillin-, cephalosporin-, ciprofloxacin- and carbapenem-resistant enterobacteriaceae
- Acylureidopenicillin, cephalosporin- and ciprofloxacin-resistant *Acinetobacter* spp.
- Acylureidopenicillin, cephalosporin-, ciprofloxacin- and carbapemen-resistant *Acinetobacter* spp.
- Acylureidopenicillin, cephalosporin- and ciprofloxacin-resistant *Pseudomonas aeruginosa*

- Acylureidopenicillin, cephalosporin-, ciprofloxacin- and carbapemen-resistant *Pseudomonas aeruginosa*
- Vancomycin-resistant *Enterococcus faecium*
- Vancomycin- and linezolid-resistant *Enterococcus faecium*

Protective equipment should be implemented according to the results of risk assessment, e.g. masks are only needed in the case of aerosols or as contact protection for nose and mouth.

Risk assessment includes the following questions:
- Where on the patient or in the patient is the pathogen located?
- Which antibiotics are available in a worst case infection?

The following measures are required:

Utensils used, as well as those medicines and antiseptics which have been applied, should be used for one patient only. There is no need for separate waste disposal, but containers should be disinfected when taken out of the room.

Laundry is collected in the patient's room in a laundry bag which is then inserted into a plastic sack. There is no need for separate transportation of dishes; using hot water of 60 °C will eliminate any germs.

Dry wound dressings, especially when used with antiseptics, are protective, so no isolation of the patient is required with a single wound if the patient is not changing his/her own dressings.

Laundry should be transported in marked sacks; dishes can be cleaned as usual with a recommended temperature over 65 °C.

Barrier care in case of hepatitis B, hepatitis C and HIV-infection

In this case, self-protection is mandatory. Gloves are therefore used in combination with the non-touch technique, if possible. In some countries, dressings drenched in blood have to be disposed of in separate containers.

Wound care of patients with acute infections

Generally, for each type of infection, a specific process is described in the hygiene handbook of the various institutions. Communication about new diagnoses is essential, especially in ambulant institutions such as homecare.

6.9 Conclusion

Wound care is possible in almost every health care facility. However, hygiene measures must then be implemented based on risk assessments, as well as for the protection of other patients and staff.

REFERENCES

Kommission für Krankenhaushygiene und Infektionsprävention. Anforderungen an die Hygiene bei der Aufbereitung von Medizinprodukten. 2012. www.rki.de/Infektionsschutz/Krankenhaushygiene/ (last accessed 12 October 2020).

Kommission für Krankenhaushygiene und Infektionsprävention. Händehygiene in Einrichtungen des Gesundheitsdienstes. 2016. www.rki.de/Infektionsschutz/Krankenhaushygiene/ (last accessed 12 October 2020).

Kommission für Krankenhaushygiene und Infektionsprävention. Prävention postoperativer Wundinfektionen. 2018. www.rki.de/Infektionsschutz/Krankenhaushygiene/ (last accessed 12 October 2020).

Kommission für Krankenhaushygiene und Infektionsprävention. Prävention der Infektion durch Enterokokken mit speziellen Antibiotikaresistenzen. 2018. www.rki.de/Infektionsschutz/Krankenhaushygiene/ (last accessed 12 October 2020).

Schwarzkopf A. Hygiene in der Arztpraxis. 4th ed. Wiesbaden: mhp publisher, 2018.

Schwarzkopf A. Multiresistente Erreger im Gesundheitswesen. 2nd ed. Wiesbaden: mhp publisher, 2016.

7

Sabine Eming, Stephan Schreml

Physiology and pathology of wound-healing

7.1 Efficient complexity of wound-healing
Sabine Eming

───────────────────────── **Key notes** ─────────────────────────

- During wound-healing, different cell populations have to fulfil their task in a coordinated manner through a complex network of various factors.
- For the wound-healing process, nature uses molecular and cellular mechanisms, which in principle are also observed in other physiological (e.g. embryonic development) and pathological processes (e.g. fibrosis, tumour growth, metastasis).

- There are a large number of underlying systemic diseases that must be considered with a differential diagnosis as causes of a poorly healing wound.
- The imbalance between increased activity of inflammatory mediators, proteolytic enzymes and decreased activity of their inhibitors is considered to be a significant local disruptive factor in chronic wounds.

The process of tissue repair is a cell-biologically complex process to restore the barrier function of the skin as quickly as possible. During wound-healing, different cell populations have to perform their tasks in a complex network of various factors coordinated in time and space. The cells receive the required signals mainly through cell-cell interactions, cell-matrix contacts or cytokine-mediated interactions.

In wound-healing, a fundamental distinction is made between tissue regeneration and tissue repair. During restoration, a restitution of the damaged tissue and function is achieved, and the process of repair by replacement of the damaged tissue with scarring leads to wound closure. Although the skin is characterised by its natural defensive and protective function and in principle by a large reparative capacity, it has only limited abilities for regeneration, i.e. for scarless healing and new formation of the skin appendages. As a rule, the healing process for each ulcer is completed with scarring and loss of the skin appendages. A scar is always functionally inferior to healthy, uninjured skin. Scar-free wound-healing is only possible in cases of skin damage limited to the epidermis; these wounds are referred to as erosions

('abrasions'). On the other hand, mucous membranes are characterised by high regenerative capacity and low scarring.

7.1.1 Phases of wound-healing

Physiological wound-healing is a process that is stringently controlled in terms of time and location. Several phases are differentiated, which overlap in a specific sequence in time and space (➤ Fig. 7.1) to simplify the presentation. In recent years there has been considerable progress in a better understanding of the molecular and cellular control mechanisms underlying a successful healing process. Initially, a pronounced inflammatory reaction occurs, leading to the elimination of defective tissue and germs. This is followed by the induction of the formation of new vessels and the activation of keratinocytes and fibroblasts. Finally, new tissue is formed in the dermis, and the wound is epithelialised. The wound closure is followed by scarring and adaptation of the replacement tissue to biomechanical requirements.

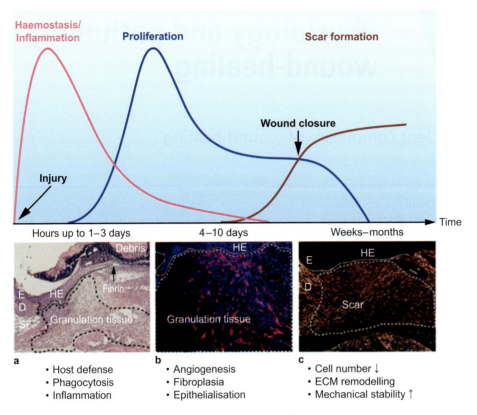

Fig. 7.1 The phases of physiological wound-healing that overlap spatially and temporally: **a** inflammatory phase, H&E staining; **b** proliferative phase with angiogenesis, CD31 immunohistochemistry; **c** scar, Sirius red staining and analysis in polarised light; E = epidermis, D = dermis; HE = proliferating epithelial wound margin; SF = subcutaneous fat tissue. [P591/I231]

Coagulation and inflammation phase

The immediate consequence of any injury beyond the epidermis is the activation of the coagulation cascade. Cross-linked fibrin molecules, fibronectin, vitronectin and thrombospondin then serve as essential lead structures for immigrant cells (> Fig. 7.1a). Thrombocytes in the fibrin clot release a multitude of different growth factors, e.g. VEGF, PDGF, TGFβ and amphiregulin, which initiate subsequent wound-healing processes. At the same time, vascular dilatation and an increase in vascular permeability lead to an increased accumulation of blood plasma in the interstitium. This process supports wound cleansing by washing out cell debris, foreign bodies and bacteria. Neutrophilic granulocytes migrate into the wound area and ensure the defence against invading microorganisms via phagocytosis

and the formation of reactive oxygen species (ROS). The production of highly potent proteases such as leukocyte elastase, cathepsin G, proteinase 3, uPA and matrix metalloproteinases (MMP) 8 and 9 causes endogenous debridement. Proinflammatory cytokines (IL-1α, -β, TNFα) stimulate downstream mediator systems such as KGF, IL-6, IL-8 and MCP1. Monocytes recruited from the blood migrate into the wound tissue after two to three days and differentiate into wound macrophages; they act as central effectors of angiogenesis and fibroblast proliferation.

The monocytes/macrophages infiltrating the wound tissue react to a multitude of environmental signals from the injured tissue and integrate them into a repair response. The specific molecular factors that control the functional plasticity of macrophages during a healing process have not yet been fully elucidated. In particular, primary research studies in the past decade have contributed to deciphering the mechanisms of monocyte/macrophage plasticity in wound tissue. In the meantime, clinical studies have confirmed the concept that modulation of macrophage activation can intervene in tissue-destroying inflammation and promote the restoration of tissue integrity. Monocytes/macrophages have been proven to be an essential therapeutic target in wound-healing disorders and the promotion of wound-healing.

Granulation phase

The vascular-rich granulation tissue, which is functionally cross-linked via media circuits, sprouts along with the temporary extracellular matrix into the tissue defect (➤ Fig. 7.1b). Necrotic tissue is degraded at the immigration front, and newly formed extracellular matrix (ECM) is deposited at the transition to healthy tissue. The cell count increases significantly, and keratinocytes migrate over the granulation tissue. In this phase, the epithelium is fragile and very susceptible to shear forces, e.g. during dressing changes. On the migration front, the keratinocytes produce interstitial collagenase (MMP-1) and as components of the basement membrane fibronectin and laminin-332. Distally located keratinocytes are involved in the regeneration of the basement membrane zone together with mesenchymal cells of the granulation tissue. In this phase of close interaction between epithelium and mesenchyme, the temporal and spatial balance of the individual factors is decisive. While the initiation of granulation tissue formation takes place without epithelial influence, keratinocytes need stimuli from the wound bed to stimulate their growth.

Epithelialisation

Keratinocytes originating from the skin appendages migrate over the granulation tissue and lead through mitosis and cell differentiation to the restoration of the epithelial barrier. Epithelialisation completes wound-healing. At the same time, the collagen fibres and the extracellular matrix mature and the tissue contracts. The granulation tissue increasingly loses water and vessels, decreases in elasticity and transforms into scar tissue.

Early and late scar tissue

After epithelial wound closure, the barrier function of the skin is mostly restored. The epidermal hyperproliferation and the keratinisation typical for wound-healing – characterised for instance by the gene expression of keratin 6 and 16 – normalise. In the connective tissue underneath, restructuring processes still take place for a long time, which transform the cell-rich, matrix-poor granulation tissue into a cell-poor, matrix-rich scar tissue (➤ Fig. 7.1c). Cells of the previous granulation tissue or the old scar may die by programmed cell death (apoptosis). The signals triggering cell death and possible consequences for the quality of scar formation are so far insufficiently defined and the subject of current investigations.

7.1.2 Pathology of wound-healing

The physiological wound-healing mechanisms can be hindered by a variety of local disruptive factors or underlying systemic diseases as well as ageing processes. In recent years, new findings in stem cell biology, gene expression and regulation, cell culture techniques and animal model development have significantly improved our understanding of the physiology and pathology of tissue repair. Modern local therapy of chronic wounds, in particular, is derived from the combination of new findings from basic research and classical therapeutic principles. To identify the underlying local and systemic disruptive factors of wound-healing and to initiate causal therapies, large differential diagnostic considerations – often with an interdisciplinary approach – are usually necessary.

7.1.3 Wound-healing at the interface of carcinogenesis

There has been a consensus since Rudolf Virchow's early observations that the underlying cellular mechanisms described above, which regulate tissue formation in physiological wound-healing, in principle also control the growth and metastasis of malignant tumours. Parallel processes between wound-healing and carcinogenesis are particularly evident in the development of neoplasias in the context of chronic inflammation.

A chronic wound without a tendency to heal must, therefore, always be thought of as a neoplastic event. For example, squamous cell carcinomas can develop as Marjolin ulcers in the area of persistent ulcers, older scars, burns or radiation fields. Also, blister formation, wound-healing disorders of the skin and the predisposition to carcinoma development characterise the clinical picture of hereditary epidermolysis such as dystrophic epidermolysis bullosa and Kindler syndrome. Thus, the following principle applies: If there is a clinical suspicion of a neoplastic change, a bioplastic clarification is necessary. Delays in diagnosis lead to a worsening of the prognosis and an increased risk of metastasis. Therefore, for all chronic wounds that do not respond to adequate therapy within eight weeks, sample biopsies should be taken from the wound margin and wound bed. An exophytic-growing or irregular wound margin, an unusually high bleeding propensity or pain may indicate neoplastic changes and should be the reason for histological clarification.

REFERENCES

Braun A, Tantcheva-Poor I, Eming SA. Parallelen zwischen Wundheilung, chronisch entzündlichen Dermatosen und Neoplasien – Wissenswertes für die Praxis. Hautarzt 2014; 65: 934–943.

Dissemond J, Augustin M, Eming SA, et al. Modern wound care – practical aspects of non-interventional topical treatment of patients with chronic wounds. J Dtsch Dermatol Ges 2014; 12: 541–554.

Eming SA, Wlaschek M, Scharffetter-Kochanek K. Wundheilung bei älteren Menschen. Hautarzt 2016; 67: 112–116.

Eming SA, Martin P, Tomic-Canic M. Wundreparatur und Regeneration: Mechanismen, Signalisierung und Übersetzung. Sci Transl Med 2014; 6: 265sr6.

Löhrer R, Eming R, Wolfrum N, Krieg T, Eming SA. Autoentzündliche Erkrankungen als Ursache von Wundheilungsstörungen. Hautarzt 2011; 62: 524–533.

Martin P. Wundheilung – mit dem Ziel einer perfekten Hautregeneration. Wissenschaft 1997; 276: 75–81.

Schäfer M, Werner S. Krebs als überheilende Wunde: eine alte Hypothese, die erneut aufgegriffen wurde. Nat Rev Mol Cell Biol 2008; 9: 628–638.

Willenborg S, Eming SA. Macrophages – sensors and effectors coordinating skin damage and repair. J Dtsch Dermatol Ges 2014; 12: 214–223.

7.2 pH value and wound-healing

Stephan Schreml

Key notes

- Although the mechanisms of wound-healing at the cellular level have been scientifically investigated in detail, the state of knowledge regarding basic clinical parameters, e.g. the pH value or also pO_2 and H_2O_2, is still insufficient.
- Wound-healing is strongly regulated by changes in the pH value, as these regulate enzyme activity (e.g. matrix metalloproteinases), alter cell proliferation and migration (e.g. keratinocytes, fibroblasts) and influence the activity of therapeutically used enzymes (e.g. streptokinase).

- The cellular processing of pH changes in the extracellular space is mediated by proton-sensitive G-protein-coupled receptors (pH-GPCRs).
- pH shifts alter the microbiome on wounds, which can be a problem in the healing of chronic wounds.
- The pH value is rarely considered in current treatment regimes. Knowledge about the pH value of wounds and a correspondingly adapted wound therapy could improve the healing of chronic wounds in the future.

7.2.1 Introduction

The healing process of cutaneous wounds depends on local wound factors, systemic mediators, possible underlying diseases such as diabetes mellitus, circulatory disorders and the type of skin injury. Depending on the balance of the factors involved, the wound-healing process is either physiological (acute wounds) or pathologically delayed (chronic wounds). Chronic wounds are characterised by inadequate repair mechanisms that prevent the achievement of lasting anatomical and functional results within a reasonable period. Chronic wounds are, therefore, a significant challenge in interdisciplinary treatment.

The healing of acute (physiological) wounds consists of three temporally and spatially overlapping phases (➤ Chap. 8.1):
1. Inflammation
2. Proliferation (neoangiogenesis, granulation, re-epithelialisation)
3. Tissue structuring (tissue remodelling), e.g. organisation of the extracellular matrix (ECM)

The initial inflammatory phase after a skin injury causes the release of cytokines, chemokines, growth factors and hydrogen peroxide (H_2O_2).

These chemoattractive factors recruit different cell types, such as granulocytes and macrophages into the wound, and thus initiate wound-healing. The pH gradients of the wound environment also have a significant effect on cellular functions such as proliferation and migration.

The subsequent proliferation phase begins with temporal overlap. This phase is characterised by neoangiogenesis, the formation of granulation tissue and extracellular matrix as well as reepithelialisation. Neoangiogenesis is essential for the supply of nutrients, oxygen and other factors due to the increased metabolic activity. Fibroblasts proliferate, and collagen synthesis and deposition are highly regulated. After the formation of the actual wound bed, the wound surface is covered with an epithelial layer. Reepithelialisation is based on the differentiation, proliferation and migration of epidermal keratinocytes, which are activated and migrate from the wound edges to the centre of the wound. It has recently been shown that the pH value is decisive for the centripetal migration of keratinocytes and their proliferation at the wound margins.

Tissue structuring begins a few days after skin injury and can take up to two years. In this phase, several proteinases contribute to coordinated wound-healing. The activity of these proteinases is modified by the wound environment, e.g. by changes in the pH value in the various stages of wound-healing. Changes in the pH value in the wound environment have a massive influence on the activity of the enzymes involved in these processes, such as matrix metalloproteinases (MMPs).

In contrast to acute wound-healing, chronic wounds are not subject to the clearly defined gradual healing process of acute wounds but are characterised by uncontrolled permanent inflammation, which impairs the formation of anatomical and functional integrity within a reasonable period.

For a more detailed insight into the pathophysiological relationship between pH and wound-healing, the following sections focus on factors affecting the skin surface or wound pH and the effect of changes in pH on the wound-healing process.

7.2.2 Influence of various factors on the pH value of the skin

The pH value of the skin surface must not be confused with the pH value of the different skin layers. The pH value of the stratum corneum gradually increases with increasing depth from the skin surface. Due to the absence of the stratum corneum and the deeper skin layers, the pH value of skin wounds must be considered separately. The average pH value of the skin surface is usually measured on the volar forearm. The spectrum described in the literature ranges from 4.0 as the lowest value to about 6.5. Often, the range on the volar forearm is between about 4.5 and 5.5 under standardised conditions (temperature, humidity, no washing of the skin for 24 hours up to several days before measurement), which we were able to prove in several studies.

It is suspected that many different factors affect the pH of the skin surface; however, the results of the studies are often contradictory. In the literature, the differences in skin pH value depending on localisation were described, which – except for intertriginous regions – could usually not be confirmed in other studies. Besides, a circadian rhythm of pH on the forearm was described with about 5.3 in late afternoon and 4.9 at night. Some authors reported a lower pH of the skin surface in men than in women, while other authors found no gender-specific differences. One reason for these contradictions could be the different and non-standardised conditions in the various studies. Standardised conditions are essential for skin surface pH studies because routine procedures such as dousing with tap water increase the pH for many hours. It should be noted that tap water has a pH value of 8 in many European countries.

Several endogenous signalling pathways have been identified that contribute to the acidity of the stratum corneum:

- Production of cis-urocanic acid (cUCA) from filaggrin
- Generation of free fatty acids from phospholipids catalysed by secretory phospholipase A2
- Acidification by the sodium proton exchanger NHE1 (see below)

Other proton transporters such as monocarboxylate transporters (MCTs) seem to play less of a role here. Due to the lack of stratum corneum, higher pH values were measured in acute and chronic wounds than on an intact skin surface. In acute wounds, initial pH values of 7 to over 8 are present, and high values of on average over seven can also often be found on chronic venous ulcers.

7.2.3 pH value of the stratum corneum and regulation of the skin barrier

For a more detailed description of the physiology and pathophysiology of the skin barrier, we refer to an article by Madison (2003). The lamellar corpuscles and the fat composition in the stratum corneum are essential components of the skin barrier. These are regulated by epidermal iron and calcium gradients, which depend on changes in the pH of the stratum corneum. The direct regulation of epidermal barrier homeostasis and the integrity of the stratum corneum by its pH is well understood. Both the degradation of corneodesmosomes caused by a serine protease (e.g. also desmoglein 1) and the β-glucocerebrosidase activity (important for the processing of lipids) are affected by changes in pH.

Molecular evidence for the importance of proton production for the restoration of the skin barrier was found in studies of the sodium proton exchanger NHE 1. NHE 1 is a specific sodium proton exchange resin that regulates the pH of the stratum corneum and on the skin surface. Compared to wild type mice, NHE 1(−/−) mice showed significantly delayed skin barrier restoration.

In our work, we were able to show that in the course of acute wound-healing from split skin removal sites at the margins, the expression of NHE1 increases continuously and thus contributes to the restoration of the pH value or the epidermal barrier. In chronic venous wounds, we found a significantly increased NHE expression at the wound margin compared to the wound centre, which may explain the low pH values found at the wound margin (about 6.5) compared to the high values found at the wound centre (about 7.5). We also found that these pH gradients could impede the proliferation of keratinocytes at the wound margin and their centripetal migration, and could thus be a reason for the persistence of chronic wounds (see below). Changes in the expression of other investigated proton transporters such as monocarboxylate transporters (MCTs) were not observed. This shows the importance of a precisely regulated pH value for wound-healing.

7.2.4 Cellular processing of the signals by altered extracellular pH values

Four proton-sensitive G-protein-coupled receptors (GPCRs) are known: GPR4 (GPR19), TDAG8 (GPR65, T Cell Death-associated Gene 8), OGR1 (GPR68, Ovarian Cancer GPCR 1) and G2A (GPR132, G2 Accumulation Protein). These GPCRs are expressed differently in different tissues, but very little is known about their expression in skin and wounds. These GPCRs are mainly activated by the protonation of different histidine residues as soon as the extracellular pH falls below the physiologically present value, e.g. the pH we have found in the margins of chronic wounds. It is known that these proton-sensitive GPCRs play a role in tumour cell proliferation, apoptosis, metastasis, angiogenesis, immune cell function and inflammatory processes. This is particularly interesting because tumours and wounds have a lot in common, which is regulated by fluctuations in the extracellular pH value ➤ Table 7.1).

Positive or negative modulation of a multitude of other GPCRs is already a successful instrument for the treatment of many diseases, such as allergies, gastric ulcers and high blood pressure – more than 50% of the pharmaceuticals on the market act directly or indirectly via GPCRs.

In addition to proton-sensitive GPCRs, it is known that acid-sensing ion channels (ASICs) register fluctuations in extracellular proton concentrations in the central nervous system. Neither the expression nor the possible role of such ASICs in wounds has

Table 7.1 Common features of tumour growth and wound-healing concerning pH value

	Neoplasm	Wounds
pH dysregulation	Inverse cellular pH gradient pH_e ~6.2–7,0 < pH_i ~7.2–7.7	Changed pH_e on the wound surface **Acute wounds:** • Day 1 postoperative: pH_e ~8.0–8.5 • Day 14 postoperative: pH_e ~6.0–6.5 **Chronic wounds:** • Wound margin pH_e ~6.5 • Wound centre pH_e ~7.5
Activation of proton-sensitive GPCRs	By lowered pH in the tumour microenvironment: pH_e ~6.2–7.0	**Acute wounds:** • Inactivated: pH_e initial ~8.0–8.5 **Chronic wounds:** • Activated at wound edge: pH_e ~6.5 • Inactivated in wound centre: pH_e ~7.5
Changed enzyme activity	Due to changes in pH_i and pH_e in tumour micro-environments (e. g. MMPs)	Due to changes in the pH_e on the wound surface (e. g. MMPs)
Cell proliferation	Increased (Influence of pH_e varies depending on tumour entity, few data?)	• Acute wounds: raised (pH_e ~8.0–8.5) • Chronic wounds: degraded (wound margin pH_e ~6.5, wound centre pH_e ~7.5)
Cell migration	Increased (influence of pH_e varies depending on tumour entity, few data?)	• Acute wounds: raised (pH_e ~8.0–8.5) • Chronic wounds: degraded (wound margin pH_e ~6.5, wound centre pH_e ~7.5)
Protein synthesis	Increased (influence of pH_e?)	• Acute wounds: raised • Chronic wounds: degraded
Changes in the extracellular matrix	During tumour growth (varied influence of pH_e on the various MMPs)	During 'tissue remodelling phase' (distinct influence of pHe on different MMPs)

pH_e = extracellular pH value; pH_i = intracellular pH value

been investigated. Other proton-sensitive proteins are TRPVs 1 and 4 (Transient Receptor Potential Channel Vanilloid Subfamily), which play a role in nociception and tumour growth. The purpose of these TRPVs in wound-healing is also still unknown.

7.2.5 Influence of pH on cell proliferation and migration

A few studies investigated the effect of pH changes on the proliferation and migration of keratinocytes and fibroblasts. Interestingly, it was found that high pH values above 7 to sometimes above 8 are optimal for the migration of keratinocytes. The proliferation activity of keratinocytes remained almost constant in a high pH range from about 7 to over 8, whereas fibroblasts only actively proliferate in a narrow pH range around 7.5. Interestingly, fibroblasts in chronic wounds even show properties of cellular senescence, e. g. reduced growth rate and increased expression of SA-β-Gal (senescence-associated β-glucocerebrosidase). These results are fascinating because the proliferation activity of fibroblasts and keratinocytes must change during the different phases of wound-healing to meet the requirements of a coordinated gradual wound-healing process. In recent studies, we have further demonstrated, as discussed above, that pH gradients in chronic venous wounds (wound margin about 6.5, wound centre about 7.4) may impede the proliferation of keratinocytes at the wound margin and their centripetal migration, and thus contribute to the maintenance of ulcerations.

7.2.6 Influence of pH on enzymes and proteins in wounds

Changes in pH also lead to changes in enzyme activity, which play a central role in the complex network of cutaneous wound-healing. MMPs are important factors in wound-healing, and the activity of the various members of this protein family is known to be regulated by changes in pH. For example, β-glucocerebrosidase (processing of lipids for homeostasis of the skin barrier) has an optimal pH of 5.6, while the ideal pH of cholesterol sulphatase (regeneration of cholesterol) is 8.0.

The pH value also influences the activity of exogenously applied enzymes in the treatment of chronic wounds. Collagenase has a narrow pH range of 6.0 to 8.0, which provides sufficient activity. Papain, on the other hand, is active over a wide pH range from 3.0 to over 12.5. For this reason, an unfavourable pH value of the wound environment can lead to complete inhibition of endogenous and therapeutically applied wound enzymes. Using 2D luminescence imaging, we were able to show very high pH values of approx. 8 to 8.5 (averaged over the entire wound surface) at split skin removal sites (as a model for acute/physiological wound-healing) on day one postoperatively, which then dropped to values of approx. 6.5 by the 14th postoperative day. In chronic wounds, a pH gradient of pHe 6.5 was observed at the margins and about 7.5 in the wound centre. These data are of particular importance for wound-healing concerning the application of proteolytic enzymes: DNAse is active in a pH range from 4.5 to 5.5, streptokinase from 7.3 to 7.6. Both enzymes are used in the treatment of chronic wounds. These examples demonstrate the importance of actual knowledge of changes in pH during the different phases of wound-healing to predict which enzymes might be beneficial for the patient.

Of course, wound-healing can also be affected by structural changes of proteins due to pH shifts. For example, it has been shown that changes in the pH value alter the structure of the extracellular matrix protein vitronectin, thereby altering the binding of endothelial cells. This fact may be necessary for neo-angiogenesis during the proliferation phase. Vitronectin also interacts with other ECM proteins, such as osteonectin, which interferes with fibroblast proliferation and collagen production.

7.2.7 Bacterial colonisation and pH in wounds

It has been shown that high pH values in chronic wounds alter the local microbiome and vice versa. The exact significance of these changes and their effects on the healing process of wounds are the subject of current research. However, the correlation between the pH value and the various bacterial colonisation patterns has already been investigated in experiments.

It could be shown that Staphylococcus epidermidis grows optimally at low pH values (about 4.7) and that colonisation with *Staphylococcus aureus* is suppressed at high pH values (about 7). Also, the pH value in wounds influences the colonisation with fungi. Here, too, research is currently being carried out into the significance of mycotic colonisation for the microbiome and healing.

7.2.8 Therapeutic changes in pH in wounds

Changes in the pH value of wounds represent promising, cost-effective and straightforward strategies for wound treatment. Changes in the pH value of a wound could, for example, be an effective means of modifying bacterial colonisation. Such therapeutic approaches are also aimed at disrupting the transmembrane pH gradients of bacteria. The efficacy of topically applied azelaic acid on *Propionibacterium acnes* and *Staphylococcus epidermidis* is based on the disturbance of the transmembrane pH gradients. Already decades ago, Leeven et al. used the chemical acidification of chronic wounds for the treatment of bacterial colonisation. Two methods were successful:

1. Occlusive polyethene reduces the loss of CO_2 from the wound (pH decreases).
2. Topically applied acetic acid immediately eliminated the colonisation with Pseudomonas aeruginosa.

In recent years, an interesting group of endogenous antimicrobial substances has been discovered: antimicrobial peptides such as cathelicidin (LL-37, a C-terminal fragment of human cathelicidin). Interestingly, LL-37 affects the proliferation rate and migration of keratinocytes as well as the production of cytokines and chemokines. Since chronic wounds usually show bacterial colonisation, it is reasonable to speculate about the future potential of treatment regimens with LL-37. Therapeutic changes in LL-37 expression are conceivable, e.g. by short-chain fatty acids such as butyrate.

Another strategy based on changes in the pH of wounds is the use of biodegradable polymers that release growth factors such as fibroblast growth factor-2 (FGF-2) depending on the pH of the wound. FGF-2 is essential for the proliferation and collagen production of fibroblasts during the proliferation phase of cutaneous wound-healing. Drug delivery systems and other test methods have already been developed in vitro. These strategies are promising, even if these methods still have to be transferred from research to practice.

Influencing the activity of the NHE1, as mentioned above, would also be a strategy for modifying the wound pH value.

7.2.9 Measurement of the pH of the skin surface and in wounds

Although there is a lack of approval and hygiene problems during reprocessing, glass microelectrodes are still the gold standards for clinical measurement of the pH value on the skin surface and in wounds. However, other methods are required for a two-dimensional representation of the spatial pH changes. Luminescence-based reversible 2D sensors, such as those we have developed in recent years, are suitable for this purpose.

7.2.10 Conclusion

Although it is known that pH has a significant effect on numerous cellular functions (proliferation, migration), enzyme activity (e.g. MMPs and therapeutic enzymes), protein expression, microbial activity and skin barrier function. The exact role of its changes in acute and chronic wounds is still unclear. Further studies on the effect of the pH value of wounds on the wound-healing process and possible treatment options are, therefore, indispensable. Since the first experimental studies on pH in wounds and wound-healing was conducted decades ago, it is difficult to understand that our knowledge in this field has not expanded enough over many decades to understand and effectively change the underlying processes.

REFERENCES

Behne MJ, Meyer JW, Hanson KM, et al. NHE1 regulates the stratum corneum permeability barrier homeostasis. Microenvironment acidification assessed with fluorescence lifetime imaging. J Biol Chem 2002; 277: 47399–47406.

Hunt TK, Twomey P, Zederfeldt B, Dunphy JE. Respiratory gas tensions and pH in healing wounds. Am J Surg 1967; 114: 302–307.

Haverkampf S, Heider J, Weiß KT, et al. NHE1-expression at wound margins increases time-dependently during physiological healing. Exp Dermatol 2017; 26: 124–126.

Leveen HH, Falk G, Borek B, et al. Chemical acidification of wounds. An adjuvant to healing and the unfavorable action of alkalinity and ammonia. Ann Surg 1973; 178: 745–753.

Madison KC. Barrier function of the skin: "La raison d'être" of the epidermis. J Invest Dermatol 2003; 121: 231–241.

Neri D, Supuran CT. Interfering with pH regulation in tumours as a therapeutic strategy. Nat Rev Drug Discov 2011; 10: 767–777.

Schneider LA, Körber A, Grabbe S, Dissemond J. Influence of pH on wound-healing: a new perspective for wound-therapy? Arch Dermatol Res 2007; 298: 413–420.

Schreml S, Meier RJ, Wolfbeis OS, Landthaler M, Szeimies RM, Babilas P. 2D luminescence imaging of pH in vivo. Proc Natl Acad Sci USA 2011; 108: 2432–2437.

Schreml S, Meier RJ, Kirschbaum M, et al. Luminescent dual sensors reveal extracellular pH-gradients and hypoxia on chronic wounds that disrupt epidermal repair. Theranostics 2014; 4: 721–735.

Webb BA, Chimenti M, Jacobson MP, Barber DL. Dysregulated pH: a perfect storm for cancer progression. Nat Rev Cancer 2011; 11: 671–677.

Weiß K, Fante M, Schreml J, et al. Proton-sensing G protein-coupled receptors (GPCRs): potential linkers of tumour growth and wound-healing? Exp Dermatol 2017; 26: 127–132.

II

Disease patterns

Joachim Dissemond

8

Systematic diagnosis of chronic wounds: the ABCDE rule

Key notes

- The ABCDE rule helps to carry out the diagnosis for patients with chronic wounds in a structured manner.
- The acronym ABCDE stands for: A = Anamnesis; B = Bacteria; C = Clinical examination; D = Defective vascular system; E = Extras.

- For an individual diagnosis it is not automatically necessary to clarify all points for all patients.

8.1 Introduction

Diagnostics should always be the basis for a successful treatment strategy. The ABCDE rule should help to plan the concept of an individualised diagnosis for patients with chronic wounds in a structured way (➤ Table 8.1).

Table 8.1 ABCDE rule for the structured diagnosis of the causes of chronic wounds

A	Anamnesis
B	Bacteria
C	Clinical examination
D	Defective vascular system
E	Extras

8.2 Definitions

A – Anamnesis   The anamnesis is always the first step in diagnostics. Patients and their relatives are interviewed about the current wound, past wounds, comorbidities and family history (➤ Table 8.2).

B – Bacteria   Bacteria are rarely the sole cause of chronic wounds (➤ Table 8.3). Superficial bacteriological smears are usually taken for screening examinations, in particular for the detection of multi-re-

sistant organisms (MRO) such as methicillin-resistant *Staphylococcus aureus* (MRSA).

Table 8.2 Anamnestic data of the patients, which can be a first indication of the underlying causes

Artificial ulcer	'Occurrence overnight'
CVI	'Tired and heavy' legs in the evenings
Pressure ulcer	Immobility, polyneuropathy
Diabetes	Polyneuropathy, lack of painfulness
Graft-versus-host	Condition following bone marrow transplantation
Calciphylaxis	Renal insufficiency, dialysis obligation
Leishmaniasis	A stay abroad, e.g. in the tropics, eastern Africa
Livedoid vasculopathy	Recurrent occurrence
Drugs	Intake of, e.g., hydroxycarbamide, phenprocoumon, sirolimus
Necrobiosis lipoidica	Comorbidity diabetes mellitus
PAD	Intermittent claudication
Pyoderma gangrenosum	Starts as 'insect bite', or 'abscess', after trauma, e.g. operation
Hypertensive ischaemic leg ulcer	Insufficiently adjusted arterial hypertension
CVI = chronic venous insufficiency; PAD = peripheral artery disease	

Table 8.3 Bacteria are rarely the cause of chronic wounds. There are however bacterial diseases that can lead to chronic wounds

Chlamydia trachomatis	Lymphogranuloma venereum
Corynebacterium diphtheriae	Diphtheria
Haemophilus ducreyi	Ulcer molle
Klebsiella granulomatis	Granuloma inguinale
Mycobacteria	Buruli ulcer, Lupus vulgaris
Treponema pallidum	Lues (maligna)

Table 8.4 Predilection sites of chronic wounds

CVI	Malleolus medialis
Pressure ulcer	Sacral, heels
Diabetes mellitus	Plantar/forefoot, toes
Necrobiosis lipoidica	Tibia, arch of the foot
PAD	Toes, forefoot
Systemic sclerosis	Fingertips
Thromboangiitis obliterans	Toes
Hypertensive ischaemic leg ulcer	Dorsolateral lower leg

CVI = chronic venous insufficiency; PAD = peripheral artery disease

Table 8.5 Pathological changes of periwound area or wound margin

Atrophie blanche	CVI, livedoid vasculopathy, hydroxycarbamide
Hairless legs	PAD, thromboangiitis obliterans
Eczema	CVI (congestive dermatitis), allergic/toxic contact eczema
Hyperkeratosis	Polyneuropathy, squamous cell carcinoma
Cool and atrophic	PAD
Livid erythaema	Pyoderma gangraenosum, vasculitis, vasculopathy, hypertensive ischaemic leg ulcer, calciphylaxis
Sclerosis	CVI (lipodermatosclerosis), systemic sclerosis, graft-versus-host disease

CVI = chronic venous insufficiency; PAD = peripheral arterial disease

Table 8.6 Basic diagnosis of the vascular system of the lower extremities

Arteries	Foot pulse palpation, ankle-brachial-index (ABI)
Veins	Doppler or duplex sonography

C – Clinical examination   During the clinical examination, apart from the anatomical location of the wounds (➤ Table 8.4), the edge of the wound as well as the wound surroundings are also important, as essential indications of the underlying causes and complications can be diagnosed here (➤ Table 8.5).

D – Blood circulation   In the case of wounds on the lower extremities, both the venous and arterial vascular systems should be examined to clarify the circulatory situation. The arterial diagnosis begins with the palpation of the foot pulse. Also, the ankle-brachial index (ABI) should always be determined by Doppler sonography. The primary diagnosis in cases of suspected chronic venous insufficiency (CVI) includes directional Doppler sonography or, preferably, a colour-coded duplex sonography of the leg veins (➤ Table 8.6).

E – Extras   In particular, if the genesis of the wounds cannot be unambiguously clarified with basic diagnostics, numerous advanced diagnostic procedures can be used in a targeted manner (➤ Table 8.7). In this context, a biopsy, which should usually be taken from the periwound area, is often the most critical procedure.

Table 8.7 Advanced diagnosis

Biopsy	Neoplasia, vasculitis, vasculopathy, leishmaniasis, necrobiosis lipoidica
Genetic analyses	Klinefelter syndrome, factor V Leiden mutation
Capillary microscopy	Systemic sclerosis
Pathergy test	Pyoderma gangrenosum, Behçet's disease
Polyneuropathy diagnosis*	Diabetes mellitus
Rumpel-Leede phenomenon	Vasculitis, clotting disorder
Serology	Vasculitis, calciphylaxis

* Touch sensitivity → 10 g monofilament, vibration sensation → tuning fork test

8.3 Conclusion

The targeted diagnosis of patients with chronic wounds is usually extensive and cost-intensive. The ABCDE rule is intended to help carry out the individually planned diagnosis in a structured manner. Here it becomes clear that interdisciplinary networking is essential for optimal diagnostics in patients with different kinds of chronic wounds.

REFERENCES

Dissemond J. ABCDE rule in the diagnosis of chronic wounds. J Dtsch Dermatol Ges 2017; 15: 732–734.

Dissemond J, Bültemann A, Gerber V, Jäger B, Kröger K, Münter C. Diagnosis and treatment of chronic wounds: current standards of Germany's Initiative for Chronic Wounds e.V. J Wound Care 2017; 26: 727–732.

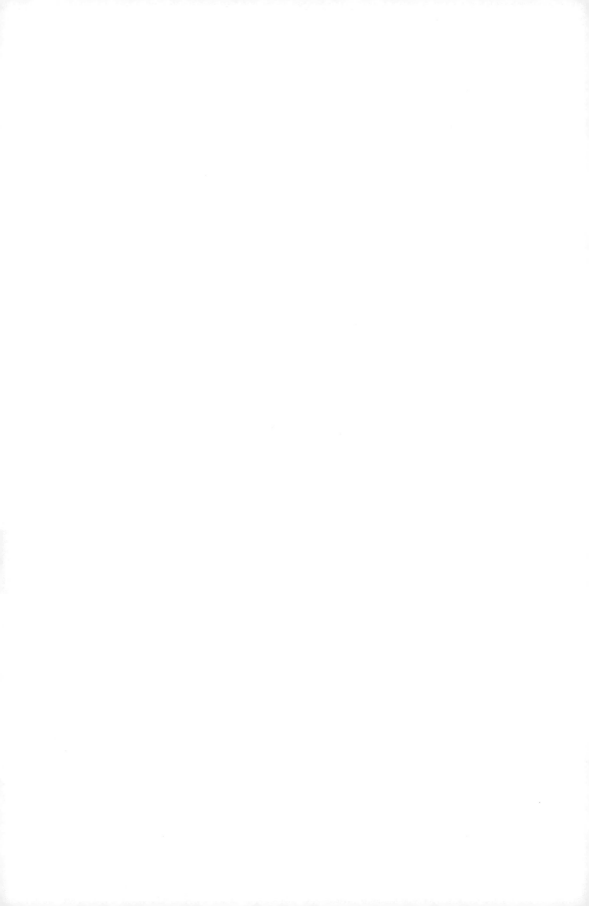

Knut Kröger

9 Disease patterns of peripheral artery disease (PAD)

Key notes

- Many patients with chronic wounds suffer from peripheral artery disease (PAD), which is either the main cause of the wound or at least significantly influences the healing process.
- Clarification of the arterial circulation condition and its targeted therapy are an essential part in the treatment of people with chronic wounds.
- More recent classifications do not classify the PAD patient into stage I to IV based on the

symptoms of their legs, but according to the prognosis for life expectancy and preservation of the limbs into either the more favourable stage of stable intermittent claudication or the prognostically unfavourable stage of critical limb ischaemia (CLI).
- In patients with CLI, successful revascularisation is the most critical prerequisite for wound-healing.

9.1 Introduction

Peripheral artery disease (PAD), also called peripheral arterial occlusive disease (PAOD), describes the clinical symptoms caused by stenoses or occlusions of the iliac arteries, starting from the infrarenal abdominal aorta. In addition to atherosclerosis – by far the most common cause of PAD – embolisms, inflammatory vascular diseases, such as thromboangiitis obliterans (Buerger's disease), accident-related vas-

cular damage or dissections must be considered as causes.

9.2 Definition

Classically, the PAD in German-speaking countries has so far been divided into four stages according to the Strasbourg surgeon René Fontaine (➤ Table 9.1).

Table 9.1 Clinical classification of the stages of severity of PAD according to Fontaine and Rutherford

Classification by Fontaine		Classification by Rutherford	
Stage	Clinical picture	Stage/Category	Clinical picture
I	Asymptomatic	0/0	Asymptomatic
II	Intermittent claudication • Walking distances > 200 m (Stadium IIa) • Walking distances < 200 m (Stadium IIb)	I/1	Mild claudication
		I/2	Moderate claudication
		I/3	Severe claudication
III	Ischaemic rest pain	II/4	Ischaemic rest pain
IV	Ulceration, necrosis or gangrene	III/5	Ischaemic ulceration (minor tissue loss)
		III/6	Ischaemic gangrene (major tissue loss)

In the English-speaking world, the classification made by Rutherford into four stages and six categories is widespread (➤ Table 9.1).

Many wound patients, e. g. people with a diabetic foot syndrome, have simultaneous polyneuropathy and therefore have little or no symptoms until necrosis occurs. Neither classification sufficiently describes their condition. Newer classifications, therefore, do not differentiate between the clinically predominant leg complaints, but rather between the prognoses of life expectancy and limb preservation. Thus, the current literature differentiates PAD into a prognostically more favourable stage of stable intermittent claudication and a prognostically unfavourable stage of chronic critical limb ischaemia (CLI). CLI must not be confused with the clinical picture of acute ischaemia on the basis of an acute embolism or an acute bypass occlusion, which must be immediately revascularised. The term CLI is intended to express that, in contrast to claudication, this is a long-term, critical clinical situation.

People with PAD-induced wounds are, therefore, always in the CLI stage. The decision is made based on laboratory or technical criteria and also on an absence of pain due to polyneuropathy. At the CLI stage, arterial hypoperfusion is the most important cause of chronic wounds or of delayed healing. Revascularisation is, therefore, the first-line treatment.

9.3 Epidemiology

The epidemiology of PAD has been studied extensively over the last 20 years. Nevertheless, there are very few reliable study results. If patients are only asked about leg complaints, the prevalence of symptomatic PAD ranges from about 1% in people less than 50 years of age to 5% in 80-year-olds. If one systematically searches for PAD using recognised measurement methods, the prevalence is 3–5% in 50-year-olds and 15–40% in 80-year-olds.

The most usual method for screening larger populations for PAD is to determine the ankle-brachial index (ABI, a quotient of systolic ankle artery pressure and systolic system pressure; ➤ Fig. 9.1). An ABI ≤ 0.9 is considered pathological. There are various suggestions for calculating ABI. For wound-healing, the calculation of ABI using the higher of the two systolic ankle artery pressures has been more prevalent. It indicates how well the residual perfusion of the leg is preserved. Cardiology is interested in ABI as a marker for coronary heart disease or coronary mortality. Therefore, it is not the residual perfusion that is of interest here, but the fact that a lower leg artery is occluded. The lower of the two ankle artery pressures is then used to calculate the ABI. Reduced ABI, which is calculated using the lowest of the two ankle artery pressures, is a risk factor for increased cardiovascular mortality, not for wound-healing disorder.

The most recent data on the prevalence of PAD in Germany come from the German epidemiological

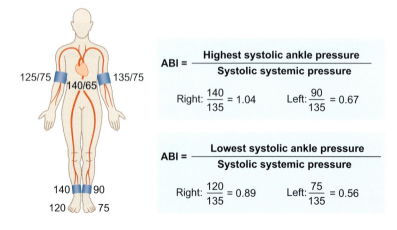

$$ABI = \frac{\text{Highest systolic ankle pressure}}{\text{Systolic systemic pressure}}$$

125/75   140/65   135/75

Right: $\frac{140}{135} = 1.04$ Left: $\frac{90}{135} = 0.67$

$$ABI = \frac{\text{Lowest systolic ankle pressure}}{\text{Systolic systemic pressure}}$$

140   90
120   75

Right: $\frac{120}{135} = 0.89$ Left: $\frac{75}{135} = 0.56$

Fig. 9.1 A sample representation of determining the ankle-brachial index (ABI) in a patient with left-sided claudication. The ABI can be calculated from the higher or lower systolic ankle artery pressure, depending on the clinical issue. [O1089/L231]

trial on ankle brachial index (getABI study) and the Heinz-Nixdorf-Recall (HNR) study. The getABI study is a cross-sectional study of 6,880 unselected people aged 65 and over who were included through their family doctor. The prevalence of PAD in this non-population-based group of people was 19.8% in men and 16.8% in women. The HNR study is a prospective population-based observational study that included 4,735 individuals aged 45–75 from the cities of Essen, Bochum or Mülheim in Germany. The prevalence of PAD was 8.2% for men and 5.5% for women. In all age groups, men were affected more frequently than women. The differences increased significantly from the age of sixty. In the 70- to 75-year-old age group, 18.2% of men and 10.8% of women suffered from PAD. This corresponds to approx. every fifth man and every tenth woman in this age group.

The CLI is not defined by the ABI, but by the absolute pressure values. If an absolute ankle artery pressure < 50–70 mmHg is measured in a patient with a leg wound or rest pain, a CLI is present by definition. Alternative diagnostic criteria are the absolute systolic toe pressure < 30–50 mmHg or transcutaneous oxygen partial pressure < 30 mmHg. Little is known about the prevalence of CLI, as the existing epidemiological studies on PAD have not yet taken CLI into account. The figures for people older than 45 years vary between 450 and 650 per 1 million inhabitants per year. Also in the registration of chronic wounds, the wounds individually attributable to PAD are generally not recorded separately, since the coincidence of PAD and diabetes mellitus is high and a distinction is not always possible without systematic diagnostics.

9.4 Diagnosis of PAD

Only a small proportion of PAD patients make typical complaints. Therefore, a systematic search for PAD is necessary. With all leg complaints, PAD should be considered for differential diagnosis, regardless of age (➤ Fig. 9.2). An unremarkable pulse palpation finding does not rule out PAD. Patients with well-developed collateral vascular occlusions may have a normal palpation finding at rest. If PAD is suspected, it must first be excluded or confirmed non-invasively by determining the ABI. If this does not work or if the results are doubtful, further haemodynamic examinations or imaging procedures should be used to confirm the diagnosis.

9.4.1 Ankle-brachial index (ABI)

Pressure measurement in the ankle arteries has become standard in the initial evaluation of patients with suspected PAD. Systolic pressure in the posterior and dorsal tibial arteries of each leg is measured, using

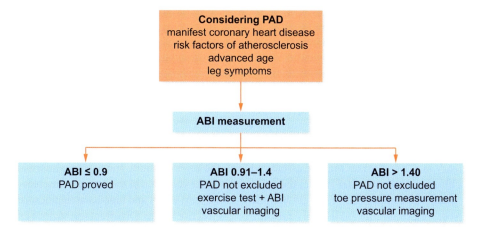

Fig. 9.2 Recommendation for ABI determination in case of suspected PAD and an evaluation of these values. [O1089/L231]

a 10–12 cm wide pressure cuff placed immediately above the ankle, and a Doppler instrument. A value of ≤ 0.9 is considered proof of PAD. The lower the ABI, the more severe the PAD. The patient should have rested for 10–15 minutes before these measurements so that the conditions for the circulatory system are the same for all analyses. Depending on the severity of the wounds, it may not be possible to apply the cuff to the distal lower leg. In these cases, the blood pressure cuff can also be applied further proximally (this should be documented accordingly), or it can be switched to pressure measurement of the toe artery.

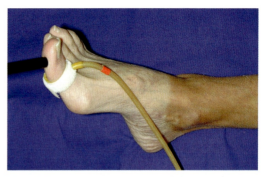

Fig. 9.3 Toe artery pressure measurement is a recognised alternative for the detection of PAD. It is performed with a narrow cuff of 1.5–2.0 cm and an 8 MHz Doppler probe or optical sensor. [O1089]

9.4.2 Stress test to confirm the diagnosis of PAD at ABI ≤ 0.9

Since a normal ABI does not exclude a PAD with certainty, in cases of doubt the PAD must be exposed with a stress test. During stress, the arterial flow obstacle (occlusion or stenosis) gets in the way of the physiological adaptation of the arterial blood circulation. If there is no increase in blood volume, metabolic dilatation leads to a decrease in blood pressure in the distal vascular bed. The ABI decreases immediately following the stress in the recovery phase, and a reduction of 15–20% is indicative of PAD. For clinical studies or comparable pre- and post-intervention measures of stress, a standardised treadmill should be used (speed 3.2 km/h and inclination 10–20% degrees). In everyday clinical life, stress due to climbing stairs or walking down the corridor is entirely sufficient for confirmatory diagnosis. Typically, stress is displayed until claudication occurs. But even if no claudication occurs, the stress of a PAD patient leads to a decrease of the ABI and thus helps in the differential diagnosis.

9.4.3 Diagnostic reliability at very high ABI values (ABI > 1.4)

In some patients with diabetes mellitus, renal insufficiency or other diseases that are associated with calcification of the vascular media, the ankle arteries cannot be compressed or cannot be fully compressed. As a result, the ankle artery pressure is incorrectly measured as too high, and ABI values > 1.4 are calculated. For these patients, a stress test is of no help, as the arteries cannot be compressed even after the stress, and therefore the pressure values cannot be assessed. For patients with such high ABI values, additional diagnostic tests are necessary to exclude or prove PAD. Alternative tests are the systolic pressure values at the toes (➤ Fig. 9.3), oscillography, transcutaneous oxygen measurement or Doppler sonography. If one of these examinations reveals pathological findings, a diagnosis of PAD may be made.

9.4.4 Imaging techniques

The diagnosis of PAD is made clinically, with a physical examination and an ABI determination. As a rule, the imaging only serves to identify the arterial flow obstacle and not the actual detection of PAD. However, the identification of the arterial flow obstacle is an essential basis for the planning of revascularisation using endovascular or open surgical techniques. Colour-coded duplex sonography, angiography, MR angiography and CT angiography are currently available for imaging.

- **Colour duplex sonography** as a safe and inexpensive method should be used as the first further diagnostic measure. A skilled practitioner can use sonography to visualise all arteries of the lower extremity and to obtain information on the condition of the arterial walls, blood flow velocity, extent and functional significance of obstructive lesions. Disadvantages include examiner dependency, impairment by vascular calcification and poor documentation of findings.

- **Angiography** involves the risks of severe contrast agent reactions (0.1%) and mortality (0.16%) from vascular injury and bleeding. Nevertheless, in many cases, a complete angiography with visualisation from the exit of the renal arteries to the foot arteries is still the procedure of choice. Digital subtraction angiography (DSA) is mostly used because it enables high-contrast images without needing to use a contrast medium or an x-ray. It should be noted, however, that the subtraction technique does not take natural calcium into account and can produce blurred images of septal stenoses due to the pulsatile movement of the stenosis.

- In many medical centres, **magnetic resonance angiography** (MRA) has become the preferred method for diagnosis and treatment planning in patients with PAD. The advantages of the MRA include its safety and the rapid generation of high-resolution, three-dimensional images of the entire abdomen, pelvis and lower limb in a single examination. Due to the high magnetic field strength, patients with defibrillators, spinal cord stimulators, intracerebral shunts, cochlear implants, etc. cannot be examined by MRA. However, acceptance of the method is hindered by the fact that sometimes quite old MR devices are used, and colleagues who are less proficient with MRA prepare the findings without knowing the patient themselves. Therefore, MRA findings should only be interpreted in light of the patient's complaints and non-invasive findings. Also, further treatment planning should not be based solely on the reconstructed angiography images, but only on the original data set, which makes the evaluation difficult for the surgeon and angiologist.

- **Multidetector Computed Tomographic Angiography** (MDCTA) is widely used in English-speaking countries for the initial diagnostic evaluation and treatment planning of PAD. The multi-layer MDCTA enables rapid visualisation of the entire lower limb and abdomen in the event of a respiratory stop with isotropic voxel resolution in the submillimeter range. The main limitations of MDCTA are the use of iodised contrast media (about 120 ml/examination), radiation exposure and the presence of calcium. Radiation exposure, in particular, makes these methods unsuitable for initial or follow-up investigations.

The question of the optimal imaging procedure must always be evaluated with the clinical findings, the availability of procedures and the questions, which need to be answered. DSA is the standard method for distal PAD and the question of revascularisability, as MRA and CTA used traditionally as overview procedures do not optimally represent the lower leg and foot in most cases. The antegrade puncture of the inguinal arteries is useful for this, and catheter presentation for the contrast medium application up to the popliteal artery is indicated.

9.5 Therapy of PAD

In the therapy of PAD, the patient's wish for a better walking distance or the healing of their gangrene or wound is paramount. The patient is often unaware that the high cardiovascular morbidity and mortality associated with PAD poses a much higher risk (➤ Fig. 9.4). In patients with PAD, long-term studies show that within five years after clinical manifestation of the disease, about 30% of patients die and about 1–3% suffer amputation. In patients with CLI, the primary amputation rate within the first 6–12 months is 10–40%. Their mortality rate is 20% after one year and 40–70% after five years.

Due to this high mortality rate, secondary prevention of systemic atherosclerosis is of great importance. Only this can increase the life expectancy of PAD patients. The modification of risk factors should, therefore, always be at the forefront of therapeutic efforts, except in vascular emergencies.

In addition to the modification of the risk profile, anti-aggregation is the second crucial therapeutic measure to reduce cardiovascular and cerebrovascular mortality in PAD patients. By taking acetylsalicylic acid (ASA), the risk of myocardial infarction, stroke and vascular death can be reduced by 25%. Internationally, the dose of 100 mg/day has now become established. Higher doses have no better effect. Clopidogrel was investigated in the CAPRIE study (clopidogrel vs. ASA in patients at risk of ischaemic events). Surprisingly, clopidogrel showed the highest

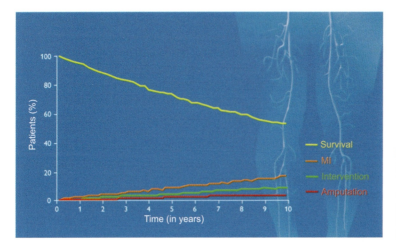

Fig. 9.4 Risks associated with PAD over a period of ten years. This rate of risk underlies the selection of current therapeutic strategies for the treatment of PAD patients. MI = myocardial infarction. [O1089]

risk reduction in the group of patients with symptomatic PAD, which led to clopidogrel approval for secondary prevention in patients with PAD.

The current best data shows the combination of ASA 100 mg/day with rivaroxaban 2 × 2.5 mg/day. In the COMPASS study, both significantly fewer cardiovascular and peripheral vascular events, including amputations, occurred with this combination therapy compared to monotherapy with ASA 100 mg/day.

9.6 Therapy of claudication

For the therapy of claudication, conservative therapy with walking exercise is the priority. In everyday clinical practice, however, this procedure is not widely accepted by patients and doctors, and even the current literature does not generally require such therapy ahead of other invasive measures, so that many patients are revascularised even in the claudication stage. In the TASC paper from 2000 it was still stated: *'Before an invasive revascularising therapy is offered to a patient with claudication, the failure of adequate walking training with pharmacological support should either have been observed or at least be expected from the overall situation.'* The 2007 TASC II now states: *'In patients with a suspected proximal lesion (buttock claudication, attenuated or missing femoral impulse), revascularisation can be considered without first undergoing broad conservative therapy.'*

Walking exercise should be supported by the intake of vasoactive medications such as naftidrofuryl or cilostazol. However, in people with an active diabetic foot syndrome (ulcers or an acute Charcot foot) walking exercise is generally not appropriate.

9.7 Therapy of chronic critical limb ischaemia

The primary treatment goal in patients with critical limb ischaemia (CLI), as in patients with stable claudication, is to reduce cardiovascular mortality. However, the preservation of the extremity at risk of amputation also places unique demands on the treatment. The following therapy goals should be pursued step by step:
- Relief of ischaemic pain
- Healing of ischaemic ulcers
- Prevention of limb loss
- Improvement of the patient's function and quality of life
- Prolongation of survival

Pain therapy for patients with CLI improves the quality of life and makes the patient more manageable for diagnosis. It must also be taken into account that ischaemia pain is an alarm sign of tissue destruction. A pain therapy that takes these alarm signals away simultaneously promotes tissue destruction. In this respect, an individual and step-by-step procedure should be discussed with pain therapists. Often, morphine derivatives are necessary, of which the side effects such as fatigue and confusion with the risk of falling are to be kept in mind for older multimorbid patients.

In CLI, revascularising measures are much more critical than in claudication (➤ Fig. 9.5, ➤ Fig. 9.6).

They are necessary for wound-healing and thereby for maintaining a functional and pain-free extremity. Therapeutic efforts should persist until the occlusion situation has been definitively elucidated with optimal imaging. The chosen treatment then depends on the premorbid condition of the patient and their extremity as well as on the presumed risk of the intervention,

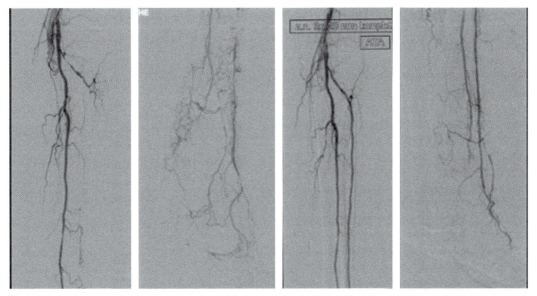

Fig. 9.5 Long-distance endovascular recanalisation of the left anterior tibial artery. The images show the occlusion situation before (left) and after the reopening of the anterior tibial artery. [O1089]

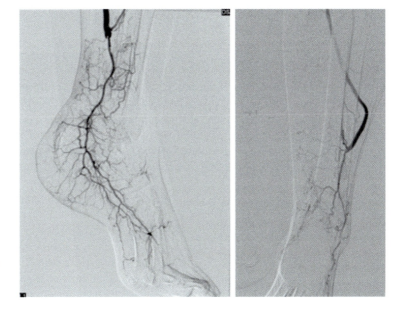

Fig. 9.6 On the left, the bypass supply to the distal tibial artery posterior and good outflow into the hollow arch of the foot and, on the right, to the distal fibular artery, which fills the distal tibial artery posterior and anterior via anastomoses. [O1089]

regarding the concomitant diseases and the expectant reopening. The primary therapeutic outcome would be wound-healing with amputation-free survival. For individual patients with CLI and advanced tissue destruction, patients with severe concomitant diseases and a minimal chance of successful revascularisation, primary amputation may be the most suitable therapy option.

If the necessity of revascularisation is recognised, any further loss of time is dangerous for the patient ('time is tissue'). Before revascularisation, wound-healing is less critical than avoiding wound deterioration due to continued pressure and florid infection. The leg should not bear any strain and the wound or gangrene covered with a non-adhesive wound dressing. When reducing the strain, care should be taken to use appropriate aids (knee-high, preferably non-removable). The prevention of pressure sores on the heels requires great attention in patients who are predominantly prone. This need for prophylaxis is also important postoperatively when the patient is completely capable of spontaneous change in position again, and there is no more analgesia-induced lack of pain awareness. If there are clinical signs of infection or radiologically documented osteomyelitis, a systemic antibiotic treatment should be initiated. Deep infections should be opened up, and the necroses which maintain the infection should be eliminated. Interventional procedures of proximal vascular lesions can also be carried out for local infections. Surgical revascularisation should not be performed until the acute infection is under control.

As a rule, in patients with CLI, revascularisation can achieve a significant improvement in arterial perfusion, but not normalisation. Therefore, wound-healing represents a further challenge after revascularisation. The focus is on the removal of necrotic and fibrotic parts of the ulcer, a moist wound environment and the avoidance of harmful substances that inhibit wound-healing, such as local pressure, reinfections, disinfectants that inhibit wound-healing, etc. The main focus is on the removal of the necrotic and fibrotic parts of the ulcer. The basic principles of wound hygiene must also be discussed with the patients and their caring relatives so that the wound is not exposed in the bathtub or shower and the dressing change must be carried out in a sterile process separately from the rest of the personal hygiene.

A causal therapy of CLI is open or endovascular revascularisation. It can only be supported by medication to a limited extent or even completely replaced in the event of failure. Although secondary prevention of atherosclerotic risk factors is necessary to reduce cardiovascular comorbidity and mortality, it only makes a minor contribution to improving perfusion of the extremities. A manifestation of heart failure, a poor nutritional status, but also anaemia or polyglobulia should be treated appropriately.

According to the guidelines for PAD, prostaglandins and prostacyclins are available for the drug therapy of CLI. In a meta-analysis of placebo-controlled PGE-1 studies, PGE-1 showed significantly better ulcer-healing and pain reduction compared to placebo. A significant difference in favour of PGE-1 was demonstrated in the six-month follow-up of major amputation and mortality (22.6% for PGE-1 vs. 36.2% for placebo). The most recent Cochrane meta-analysis of prostanoid efficacy in patients with CLI showed positive effects in terms of ulcer-healing, pain reduction and reduction in amputation rate compared to placebo or active control therapies in 20 RCTs studied, with poor study quality restricting the efficacy of prostanoids. However, no long-term benefit was demonstrated in these studies.

Similarly, the ESPECIAL study, a prospective, placebo-controlled, randomised study, showed no effect of Alprostadil vs. placebo in more than 800 patients with CLI. There were no significant differences in amputation rate or mortality. However, the study has major methodological weaknesses that contrast with the proper clinical experience observed in some patients.

In an older meta-analysis, it was shown that two- to four-week treatment with iloprost reduced rest pain and ulcer size. Also, verum showed a 65% survival and leg maintenance rate compared to 45% for placebo after six months of observation.

Overall, the data on prostanoids are not at the level of evidence that would be available today. In the therapy of CLI, however, they have a firm place and an international recommendation, so that they should be considered in every patient in addition to the interventional or surgical measures. Since prostanoids cannot influence diabetic microangiopathy, it is not indicated for patients with diabetic foot syndrome. Before the administration of prostaglandins in diabetic foot syndrome, an external second opinion should ensure that there is no possibility of revascularisation. Current evaluations of the data of a large health insurance company show that too often no vascular procedures are performed in German clinics before amputation.

Directly acting vasodilators, anti-aggregates, anti-coagulants and other vasoactive substances such as naftidrofuryl, cilostazol, which can be used in claudication, are not helpful here because they primarily increase the blood supply to the nonischaemic areas.

9.7.1 Spinal cord stimulation

A Cochrane meta-analysis of six studies involving a total of 450 patients showed that spinal cord stimulation was associated with better limb preservation than conservative treatment in patients with no possibility of revascularisation. Out of 238 patients with spinal cord stimulation, 72 were amputated within 12 months; out of 195 patients without this stimulation 81 were amputated. It should be critically noted that these were always open studies and that the inclusion criteria were not clearly defined in some cases.

9.7.2 Neoangiogenesis

The stimulation of new vessel formation is a promising approach to improve blood flow in patients with non-revascularisable vascular occlusions, which is being intensively investigated in clinical studies. However, so far, no convincing results are available that would make broad clinical use likely soon. There are three types of vascular growth:

- Vasculogenesis is characterised by the involvement of precursor cells in the development of vessels and takes place predominantly, but not exclusively, in the embryo.
- Angiogenesis, in its classical form, describes the process of sprouting and maturation of new vessels from existing ones.
- Collateral growth describes the growth of pre-existing collateral vessels and does not represent neoangiogenesis in the narrower sense.

Ultimately, neoangiogenesis is used to initiate and accelerate the physiological processes that take place during the recruitment of already created small collateral vessels (biological bypasses) or wound-healing.

9.7.3 Growth factors and gene transfer

Another therapeutic option is to enhance the growth factors expression which stimulates the processes of angiogenesis and arteriogenesis. It has been shown that therapy with genes for growth factors is much more effective than the use of their proteins themselves. Also, intramuscular injection into the skeletal muscle has become widely accepted compared to other application pathways. However, it has not yet been clarified which growth factor is best suited for this therapy. Only genes belonging to the growth factors vascular endothelial growth factor (VEGF) and fibroblast growth factor (FGF) have been tested in the Phase 2 studies completed to date. It is also not yet clear whether monotherapy is sufficient because angiogenesis and arteriogenesis are regulated by several factors, sometimes at different times. In the case of combination therapy, the questions of the optimal combination and timing still need to be clarified.

9.7.4 Progenitor cells

Since the discovery of endothelial progenitor cells in adult organisms, the involvement of these cells in vascular growth in adults – and thus a form of adult vasculogenesis – has been demonstrated several times. In contrast to the initial idea that these progenitor cells contribute to vascular growth mainly through direct incorporation into the vascular wall, recent data seem to indicate that they are indirectly involved in the formation of new vessels through extravasation and production of angiogenic substances at sites of neoangiogenesis and thus through the creation of a proangiogenic milieu.

9.7.5 Autologous bone marrow stem cell transplantation (SCT)

Transplanted stem cells from the bone marrow make a microenvironment through the release of various mediators such as MCP-1, VEGF, FGF, IL-6 etc., which stimulates both angiogenesis and the growth of preformed collateral connections. In an analogy to corresponding cardiological studies, such monocytic bone marrow cells were also transplanted in PAD patients with CLI without the possibility of invasive or surgical revascularisation. In the TACT study, 47 patients with advanced ischaemia of the extremities were treated with autologous bone marrow SCT in two strata. Overall, this resulted in an improvement in blood circulation, an extension of the walking distance, an increase in tissue oxygen saturation, a significant reduction in pain and accelerated wound-healing.

9.8 Conclusion

Many patients with chronic wounds have PAD, which is either the leading cause of the wound or at least has a significant influence on healing. The clarification of the arterial circulation situation and its targeted therapy are, therefore, an essential component in the diagnosis and treatment of people with chronic wounds.

REFERENCES

Dormandy JA, Rutherford RB. Management of peripheral arterial disease (PAD). TASC Working Group. TransAtlantic Inter-Society Consensus (TASC). J Vasc Surg 2000; 31: S1–S296.

Farber A, Eberhardt RT. The current state of critical limb ischemia: A systematic review. JAMA Surg 2016; 151: 1070–1077.

Norgren L, Hiatt WR, Dormandy JA, et al. Inter-Society Consensus for the management of peripheral arterial disease (TASC II). J Vasc Surg 2007; 45 (Suppl.): 5–67.

Shiraki T, Iida O, Takahara M, et al. Predictors of delayed wound-healing after endovascular therapy of isolated infrapopliteal lesions underlying critical limb ischemia in patients with high prevalence of diabetes mellitus and hemodialysis. Eur J Vasc Endovasc Surg 2015; 49: 565–573.

TASC Steering Committee, Jaff MR, White CJ, et al. An update on methods for revascularization and expansion of the TASC lesion classification to include below-the-knee arteries: A supplement to the inter-society consensus for the management of peripheral arterial disease (TASC II). J Endovasc Ther 2015; 22: 663–677.

10

Stephan Morbach, Gerhard Rümenapf

Disease patterns in diabetes mellitus

Key notes

- The stress symptom of a person with neuropathy is the foot ulcer, while that of a person without neuropathy is pain.
- Peripheral artery disease (PAD) is often clinically silent when neuropathy is present at the same time, and its relevance is underestimated.

- Before any amputation, the possibility of revascularisation should be considered. Every patient should also be entitled to a qualified second opinion before an amputation.
- Preservation of quality of life, mobility and independence are the overriding goals in the care of people with diabetic foot syndrome.

10.1 Introduction

Diabetic foot syndrome (DFS) is a lifelong complication of diabetes mellitus that threatens the lives and mobility of those affected. The term covers all pathological changes in the foot of people with diabetes mellitus and diabetic polyneuropathy. Ulcers or necrosis usually develop as a result of repetitive stress with limited pain sensation. In more than 50% of cases, a relevant peripheral artery disease (PAD) is also present.

Delayed or ineffective treatment may result in the loss of an entire limb. Such progressions could be avoided if patients with DFS were treated at an early stage with an interdisciplinary therapy concept as part of a cross-sectoral approach, in which the improvement of the arterial blood circulation is a central component. Given that recurrence rates for DFS are between 25–100% in the first year, one should not talk about healing in order to avoid sending false safety signals to patients, their relatives and occupational groups involved in care. Preferably, the terms 'transition to remission' or 'active and inactive phases of DFS' should be used.

10.2 Epidemiology

DFS plays a prominent role among chronic wounds. In addition to venous leg ulcers and pressure ulcer, foot lesions in people with diabetes are among the most common causes of poorly healing wounds in Europe. The prevalence of foot lesions in diabetes mellitus is 4–10%, with the annual incidence about 2%. Wounds caused by DFS are complex and costly.

In most patients with DFS, the cause is diabetic polyneuropathy with reduction or loss of protective sensation. Due to an ageing society and a steadily increasing number of people with diabetes, the frequency of PAD occurrence in these patients is also increasing. Chronic critical limb ischaemia (CLI) due to PAD of the pelvic and leg arteries is the leading cause of the non-healing of foot wounds and the high number of major amputations.

As a result of intensive efforts in many medical specialities to prevent, diagnose, use modern wound treatment methods and revascularise in time, the number of major amputations, i. e. amputations above the ankle joint, which ten years ago was still over 20,000 in people with diabetes in Germany alone, is continuously decreasing. However, many of the remaining transfemoral and transtibial amputations could also be avoided if internationally proven, guideline-compliant interdisciplinary therapy concepts, especially concerning timely revascularisation in PAD ('time is tissue'), were followed more consistently.

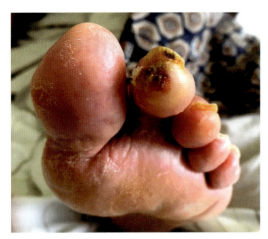

Fig. 10.1 Hammer toe with toe tip ulcer in a patient with diabetic neuropathy, hyperextension of the toes and failure of the intrinsic foot muscles. [P575]

10.3 Pathophysiology and pathogenesis

Chronic wounds on the feet of a person with diabetes differ from other chronic wounds in their specific pathophysiology and pathogenesis, i.e. in the individual functional mechanisms of the legs under the pathological conditions associated with long-term diabetes mellitus. Ulceration, infection and destruction of tissue on the feet of people with diabetes, accompanied by pre-existing neurological deficits or various degrees of severity of PAD, characterise DFS. By far, the most critical cause for its development is diabetic polyneuropathy in combination with abnormal pressure (➤ Fig. 10.1).

In principle, the pressure load on the feet is very high in humans, caused by the upright gait. Pressure-induced foot lesions can also occur in healthy people under certain circumstances, but they heal quickly due to the proper protective mechanisms (pain, good arterial perfusion, good wound-healing). In people with diabetes, these are disturbed by the pathologies listed below, which interact as possible **resistance-reducing conditions** for the development of foot lesions associated with diabetes (**'why is there an ulcer at all?'**):

- Diabetic neuropathy
- Micro- and macroangiopathy (PAD)
- Soft tissue oedema

- Atrophy of the plantar fat pad
- Calluses of the cornea, hyperkeratoses
- Impaired immune defense
- Partial loss of body perception (asomatognosia, 'Leibesinselschwund') depression

Direct **localised reasons** for foot lesions are therefore mostly changes of the normal biomechanics or trivial trauma, which lead not to the emergence of pain but local tissue defects due to neuropathy (**'why in this exact spot?'**):

- Inappropriate footwear, not suitable for persons with diabetes
- Objects in the shoe, e.g. nails, Lego bricks, coins, etc.
- Overweight
- Walking barefoot
- Improper foot care
- Burns, e.g. from heating pads with inherently cold feet
- Foot and toe deformities, limited joint mobility
- Shortening of the calf muscles with dropfoot or bunions
- Falls, accidents, fractures with Charcot's foot

Finally, causes for the non-healing of ulcers are particularly:

- Disregard of PAD with CLI
- Inadequately treated bacterial infections
- Lack of pressure relief of the lesions
- Activity level too high
- Insufficient therapy adherence of the patient

In summary, it can be said that with DFS, the wound itself is not chronic, but rather those conditions which reduce resistance and lead to the formation of the wound. If all rules of modern wound treatment are followed, as well as revascularisation being carried out as required, and pressure is relieved consistently, the expected treatment result for people with diabetes is not significantly worse than for persons without diabetes. According to the predominant underlying condition, lesions on the foot of a person with diabetes are divided into neuropathic (➤ Fig. 10.2), neuroischaemic (➤ Fig. 10.3) and predominantly ischaemic lesions, which are however very rare. While the proportion of purely neuropathic foot lesions is overestimated, the simultaneous presence of ischaemia is underestimated. On the other hand, the overall frequency of diabetic polyneuropathy is underestimated, which explains the often fatally long delays in the diagnosis of DFS patients (*'if it doesn't hurt, we don't look'*).

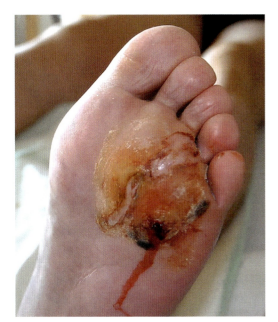

Fig. 10.2 Neuropathic foot ulcer according to Wagner-Armstrong stage 2B. [P575]

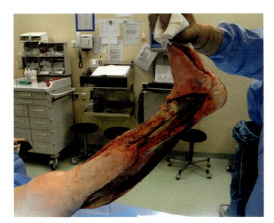

Fig. 10.3 'Foot attack' in a person with diabetes and a neuroischaemic foot. The dorsal foot phlegmon developed painlessly within two days. [P575]

10.3.1 Sensorimotor diabetic polyneuropathy with DFS

Neuropathic ulcers

Distal sensory polyneuropathy is distributed symmetrically distally (stocking-shaped) and leads to a reduced sensation of vibration, touch, pressure, pain and temperature. Discomfort and paraesthesia

is frequently reported ('painful-painless foot'). Mechanical, chemical or thermal trauma (e.g. scalding from hot water bottles or heating pads) are not perceived by the patient and lead to injuries or wounds. The foot pulses are usually palpable.

Due to the motor components of neuropathy, the inner muscles of the foot (intrinsic musculature) atrophy and the relative strength of the lower leg muscles change to the disadvantage of the dorsal flexors. This results in ball foot or pointes foot with an overload of pressure on the forefoot. Also hammer and claw toes develop, which are susceptible to local pressure ulcers. The atrophy of the fat on the sole also leads to excessive pressure on the metatarsal heads. Autonomous neuropathy leads to vasodilatation, reduction of sweat secretion, and dry, cracked and vulnerable skin, which is prone to callus formation on the sole and trophic changes of the toenails (➤ Fig. 10.1, ➤ Fig. 10.4). The skin of these 'autosympathectomised' feet is warm and simulates good blood circulation. The arterial blood is guided past the terminal vessels via pathological arteriovenous shunts, which leads to reduced blood flow to deeper tissue ('chronic capillary ischaemia', see below).

As a result of diabetic polyneuropathy, the typical plantar neuropathic (callused) ulcer develops on the sole. It usually begins with small subcellular haemorrhages. Frequently, callus abscesses develop, which on the one hand perforate to the outside and appear to be 'punched out' (previously 'malum perforans'), and on

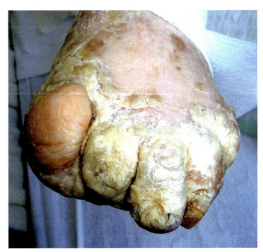

Fig. 10.4 Neuropathic diabetic foot after several minor amputations. [P575]

the other hand can seize and destroy deeper structures such as bones and joints (➤ Fig. 10.2). The fact that neuropathy cannot be cured leads to the assessment of DFS as a lifelong disease.

Diabetic neuro-osteoarthropathy (Charcot foot)

Another consequence of neuropathy is diabetic neuro-osteoarthropathy (DNOAP, Charcot arthropathy). Charcot arthropathy can be defined as progressive and destructive arthropathy of single or multiple bones or joints. The exact pathogenesis of the acute Charcot foot has not yet been clarified. All patients have peripheral neuropathy. Autonomous neuropathy of vasomotor or trophically significant nerves impairs the nutrition of affected bones (neurovascular hypothesis). The repetitive and continued traumatisation favoured by the loss of sensitivity destroys bones and joints (neurotraumatological hypothesis). This destruction is mediated by an increased release of proinflammatory cytokines, which have osteoclast-activating properties on the one hand, and the release of which is further stimulated and maintained by the resulting tissue trauma (osteolysis, fractures) on the other.

In the early stage of inflammation, which is accompanied by redness, swelling and overheating of the foot, x-rays rarely show any skeletal changes. In this phase, however, magnetic resonance imaging (MRI) can already reveal typical intraosseous oedema. Primary therapy consists of complete immobilisation.

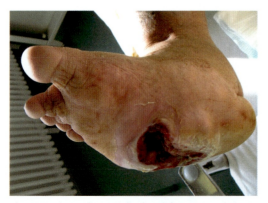

Fig. 10.5 Charcot foot with flat foot deformation and plantar ulceration in Wagner-Armstrong 3D stage with massive ischaemia in lower leg type PAD. [P575]

In cases of acute dislocation or apparent instability, conservative therapy is usually unsuccessful. Surgical treatment should be considered at an early stage after the initial swelling has subsided. In this phase, stabilisation in an anatomically correct position is much easier to achieve than in a 'healed' situation. As with the surgical treatment of the infected Charcot foot in corresponding ulcerations, these procedures should be restricted to specialised centres (➤ Fig. 10.5).

10.3.2 Critical limb ischaemia in DFS

Due to the threatening accumulation of risk factors, people with diabetes tend to develop rapidly progressive generalised arteriosclerosis, which explains their high excess mortality from cardiovascular causes. The mortality rate of patients with DFS is about 50% within five years and is therefore comparable to that of metastatic carcinoma, for example of the colon. In more than half of the cases, DFS is accompanied by relevant PAD of the pelvic and leg arteries in the sense of critical limb ischaemia (CLI). It comprises various degrees of ischaemia, ranging from pain at rest to skin defects and gangrene in people without diabetes. The prognosis of important outcome parameters (open arterial reconstruction, amputation-free survival, life expectancy) decreases with the increasing severity of ischaemia. Due to sensory diabetic neuropathy, ischaemic pain which is one criterion of the CLI, is no longer present; due to autonomous neuropathy (auto-sympathectomy), visibly reduced blood circulation of the foot is also lacking (see below). As a result, people with diabetes often reach the most severe stage of foot ischaemia with ulceration or necrosis of the foot without clinical signs. In addition to ischaemia, a general weakening of the immune defense in people with diabetes considerably increases the risk of infection (foot attack, ➤ Fig. 10.3) and the associated risk of amputation. The risk of developing gangrene is 20 to 50 times higher in diabetic patients than in non-diabetic patients.

Macroangiopathy/PAD

Typical for patients with diabetes mellitus is multilevel manifestation of PAD. (➤ Fig. 10.6). On the one hand,

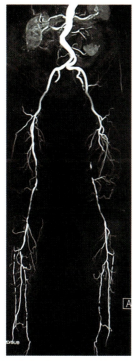

Fig. 10.6 PAD of the multistage type in a patient with diabetic foot syndrome. [P575]

about 70% of the occlusions are found below the knee, while the foot arteries are often less severely affected. In DFS, this enables successful vascular reconstructive measures down to the foot. On the other hand, simultaneous vascular medical care of several vascular floors may become necessary, for example, by hybrid interventions. In addition to macroangiopathy of the pelvic and leg vessels of the person with diabetes, further factors are added which intensify ischaemia of the foot tissue and can additionally interfere with wound-healing.

Diabetic microangiopathy

Diabetic microangiopathy is not obstructive and therefore does not lead to an increased peripheral vascular resistance. However, it is accompanied by a thickening of the capillary basement membrane, which makes the diffusion of oxygen into the tissue more difficult. There is still a widespread misconception that DFS is mainly a consequence of diabetic microangiopathy, and therefore revascularisation is not possible.

Chronic capillary ischaemia

In addition to macro- and microangiopathy, functional microcirculatory disorders occur in patients with DFS. As a result of the loss of function of sympathetic nerve fibres, arteriovenous shunt vessels are dilated in the skin so that the foot appears well supplied with blood, even if there is already severe PAD. On the other hand, the loss of function of the sympathetic fibres leads to precapillary vasoconstriction with an insufficient supply of oxygen to the tissue (chronic capillary ischaemia). The shunt-induced congestion in the venules leads to tissue oedema, which can promote the development of foot lesions in DFS.

Media sclerosis/Mönckeberg's sclerosis

Approximately 50% of DFS patients have calcification of the tunica media (media sclerosis, Mönckeberg's sclerosis), which is often visible on x-rays. It reduces the elasticity of the arterial vessel wall and promotes the development of arteriosclerosis. It is another consequence of autonomic diabetic neuropathy and signals an increased risk for the development of ulcers and amputations. Media sclerosis often results in falsely high ankle-brachial index (ABI). Severe CLI may therefore have been missed. The use of the toe-brachial index (TBI) and pulse wave analysis help to select candidates for invasive procedures: a TBI ≥ 0.75 and triphasic Doppler flow profiles largely rule out a relevant PAD.

10.4 Classification of DFS

If a lesion is diagnosed as DFS in a patient, it should be classified according to the extent of tissue destruction according to the Wagner and combined Wagner-Armstrong classification (➤ Table 10.1, ➤ Table 10.2, ➤ Fig. 10.7). While the former is limited to the extent, localisation and depth of the wound, the latter also considers pathogenesis (ischaemia and infection) and is preferably used in Germany. The PEDIS classification of the IWGDF (International Working Group on the Diabetic Foot) is also applied interna-

Table 10.1 Classification of diabetic foot ulcer (DFU) expansion depth according to Wagner

Wagner grade	Description
0	High-risk foot
1	Superficial wound
2	Wound reaching tendon or joint capsule
3	Wound with bone involvement or joint fracture
4	Necrosis of foot parts
5	Necrosis of the entire foot

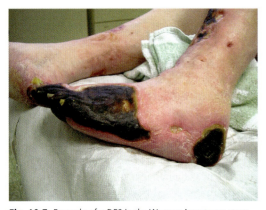

Fig. 10.7 Example of a DFS in the Wagner-Armstrong stage 4D. [P575]

tionally. It includes the parameters of blood flow (P = perfusion), wound size (E = extent/size), depth expansion (D = depth/tissue loss), infection (I = infection) and protective sensation (S = sensation). The anatomical localisation of the lesion is only considered in the SINBAD classification: it distinguishes ulcers in the forefoot area from those in the midfoot and rearfoot.

10.5 Localisation of diabetic ulcers

Although not all currently used classifications take this into account, the localisation of lesions with DFS is of significant importance for therapy planning, prognosis and, in particular, prevention of recurrence. Thus, ulcers in the metatarsal and especially in the heel area heal more slowly than toe lesions, while the healing time in plantar and non-plantar localisation does not differ. Patients with heel ulcers seem to have a higher mortality risk compared to those with forefoot ulcerations with an identical risk for major amputation. Also, the causes of foot lesions (localisation-determining causes) can often be assigned to typical localisations. For example, pressure ulcers tend to occur over bone protrusions, while venous ulcers occur in the ankle region and pressure ulcers at the heel. Thermal damage is often found in areas with no pressure-bearing, while accidental trauma is also present in the sole in non-supporting areas.

Hochlenert et al. have carried out a detailed investigation of these events and propose a systematic subdivision into so-called entities. The regular relation between localisation and causes of DFS allows standardisation of therapy options when using this concept.

Table 10.2 Description of DFS using the combined Wagner-Armstrong classification

Wagner degree						
	0	1	2	3	4	5
Armstrong stage						
A	Pre- or post-ulcerative high-risk foot	Superficial wound	Wound up to the level of tendons or joint capsules	Wound up to the level of bones and joints	Necrosis of parts of foot	Necrosis of the entire foot
B	With infection	With infection	With infection	With infection	With infection	With infection
C	With ischaemia	With ischaemia	With ischaemia	With ischaemia	With ischaemia	With ischaemia
D	With infection and ischaemia	With infection and ischaemia	With infection and ischaemia	With infection and ischaemia	With infection and ischaemia	With infection and ischaemia

10.6 Treatment of DFS

The overriding goals when treating people with a DFS are maintaining the quality of life, mobility and independence. The close and structured cooperation of all care levels, occupational groups and medical disciplines involved in the process are decisive for the best possible treatment outcome. Therapy with DFS depends on the severity of the present lesion and the dominant underlying disease (polyneuropathy, PAD), chronic venous insufficiency, neuro-osteoarthropathy or combinations thereof. Patients with relevant PAD as well as patients with severe infections are high-risk patients and should be treated in specialised inpatient facilities.

Since patients with DFS often suffer from other severe internal diseases such as coronary heart disease, chronic heart failure, cerebral arterial occlusive disease or chronic renal failure, these diseases must also be included in treatment planning. The affected patients should also receive aggressive cardiovascular risk management. Such an approach improves not only the short-term outcome of treatment for these patients considerably but also the medium-term prognosis. In addition to the consistent therapy of comorbidities, perioperative management of blood glucose levels is also essential. Significant hyperglycaemia should be avoided while at the same time minimising the risk of hypoglycaemia.

Therapy planning for very old patients with considerable limitations in mobility and cognitive functions must be particularly specific.

The primary goals of the interdisciplinary therapy with DFS are to:
- Heal ulcers
- Avoid major (and minor) amputations
- Eliminate pain
- Restore walking ability
- Maintain the quality of life, mobility and independence

The principles of interdisciplinary therapy with DFS are based on the current recommendations of the International Working Group on the Diabetic Foot:
1. Complete pressure relief to eliminate the chronic traumatisation of the wound and its environment
2. Treatment of clinically visible infections
3. Restoration of arterial blood flow as much as possible
4. Application of modern wound management to support and accelerate ulcer-healing if necessary

10.6.1 Offloading

Pressure relief plays a vital role in all stages of wound-healing. The simplest form of pressure relief is bed rest, with all the associated disadvantages. In particular, the occurrence of new pressure zones in the areas affected by lying down must be avoided. Another possibility is the temporary use of a wheelchair. For mobile patients, pressure relief can be achieved using casting techniques (total contact casting, TCC), custom-made or industrially manufactured orthoses (e.g. the Diabetic Walker) or therapeutic footwear (➤ Chap. 30.1).

10.6.2 Infection treatment

The diagnosis of infection with DFS is made clinically. The valid classifications of diabetic foot infections (PEDIS, see above; Infectious Diseases Society of America, IDSA) differentiate the severity according to the presence or absence and extent of local signs of inflammation, the involvement of deep tissue structures and the presence of systemic signs of infection. The antibiotic treatment of DFS is initially 'calculated' in the case of clinical indication and, if necessary, can be changed over to targeted therapy after receipt of the antibiotic chart. The duration of drug treatment depends on the extent of the findings. While treatment periods of 1–2 weeks are usually sufficient for soft tissue infections alone, long-term therapy of 4–6 weeks may be necessary for purely conservative treatment of the infected bone (osteomyelitis, better osteitis). In the case of extensive soft tissue infection, but especially if deeper tissue structures are affected, surgical measures such as drainage, debridement or minor amputation are often unavoidable. Further information on infection treatment can be found in ➤ Chap. 26.

10

10.6.3 Revascularisation with DFS

With DFS, PAD must always be considered. If there are signs of PAD, a vascular specialist must quickly be involved in the further diagnosis to keep the time between the occurrence of a neuroischaemic diabetic foot lesion and its treatment as short as possible. Up to 80% of major amputations can be avoided by timely revascularisation. The decision for endovascular or vascular surgical strategies depends on the complexity and length of the vascular occlusions, but also on the competence and equipment of the treating vascular specialist. The procedures should be regarded as complementary, not competitive. They can often be combined (hybrid interventions), reducing trauma through open vascular surgery and reducing periop-erative mortality. Long-term vascular surgical results with DFS remain the gold standard for endovascular techniques.

More important than perfecting the surgical tech-nique and materials, however, is the willingness to employ aggressive revascularisation and flexibility in indication and surgical tactics. Interdisciplinary communication is essential to achieve an optimal treatment result with the effort involved and the process-related risk to the patient. Adjuvant therapies, such as stem cell therapy, should currently be reserved for patients in the Wagner stage > 3 after exhaustion of all possibilities of revascularisation and in cases of imminent amputation of the extremities.

10.6.4 Local wound treatment

Local wound treatment with DFS is based on the stages of wound-healing and follows the principles of moist wound treatment.
The essential principles are:
1. Regular changes of wound dressings with inspec-tion and cleaning of the wound

2. Complete debridement for necrosis removal and reduction of germ load
3. Protection of regenerating tissue

Local treatment is selected individually, based on the current stage of wound-healing, the amount of exudate, the presence or absence of signs of infec-tion, the presence of a normal or pathological healing process, as well as application aspects, cost-benefit criteria and available clinical evidence.

At the necrosis and infection stage, necrosectomy is the most important procedure. The necessary debridement should be as radical as possible. Only at this stage, bactericidal substances are used locally. In the granulation stage, the focus is on promoting the formation of granulation tissue. In the epithelialisation stage, it is aimed at the closure of the wound surface. For this purpose, either a spontaneous covering by the growth of the epithelial layer can be anticipated or a plastic covering, such as split skin grafts or alternative procedures, can be used. Even after complete wound closure, the wound should be protected in the scarring phase (remodelling stage) by gradual pressure and optimised skincare. More detailed information on the systematics of local wound treatment can be found in ➤ Chap. 23, ➤ Chap. 24, ➤ Chap. 25 and ➤ Chap. 26.

10.7 Follow-up care, relapse prevention

The safest way to avoid amputation is to prevent the first ulcer. If reduced pain is observed with ini-tial damage and is diagnosed as a central feature of a sensory deficit in neuropathy, findings should be checked at defined intervals, with initial protective measures taken and further risk diseases searched for (➤ Table 10.3). If it is not possible to avoid the

10

Table 10.3 DFS risk categories according to IWGDF and corresponding control intervals

Risk category	Risk profile	Control interval
0	No sensory neuropathy	1 × year
1	Sensory neuropathy	1 × every 6 months
2	Sensory neuropathy and signs of peripheral artery disease or foot deformities	1 × every 3–6 months
3	History of sensory neuropathy and ulcer or amputation	1 × every 1–3 months

first ulcer event, almost 100% of those affected will develop at least one new lesion within one year after it has healed without applying protective measures. Even if they are cared for in treatment centres with a high level of expertise, one-quarter to one-third of those affected suffer a new lesion during the first year after healing. Within five years, up to 70% of patients will experience a relapse.

The permanent monitoring of patients with DFS or Charcot neuro-osteoarthropathy 'in remission' by specialised outpatient foot treatment facilities is, therefore, an essential part of the successful management of this disease. These facilities organise and coordinate the following tertiary prevention measures:

- Monitoring the progress of PAD and neuro-osteoarthropathy
- Continuous pedological care
- Protective shoe and bedding supply suitable for stage-related therapy
- Timely treatment of pre-ulcerative foot lesions
- Foot surgery, e.g. tendon lengthening for claw toes or Achilles tendon lengthening for ball foot

10.8 Conclusion

DFS is a lifelong disease comprimising active and inactive phases. Specialised outpatient and inpatient treatment facilities for patients with diabetes-related foot complications, which have established themselves in the wake of the introduction of DMP diabetes, among other things, demonstrate the potential for improving the prognosis of DFS through a structured interdisciplinary approach. A further improvement of these results could be achieved by integrating such centres into regional networks.

REFERENCES

Armstrong DG, Boulton AJM, Bus SA. Diabetic foot ulcers and their recurrence. N Engl J Med 2017; 376: 2367–2375.

Armstrong DG, Mills JL. Toward a change in syntax in diabetic foot care: prevention equals remission. J Am Podiatr Med Assoc 2013; 103: 161–162.

Boulton AJ. Diabetic neuropathy and foot complications. Handb Clin Neurol 2014; 126: 97–107.

Claessen H, Narres M, Haastert B, et al. Lower-extremity amputations in people with and without diabetes in Germany, 2008–2012 – an analysis of more than 30 million inhabitants. Clin Epidemiol 2018; 10: 475–488.

Hochlenert D, Engels G, Morbach S. Das Entitätenkonzept des diabetischen Fußsyndroms. Diabetologe 2015; 11: 130–137.

Lipsky BA, Aragon-Sanchez J, Diggle M, et al. IWGDF guidance on the diagnosis and management of foot infections in persons with diabetes. Diabetes Metab Res Rev 2016; 32 (Suppl. 1): 45–74.

Morbach S, Furchert H, Groblinghoff U, et al. Long-term prognosis of diabetic foot patients and their limbs: amputation and death for a decade. Diabetes Care 2012; 35: 2021–2027.

Rogers LC, Frykberg RG, Armstrong DG, et al. The Charcot foot in diabetes. Diabetes Care 2011; 34: 2123–2129.

Schaper NC. Diabetic foot ulcer classification system for research purposes: a progress report on criteria for including patients in research studies. Diabetes Metab Res Rev 2004; 20 (Suppl. 1): 90–95.

Schaper NC, Van Netten JJ, Apelqvist J, et al. Prevention and management of foot problems in diabetes: a Summary Guidance for Daily Practice 2015, based on the IWGDF Guidance Documents. Diabetes Metab Res Rev 2016; 32 (Suppl. 1): 7–15.

11

Markus Stücker

Disease patterns in chronic venous insufficiency (CVI)

Key notes

- Diseases of the venous system can lead to skin changes on the lower leg, often on the inner ankle area.
- Venous diseases are usually diagnosed non-invasively, with duplex sonography playing a central role.

- A wide range of therapeutic options such as crossectomy and stripping, endovenous thermal ablation, sclerotherapy, compression and venous medication allows individualised therapies, depending on the overall situation of the patient and the respective findings of the vascular system in the leg.

11.1 Introduction

Chronic venous disease is defined as a morphological and/or functional disorder of the venous system, of prolonged duration, manifested either by subjective symptoms or clinical signs to be further investigated and, if appropriate, treated. The term chronic venous insufficiency (CVI) is usually used only when clinical manifestations of chronic venous disease, such as oedema, skin changes and venous ulcerations, are already detectable.

11.2 Definition

Chronic venous diseases are classified internationally according to the CEAP system (Clinical-Etiology-Anatomy-Pathophysiology; (> Table 11.1, > Table 11.2). This system records all venous disorders and not only CVI.

The exact definition of clinical pictures is essential for the accurate description of venous diseases. This is explained in the following, according to Allegra et al., 2003.

Telangiectasias Permanently dilated intradermal venules of less than 1 mm diameter. Synonym: spider veins.

Table 11.1 CEAP classification of chronic venous diseases

C	Clinical classification	a	Asymptomatic
		s	Symptomatic
E	Etiologic classification	Ec	Congenital
		Ep	Primary
		Es	Secondary
		En	No cause identified
A	Anatomical classification	As	Superficial veins
		Ad	Deep veins
		Ap	Perforator system
		An	No venous location identifiable
P	Pathophysiologic classification	Pr	Reflux
		Po	Obstruction
		Pn	Combination of reflux and obstruction

Reticular veins Permanently dilated, bluish to greenish intradermal veins from 1 to less than 3 mm in diameter. Reticular veins usually meander. This excludes 'normal' visible veins with relatively transparent skin.

Varicose Subcutaneous, permanently dilated veins of at least 3 mm diameter in a standing position. Varicose veins are usually wavy, but refluxing veins running in a straight line can also be classified as varicose veins. This can be the case, for example, with truncal varices, but also with lateral branches.

Table 11.2 Clinical manifestations of chronic venous diseases according to the CEAP classification

Stage	Changes
C0	No visible or palpable signs of venous disease
C1	Telangiectasias and/or reticular veins
C2	Varicose veins
C3	Oedema due to venous insufficiency
C4	Changes in skin and subcutaneous tissue secondary to CVD
C4a	Hyperpigmentation or eczema
C4b	Lipodermatosclerosis or atrophie blanche
C5	Healed venous leg ulcer
C6	Active venous leg ulcer

Corona phlebectatica paraplantaris   Fan-shaped intradermal telangiectasias at the medial or lateral edge of the foot. The significance of the corona phlebectatica paraplantaris is not clear from the start. Sometimes it may be an early sign of advanced venous disease. Sometimes, however, it also occurs in legs that have simple telangiectasias or spider veins elsewhere in the legs, without the advanced venous disease (➤ Fig. 11.1).

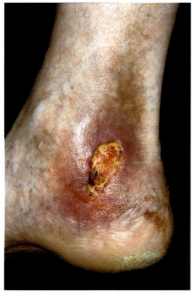

Fig. 11.1 Chronic venous ulcer. Typical localisation between inner ankle and Achilles' tendon. At the medial edge of the foot there are intradermal telangiectasias as the so-called corona phlebectatica paraplantaris. [P611]

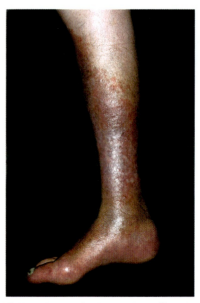

Fig. 11.2 Hyperpigmentation/purpura jaune d'ocre. Broad finding at the inner ankle. Towards the calf there is an overlay of a stasis eczema. [P611]

Oedema   Palpable increased amount of fluid in subcutaneous fatty tissue, which can be indented under pressure. It should be noted that the CEAP classification only refers to oedema caused by a venous disorder, and not to internal or another type of oedema. Venous oedema typically occurs in the ankle region but can spread to the rest of the leg and foot.

Pigment/Purpura jaune d'ocre   Brown pigmentation of the skin, usually in the ankle region, but also on the rest of the leg and foot. Pigmentation is one of the early skin changes in chronic venous diseases (➤ Fig. 11.2).

Stasis eczema   Erythematous, possibly blistering and scaly changes in the skin of the leg. Eczema is often located near varicose veins, but can also occur on the rest of the leg. Occasionally there are scattered manifestations over the whole body. The term stasis dermatitis is used synonymously with stasis eczema (➤ Fig. 11.3).

Lipodermatosclerosis   Chronic induration of the skin, sometimes associated with scarring or contractures. Lipodermatosclerosis is a sign of severe venous disease, characterised by sclerosis and chronic in-

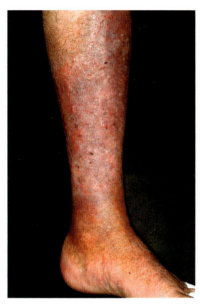

Fig. 11.3 Stasis eczema. Diffuse regional reddening and desquamation of the hyperpigmented skin at the medial lower leg and pretibial. Focal erosions. [P611]

flammation of the skin, subcutaneous fatty tissue and sometimes also the fascia.

Hypodermitis   An acute form of lipodermato-sclerosis is called hypodermitis. It is characterised by diffuse reddening of the skin due to acute inflammation and pain. Hypodermitis is also known as pseudoerysipelas and differs from erysipelas or cellulitis in that it lacks lymph node swelling and fever.

The course of hypodermitis is not as acute as that of erysipelas.

Atrophie blanche   Circumscribed, often roundish oval areas of whitish and atrophic skin, which are characterised by dilated capillaries and sometimes hyperpigmentations. Atrophie blanche is a sign of severe venous disease. It must be distinguished from the scars of healed ulcerations.

Postthrombotic syndrome   A unique form of chronic venous disease is the postthrombotic syndrome (PTS), which often leads to chronic wounds. PTS is a chronic consequence of deep vein thrombosis, which occurs after 20–40% of thromboses. It is defined by symptoms such as leg pain, heaviness, oedema, hyperpigmentation, lipodermatosclerosis and venous leg ulcers, which must persist for at least six to 24 months after acute venous thrombosis. In the first few weeks of acute venous thrombosis, symptoms are similar to leg pain and heaviness can occur without being PTS in the narrower sense. PTS is associated with a significant loss of quality of life. The American Heart Association (AHA) currently recommends the Villalta score for PTS diagnostics (➤ Table 11.3).

Scores < 5 indicate absence of PTS. A score of 5 to 9 indicates a mild PTS, a score of 10 to 14 indicates a moderate PTS, and a score of ≥ 15 or with a venous ulcer indicates a severe PTS. The Ginsberg criterion, which covers more severe PTS, must be distinguished from this. A diagnosis of a PTS is five times more

Table 11.3 Villalta score for PTS diagnostics – recommended by the American Heart Association (AHA)

	Non-existent	Mild	Moderate	Heavy
Pain	0	1	2	3
Cramps	0	1	2	3
Feeling of heaviness	0	1	2	3
Paresthesia	0	1	2	3
Pruritus	0	1	2	3
Pretibial oedema	0	1	2	3
Hyperpigmentation	0	1	2	3
Venous ectasia	0	1	2	3
Rashes	0	1	2	3
Induration of the skin	0	1	2	3
Pain with calf compression	0	1	2	3

11

frequent after the Villalta score than after the Ginsberg criterion. The Ginsberg criterion is defined as follows:

- Daily swelling and pain for at least one month
- After at least six months following diagnosis of DVT
- Worsens when standing/walking
- Improves in peace and elevation

11.3 Epidemiology

Chronic venous diseases are a widespread disease, as the 2003 Bonn Vein Study clearly showed for Germany. Every fifth woman and every sixth man has a CVI (C3–C6 according to the CEAP classification). Lower leg eczema occurs in 7.5% of people, 29% suffer from varicose veins, 0.9% have had a pulmonary embolism, 2.9% a deep vein thrombosis and 1.1% an active or healed venous leg ulcer. Only 9.6% of the population have no external signs of a venous change. Of the population, 59% have isolated telangiectasias or reticular veins. The severity of chronic venous diseases increases with age.

11.4 Diagnostics of chronic venous diseases

Among the typical symptoms of CVI are the subjective symptoms, as asked for in the Villalta score; particularly heaviness and itching, but also calf cramps and discomfort, such as tingling and restlessness, should be asked for in the anamnesis. Information on superficial or deep vein thromboses and sometimes the presence of thrombophilia are essential for the further classification of the clinical picture. Especially in the advanced stage, the clinical picture is very typical for chronic venous diseases, so that a careful inspection of the legs is of particular importance. If ulcerations are present, the ankle-brachial index (ABI) should be determined in addition to the venous diagnosis.

In apparatus-based diagnostics, functional methods such as photoplethysmography and vein occlusion plethysmography, in particular, provide information on the haemodynamic consequences of Doppler and duplex diagnostics. Today, duplex sonography is the gold standard, especially before invasive procedures. Directional Doppler sonography can, however, often offer an initial guidance. Duplex sonography should be able to give some information about the groin area, with the sapheno-femoral junction, and about the knee area, with the sapheno-popliteal junction. Also, further venous sections on the thigh and lower leg should be examined for reflux diagnostics.

Planning the therapy for chronic venous diseases requires assertions on refluxes and obstructions of the deep veins, on refluxes of the truncal veins (V. saphena magna and V. saphena parva) as well as on refluxes via larger perforating veins. In German-speaking countries, the saphenous vein insufficiency of the V. saphena magna and V. saphena parva is classified according to the stages of Hach ➤ Table 11.4).

Further examination methods such as phlebodynamometry (an invasive measurement of peripheral venous pressure), phlebography (X-ray examination using contrast medium), computer tomography and magnetic resonance imaging are procedures that are reserved for specific questions. For example, phlebography can be used to assess occlusions of the pelvic veins, nuclear spin angiography to determine complex angiodysplasia syndromes and computer tomography to diagnose pulmonary embolisms.

Table 11.4 Stage classification of saphenous varicosis according to Hach

	Saphenous vein insufficiency of the V. saphena magna	Saphenous vein insufficiency of the V. saphena parva
Stage I	Reflux only in the groin area	Reflux only in the hollow of the knee
Stage II	Reflux to proximal of the knee	Reflux up to the middle of the calf
Stage III	Reflux to immediately caudal of the knee	Reflux up to the ankle
Stage IV	Reflux to the ankle	

11.5 Therapy of chronic venous diseases

There is a medical indication for the therapy of chronic venous diseases if symptoms or complications such as heaviness, swelling or skin changes have already occurred, or if complications are imminent (e. g. increased risk of thrombosis with extensive varicosis). This can be differentiated from treatments for aesthetic disorders, such as those for spider veins on the thigh.

11.5.1 Invasive therapy of symptomatic chronic venous diseases

The aim of invasive therapy for chronic venous diseases is to eliminate refluxing veins or vein sections and thereby improve the function of the superficial venous system. It is more rarely possible to improve venous function in PTS by invasive measures such as stenting occluded pelvic veins. Various techniques are available today for the treatment of varicose veins, which are applied individually according to the patient's findings and needs. The following procedures are to be mentioned here:

Crossectomy and stripping operation

The crossectomy and stripping operation is still the procedure with the lowest recurrence rate, especially in the grain, according to the currently available meta-analyses of five-year results. It can often be performed on an outpatient basis. Comparative studies between endovenous thermal ablative procedures, crossectomies and stripping are limited to endoluminal ablative lasers with wavelengths below 1,000 nm and using bare fibre. It remains to be seen to what extent the longer wavelengths of 1,470 nm or 1,940 nm and radial fibres also lead to better effectiveness in the grain.

Sclerosing therapy

By injecting aethoxysklerol in a foam or liquid form, the treated varix is permanently transformed into a connective tissue strand. Foam sclerosing, in particular, is also suitable for large-calibre veins. Compared to the endovenous thermal-ablative procedures and the crossectomy and stripping operation, however, the five-year comparison shows lower effectiveness of foam sclerosing with more frequent recurrences. The advantage of foam sclerosing, however, is that it is a non-operative procedure. Anaesthesia is not necessary. The procedure can, therefore, be a good way of eliminating causative refluxes in the superficial venous system, especially in older adults with venous leg ulcers.

Miniphlebectomy

Lateral saphenous branch varices can be removed either by sclerosing therapy or by a miniphlebectomy. In a miniphlebectomy, the varicose vein is extracted with a small hook via small stab incisions, which is often possible under local anaesthesia. The larger the lateral branch varices are, the more likely a miniphlebectomy is used; the smaller the varices are, the more likely they are treated with sclerosing therapy.

Endovenous thermal-ablative processes

The targeted application of heat through laser catheters or radiofrequency catheters leads to damage to the venous wall and ultimately to connective tissue remodelling and degradation. These catheter-assisted procedures are particularly suitable for the V. saphena magna and V. saphena parva, but also straight sections of the V. accessoria anterior and other straight-line varicose vein sections.

Compression therapy

Compression therapy is regarded as an essential therapy in phlebology. It is especially indispensable for patients with PTS. Medical compression stockings are preferable to compression bandages after the end of the decongestion phase. This also applies to patients with venous leg ulcers for whom special ulcer compression stockings are available. Several studies have shown that

11

lower leg ulcers heal faster when using compression stockings than with compression bandages.

11.5.2 Pharmacological therapy

Extracts from red vine leaves or horse chestnut seeds and troxerutin are available for systemic evidence-based therapy of vein complaints. Externa, which do not have a proven effect on venous disorders, are to be distinguished from evidence-based effective vein medications in tablet form.

When should vein medications be used? If with symptomatic varicose veins, treatment is not possible or not desired, or if symptoms persist after appropriate treatment, compression therapy or any of the systemic pharmacotherapies mentioned above can be applied. Especially in the case of chronic venous diseases with persistent symptoms, conservative treatment should be carried out on a longterm basis. The effect of this conventional therapy should be checked regularly, e. g. by quality of life tests or symptom scores.

11.6 Conclusion

The most common cause of lower leg ulcerations in Europe is CVI. More than 50% of patients with venous leg ulcers do not have insufficiency of the deep veins, so the cause of the chronic wound can be treated by treating varicose veins. Accordingly, the typical subjective symptoms and clinical changes should be carefully examined in the venous system, which is now possible without invasive techniques.

REFERENCES

Allegra C, Antignani PL, Bergan JJ, et al. The 'C' of CEAP: suggested definitions and refinements: an International Union of Phlebology conference of experts. J Vasc Surg 2003; 37: 129–131.

Soosainathan A, Moore HM, Gohel MS, Davies AH. Scoring systems for the post-thrombotic syndrome. J Vasc Surg 2013; 5: 254–261.

Rabe E, Pannier-Fischer F, Bromen K, et al. Bonner Venenstudie der Deutschen Gesellschaft für Phlebologie. Phlebologie 2003; 32: 1–14.

Stücker M, Debus ES, Hoffmann J, et al. Consensus statement on the symptom-based treatment of chronic venous diseases. J Dtsch Dermatol Ges 2016; 14: 575–583.

12 Disease patterns in pressure ulcers

Jan Kottner

Key notes

- Pressure ulcers are caused by prolonged deformation of the skin and the underlying tissue.
- Immobility is the most critical direct risk factor for the development of pressure ulcers.
- Pressure ulcers are currently classified according to the visibly affected tissue.
- Stage 1 pressure ulcers and suspected deep tissue damage are pressure ulcers under intact skin.

12.1 Pressure ulcer aetiology and pathogenesis

According to the International Guidelines on the Prevention and Treatment of Pressure Ulcers/Injuries issued by the National Pressure Ulcer Advisory Panel (NPUAP), the European Pressure Ulcer Advisory Panel (EPUAP) and the Pan Pacific Pressure Injury Alliance (PPPIA) in 2014, pressure ulcers are localised damage to the skin and/or underlying tissue, typically over bony prominences, as a result of pressure or pressure in combination with shear. This definition indicates that mechanical deformation of the skin and subcutaneous soft tissues such as fat or muscle tissue leads to tissue damage over time. Compression and shear in the tissue always coincide. The probability that a pressure ulcer will develop increases with the duration and intensity of the deformation. Typically, the areas of the body which are particularly affected are where firm internal structures such as bones, tendons or joints are in contact with hard surfaces when sitting or lying down and they exert particular pressure on the soft tissue in between them. Depending on the body position (e.g. sitting, lying down), typical pressure ulcer predilection sites are located on the heels, the sacral region or the buttocks (➤ Fig. 12.1).

Depending on the area of the body, pressure damage can occur in all tissues. As a rule, however, muscle and subcutaneous fat tissue are particularly susceptible. The skin is much more resistant to mechanical loads. Also, the degree of mechanical deformation near the bone is higher than in the vicinity of the contact surface. ➤ Fig. 12.2 shows an example of a transverse section at pelvic level lying on a standard mattress. When lying on a hard surface, the muscles and subcutaneous fat tissue near the sacrum are compressed and sheared (➤ Fig. 12.3).

Prolonged mechanical deformation can lead to several damages. Direct muscle and fat cell death can occur if they are deformed over an extended period exceeding their natural resistance. A rupture of the cytoskeleton or plasma membrane is under discussion. In the case of severe deformation and the presence of other risk factors (➤ Chap. 13.2), this process progresses comparatively quickly, and damage can occur within a few minutes. This process is referred to as direct deformation damage.

The occlusion of blood vessels is another pathogenetic mechanism. Over time, this results in an undersupply of tissue and a local accumulation of metabolites and acidosis. However, even with more severe deformation, complete ischaemia hardly occurs due to compensatory mechanisms. Pressure-induced circulatory disorders take comparatively longer to cause tissue damage. If the blood supply to less perfused tissue is restored after an extended period of ischaemia, e.g. after off-loading reperfusion injury can occur. The previously accumulated metabolic products enter the surrounding tissue as a result of increased blood flow, triggering an inflammatory reaction.

The occlusion of lymph vessels, and the direct rupture of capillaries or traumatic shearing of tissue are under discussion as further pathophysiological mechanisms during the development of pressure ulcers. Today, it is assumed that all these mechanisms are likely to interact with and reinforce each other.

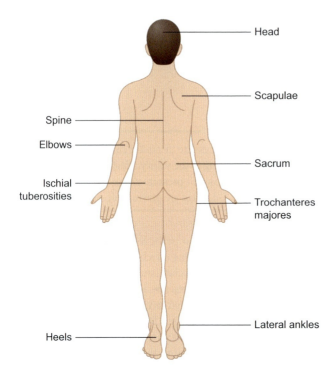

Fig. 12.1 Pressure ulcer predilection sites. [P576/L231]

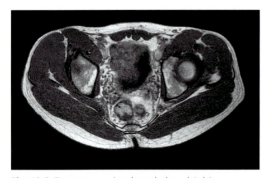

Fig. 12.2 Transverse section through the pelvis lying on a standard mattress. [T1051]

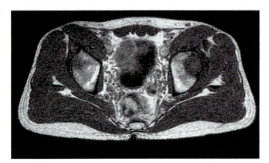

Fig. 12.3 Transverse section through the pelvis lying on an MRI examination table. [T1051]

Ways in which pressure ulcers are formed

• Direct deformation damage of cells
• Direct shear injuries
• Occlusion of blood and lymph vessels
• Reperfusion injury

As soon as the initial cell and tissue damage has occurred, there are two possible processes. One is that the affected area is small, the pressure on the tissue is reduced, and blood circulation is adequate. Over time, local necroses are resorbed, and the damaged tissue regenerates. Except for characteristic dark, livid discolouration under intact skin or pain, which may or may not be present (➤ Fig. 12.8), there are no other clinical signs. The initial pressure damage heals completely.

However, if the damaged area is large or if other factors are present that prevent healing, then undermining, tunnelling and finally, a clinically visible pressure ulcer typically occurs. From the initial damage to the appearance of a pressure ulcer can take between a few days up to two weeks. If a pressure ulcer is clinically diagnosed, it may have been caused several days previously.

12.2 Pressure ulcer risk

Hundreds of risk factors for the development of pressure sores are mentioned in the literature. However, only the **direct** risk factor of 'pressure' is clinically relevant, since only prolonged pressure can cause pressure ulcers. The practical consequence is that these patients have a high-pressure ulcer risk, who have mobility restrictions and are therefore unable to move at regular intervals. These are in particular patients who are sedated or ventilated (e.g. in the operating room, intensive care unit) or patients with paralysis (e.g. paraplegics). If their sensitivity to pressure is impaired, e.g. in diabetic neuropathy or with peridural anaesthesia, the prolonged pressure load is worse because warning signs such as pain are not perceived.

The countless other risk factors such as age, underlying diseases, physique and various medications are **indirect** risk factors. These increase or decrease the probability of pressure ulcer development only in the presence of direct risk factors. Research results of recent years suggest that intrinsic pressure ulcer risk is very variable. Thus, individual anatomy has a significant influence on the extent and type of deformation during pressure loading, and the body's ability to regenerate initially damaged tissue varies greatly.

So-called pressure ulcer risk scales have been used in clinical practice worldwide for over 50 years. Pressure ulcer risk scales consist of many items that usually measure demographic and functional aspects, e.g. incontinence, activity and nutrition. The sole use of these scales to estimate the individual risk of pressure ulcers does not correspond to the state of knowledge. A determined scale value is not a sufficient criterion for measuring or assessing the risk of pressure ulcers. Guidelines and standards today recommend a two-stage approach. During the first patient contact, it should be checked whether the risk of pressure can be excluded. If this exclusion is not possible, an in-depth, comprehensive assessment must be carried out.

12.3 Pressure ulcer diagnosis and classification

The diagnosis of pressure ulcers can only be made based on a thorough anamnesis. A pressure ulcer can develop only when there have been periods of prolonged immobility and prolonged pressure on the tissue. In principle, a pressure ulcer can develop anywhere in the body. Nevertheless, it occurs particularly frequently at the typical predilection sites (➤ Fig. 12.1). Device-associated pressure ulcers are always located where the medical device has had direct contact with the skin. Since the action of local pressure causes pressure ulcers, the resulting wounds are usually sharply limited, round to oval. Deep pressure ulcers almost always have tunnels and undermining areas. The actual tissue damage is often much higher than the skin defect suggests.

If a pressure ulcer is present, it should be classified in the next step. Comparable to other wound classifications, pressure ulcers are classified according to the visibly affected tissue. However, since pressure ulcers initially develop in deeper tissues under (initially) intact skin, the current classifications do not necessarily correspond to the degree of severity and do not imply progression. The currently relevant classifications are summarised in ➤ Table 12.1. In particular, the differences between the NPUAP-EPUAP classification and the ICD-10 code led to some intensive debates. However, both classifications are very similar. The revision of the International Classification of Diseases (ICD) was completed in 2018 and is now available as ICD-11 (https://icd.who.int/). The ICD-11 code takes into account the current state of knowledge and will be the international reference classification for the coming years.

12.3.1 Pressure ulcer stage I

This stage presents with a pronounced, longer-lasting local redness (➤ Fig. 12.4). This redness does not fade with light pressure on the skin. Also, pain or oedema may occur. The skin is intact, there is no wound, and local wound treatment is not necessary. In the presence of a stage I pressure ulcer, it cannot be ruled out that deeper tissue has already been damaged. The

12

Table 12.1 Comparison of current pressure ulcer classifications

NPUAP/EPUAP 2014	ICD-10*	ICD-11 2018
A pressure ulcer is a localised injury to the skin or underlying tissue, usually over a bony prominence, as a result of pressure, or pressure in combination with shear. Many contributing or confounding factors are associated with pressure ulcers; the significance of these factors is yet to be elucidated.	**L89 Pressure ulceration and pressure zone** Note: if the degree of a pressure ulcer cannot be determined reliably, the lower degree must be coded.	**EH90 Pressure ulceration** Pressure ulcers result from localised injury and ischaemic necrosis of skin and underlying tissue due to prolonged pressure, or pressure in combination with shear; bony prominences of the body are the most frequently affected sites; immobility and debility are major contributing factors.
Category/stage I: non-blanchable erythema Intact skin with non-blanchable redness of a localised area usually over a bony prominence. Darkly pigmented skin may not have visible blanching; its colour may differ from the surrounding area. The area may be painful, firm, soft, warmer or cooler when compared to adjacent tissue. Category/stage I may be difficult to detect in individuals with dark skin tones. May indicate 'at-risk' individuals (a heralding sign of risk).	**L89.0 Pressure ulceration stage I** Pressure zone with non-push-off redness on intact skin	**EH90.0 Pressure ulceration stage I** Pressure ulceration stage I is a precursor to skin ulceration. The skin remains intact, but there is non-blanchable redness of a localised area, usually over a bony prominence. The area may be painful, firm, soft, warmer or cooler when compared to adjacent tissue. It can be challenging to detect in individuals with dark skin, but affected areas may differ in colour from the surrounding skin. The presence of pressure ulceration stage 1 may indicate persons at risk of progressing to frank ulceration.
Category/stage II: partial thickness skin loss Partial-thickness loss of dermis presenting as a shallow open ulcer with a red-pink wound bed, without slough. May also present as an intact or open/ruptured serum-filled blister. Presents as a shiny or dry shallow ulcer without slough or bruising.* This category/stage should not be used to describe skin tears, tape burns, perineal dermatitis, maceration or excoriation. *Bruising indicates suspected deep tissue injury.	**L89.1 Pressure ulceration stage II** Pressure ulcers (sores) with: • Abrasion • Bubble • Partial loss of skin with the involvement of epidermis or dermis • Skin loss	**EH90.1 Pressure ulceration stage II** Pressure injury with partial-thickness loss of dermis. It presents as a shallow open ulcer with a red or pink wound bed without slough or as a serum-filled or serosanguinous blister which may rupture. This category should not be used to describe skin tears, tape burns, incontinence-associated dermatitis, maceration or excoriation.
Category/stage III: full-thickness skin loss Subcutaneous fat may be visible, but bone, tendon or muscle are not exposed. Slough may be present but does not obscure the depth of tissue loss. May include undermining and tunnelling. The depth of a category/stage III pressure ulcer varies by anatomical location. The bridge of the nose, ear, occiput and malleolus do not have subcutaneous tissue, and category/stage III ulcers can be shallow. In contrast, areas of significant adiposity can develop extremely deep category/stage III pressure ulcers. Bone/tendon is not visible or directly palpable.	**L89.2 Pressure ulceration stage III** Pressure ulcer with loss of all skin layers with damage or necrosis of the subcutaneous tissue, which can reach down to the underlying fascia.	**EH90.2 Pressure ulceration stage III** Pressure ulcer with full-thickness skin loss. Subcutaneous fat may be visible, but bone, tendon or muscle are not exposed. Slough may be present but does not obscure the depth of tissue loss. There may be undermining and tunnelling into adjacent structures. The depth varies by anatomical location: stage III pressure ulcers can be shallow in areas with little or no subcutaneous fat (e.g. bridge of the nose, ear, occiput and malleolus). In contrast, stage III pressure ulcers can be extremely deep in areas of significant adiposity.

Table 12.1 Comparison of current pressure ulcer classifications *(cont'd)*

NPUAP/EPUAP 2014	ICD-10*	ICD-11 2018
Category/stage IV: full thickness tissue loss Full-thickness tissue loss with exposed bone, tendon or muscle. Slough or eschar may be present on some parts of the wound bed. Often include undermining and tunnelling. The depth of a category/stage IV pressure ulcer varies by anatomical location. The bridge of the nose, ear, occiput and malleolus do not have subcutaneous tissue, and these ulcers can be shallow. Category/Stage IV ulcers can extend into the muscle or supporting structures (e. g., fascia, tendon or joint capsule) making osteomyelitis possible. Exposed bone/tendon is visible or directly palpable.	**L89.3 Pressure ulceration stage IV** Pressure ulcer with necrosis of muscles, bones or supporting structures (e. g. tendons or joint capsules).	**EH90.3 Pressure ulceration stage IV** Pressure ulcer with visible or directly palpable muscle, tendon or bone as a result of a full-thickness loss of skin and subcutaneous tissue. Slough or eschar may be present. The depth varies by anatomical location: stage IV pressure ulcers can be shallow in areas with little or no subcutaneous fat (e. g. bridge of the nose, ear, occiput and malleolus), but are typically deep and often undermine or tunnel into adjacent structures.
Suspected deep tissue injury: depth unknown A purple or a localised maroon area of discoloured intact skin or a blood-filled blister due to damage of underlying soft tissue from pressure or shear. The area may be preceded by tissue that is painful, firm, mushy, boggy, warmer or cooler when compared to adjacent tissue. Deep tissue injury may be difficult to detect in individuals with dark skin tones. While emerging, it may include a thin blister over a dark wound bed. The wound may further evolve and become covered by thin eschar. Development may be rapid, exposing additional layers of tissue, even with optimal treatment.		**EH90.4 Suspected deep pressure-induced tissue damage, depth unknown** An area of soft tissue damage due to pressure or shear, which is anticipated to evolve into a deep pressure ulcer but has not yet done so. The affected skin is typically discoloured purple or maroon and may display haemorrhagic blistering. It may be painful and oedematous. It can be either warmer or colder than adjacent tissue. Evolution into a deep ulcer may be rapid even with optimal treatment.
Unstageable: depth unknown Full-thickness tissue loss in which the base of the ulcer is covered by slough (yellow, tan, grey, green or brown) or eschar (tan, brown or black) in the wound bed. Until enough slough or eschar is removed to expose the base of the wound, the actual depth, and therefore category/stage, cannot be determined. Stable (dry, adherent, intact without erythema or fluctuance) eschar on the heels acts as a 'natural (biological) bodily protection' and should not be removed.		**EH90.5 Pressure ulceration, ungradable** Pressure ulcers with full-thickness skin loss in which actual depth of the ulcer is completely obscured by slough (yellow, tan, grey, green or brown) or eschar (tan, brown or black) in the wound bed. Until enough slough or eschar is removed to expose the base of the wound, it is not possible to determine whether the ulcer is stage III or stage IV.
	L89.9 Pressure ulceration, stage not further described Pressure ulcer (pressure ulcer) without indication of a stage.	**EH90.Z Pressure ulceration of unspecified stage** This category is an 'undefined' residual category.

* https://icd.who.int/browse10/2019/en#/L89.02019

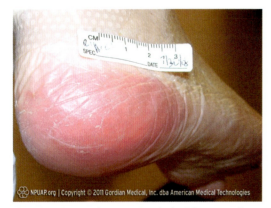

Fig. 12.4 Pressure ulcer stage I on the heel. [W1012-01]

affected body area must be relieved immediately and sustainably to prevent the pressure ulcer from worsening and promoting regeneration (➤ Chap.30.2).

12.3.2 Pressure ulcer stage II

A stage II pressure ulcer is a flat ulcer restricted to the dermis. The wound bed is red, and the wound may bleed, have fibrin deposits and scabs. Serous-filled blisters, which may rupture, are also included in this category (➤ Fig. 12.5). There are several other superficial wounds and skin damage that should be differentiated from pressure ulcers, e.g. incontinence-associated dermatitis (IAD; ➤ Table 12.1). Local wound treatment is required.

12.3.3 Pressure ulcer stage III

These are the classic pressure ulcers with deep tissue involvement. The ulcer extends into the subcutaneous structures. Depending on the structure and area of the body, these wounds can be rather small and flat, e.g. at the bridge of the nose or ear (➤ Fig. 12.6), or extended and deep. The wounds usually show undermining and necrotic coatings, and healing is protracted. In the vast majority of cases, the wound is chronic.

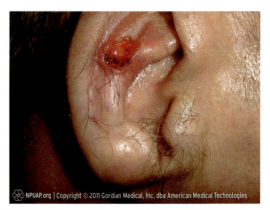

Fig. 12.6 Pressure ulcer stage III on the ear. [W1012-01]

12.3.4 Pressure ulcer stage IV

The stage IV pressure ulcer extends into the muscles, tendons, ligaments or bones (➤ Fig. 12.7). The clinical appearance is similar to that of a stage III pressure ulcer. Necroses are common and local wound treatment is required.

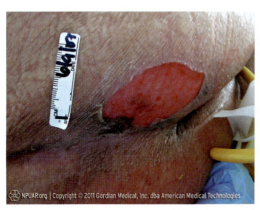

Fig. 12.5 Pressure ulcer stage II, ruptured blister. [W1012-01]

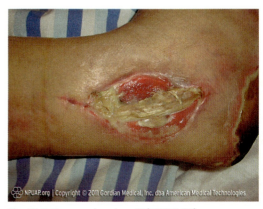

Fig. 12.7 Pressure ulcer stage IV. [W1012-01]

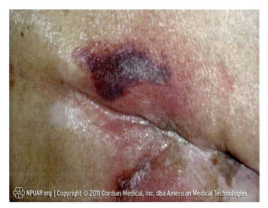

Fig. **12.8** Deep tissue injury. [W1012-01]

12.3.5 Deep tissue injury

The suspected deep tissue injury is a dark, livid to black discolouration under intact skin (➤ Fig. 12.8). It is presumed to be pressure-induced necrosis of the subcutaneous tissue. The area can be painful and clearly distinguish itself from the healthy skin. If deep tissue damage is suspected, pressure on the affected part of the body must be eased consistently (➤ Chap. 31). As no ulcer is present, wound treatment is not necessary at first. If the damage is irreversible, a stage III or IV pressure ulcer develops in the following days.

12.3.6 Unstageable

Pressure ulcers of stages III and IV often show necroses and coatings (➤ Fig. 12.9). If the wound bed is not visible due to these coatings, a distinction cannot be made between a stage III and stage IV pressure ulcer.

12.4 Therapy of pressure ulcers

The therapy begins with a comprehensive assessment of the patient and the pressure ulcer. The ABCDE rule (➤ Chap. 9) can help in wound diagnosis:
- **A**namnesis of the patient and the wound
- **B**acteria (bacteriological wound swab if necessary)
- **C**linical examination of the wound
- **D**efective vascular system
- **E**xtras – ultrasound if necessary

As with other chronic wounds, causal therapy is mandatory. This consists of consistent and permanent off-loading. If this is not possible, the duration and intensity of the mechanical loads should be kept as low as possible (➤ Chap. 30.2).

The next step is to define achievable therapy goals. As a rule, wound-healing should be pursued, but there are also exceptional situations in which healing of the pressure ulcer is not realistic, e.g. at the end of life. In these cases, alternative therapy goals should be defined, e.g. freedom from pain, prevention of wound infection or reduction of wound size.

The local wound treatment should be carried out according to M.O.I.S.T. principles (➤ Chap. 23):
- Moisture balance
- Oxygen balance
- Infection control
- Supporting strategies
- Tissue management

Adequate pain treatment must be provided before and during local wound treatment.

The healing of pronounced stage III and IV pressure ulcers with local wound therapies can be very protracted and sometimes impossible. In these cases, surgical consultation should be carried out to weigh up the advantages and disadvantages of surgical treatment, such as flap plastic surgery, and then carry this out if necessary.

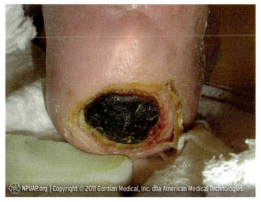

Fig. **12.9** Unclassifiable pressure ulcer of the heel. [W1012-01]

12.5 Conclusion

Pressure ulcers are pressure damage to the skin and the underlying soft tissue. Pressure ulcers typically occur under intact skin, which makes early diagnosis difficult. Pressure ulcers are classified based on visible tissue damage, but wound characteristics such as depth, size and type of exposed tissue are more critical for therapy planning. Typical deep pressure ulcers of stages III and IV are usually chronic wounds and the therapy follows the principles of modern wound treatment. Severe and non-healing pressure ulcers must be treated surgically.

REFERENCES

Kottner J, Black J, Call E, Gefen A, Santamaria N. Microclimate: A critical review in the context of pressure ulcer prevention. Clin Biomech 2018; 59: 62–70.

Kottner J, Kröger K, Gerber V, Schröder G, Dissemond J. [Recognition and correct classification of pressure ulcers: a position paper]. Hautarzt 2018; 69: 839–847.

National Pressure Ulcer Advisory Panel, European Pressure Ulcer Advisory Panel, Pan Pacific Pressure Injury Alliance. Prevention and treatment of pressure ulcers: Clinical practice guideline. 2014.

Oomens CW, Bader DL, Loerakker S, Baaijens F. Pressure-induced deep tissue injury explained. Ann Biomed Eng 2015; 43: 297–305.

13

Jonas Kolbenschlag, Adrien Daigeler, Tobias Hirsch

Disease patterns in burns

Key notes

- Burns are classified as four degrees according to the depth of damage to the skin.
- Estimating the extent of the area can be done according to the rule of nines.
- With a severe second-degree (IIb) burn or worse, surgical therapy is indicated in most cases.

- Severe burn injuries should be treated in a specialist centre.
- Systemic antibiotic therapy should only be carried out in cases of severe clinical features and, if possible, targeted.

13.1 Introduction

More extensive burns present a severe clinical picture due to the extensive tissue damage and the loss of the barrier function of the skin. To optimally treat such severely injured patients, a multidisciplinary treatment concept is required, in addition to a targeted surgical strategy. The present chapter is therefore intended to convey the basics of burn treatment with a focus on wound treatment.

13.2 Definition and classification

Two parameters are particularly important for determining the extent of a burn: the burnt surface area as a percentage and the depth of the injury (first- to fourth-degree).

The burnt skin can be estimated using the Wallace rule of nine, where each part of the body accounts for 9% or more of the total area. Thus, one arm represents 9% of the total surface area, one leg 18%, etc. Alternatively, the so-called rule of palm can be applied, whereby a palm, including the injured person's finger, represents approximately 1% of their body surface. These methods are particularly used for preclinical assessment. Clinically, drawings or software-based solutions can also be used to obtain a more accurate picture.

The depth of burn is divided into four degrees and depends on the affected tissue layer (➤ Table 13.1).

An example of a first-degree burn is classic sunburn (solar dermatitis) with redness and pain, presenting with a purely epidermal lesion which does not lead to a loss of skin integrity and heals promptly without therapy.

Second-degree burns are characterised by intradermal damage, which raises the epidermis like a blister. Lesions with a IIa-degree burn are more superficial dermal lesions in which the blood supply to the wound bed is mostly maintained. They are therefore characterised by a reddish wound bed and – due to the preserved basal cell layer – by scarfree spontaneous healing.

In lesions with a IIb-degree burn, the subdermal vessel plexus and the basal cell layer are damaged or completely destroyed, resulting in a whitish appearance of the wound bed. Due to the thermal destruction of the skin appendages, the hair can often simply be stripped off. Due to the depth of the damage, spontaneous healing no longer takes place, which is why surgical therapy is indicated in most of these cases.

Third-degree burns present with a full-thickness or transdermal damage; blister formation no longer occurs at this stage. They are characterised by their leathery aspect, and often thrombotic subcutaneous veins can be seen due to the deeper penetration of the heat.

13

Table 13.1 Classification of degrees of burns

Degree	Clinical picture	Depth of damage	Therapy
I	Redness	Epidermal	Conservative (a few days)
IIa	• Blistering • Reddish wound bed	Superficially dermal	Conservative (about 14 days)
IIb	• Blistering • Whitish wound bed • Loss of skin appendage	Deep dermal	Operative (tangential)
III	• Leathery • White-greyish • Thrombotic subcutaneous veins	Transdermal	Operative (epifascial)
IV	Charring	Subcutaneous tissue	Operative (extensive debridement)

Fourth-degree burns present with charring injuries. These are accompanied by destruction of the deeper structures and are generally rare. They can be found, for example, after high-voltage injuries or during prolonged exposure to heat.

In most cases, the less experienced tend to overestimate the area of body surface area burnt, while the depth of burn is often underestimated.

13.3 Epidemiology, genesis and pathophysiology

According to the World Health Organisation (WHO), burns were the fourth most common type of injury worldwide in 2004. The most striking feature here is the accumulation of severe burns and fatalities in countries classified by the World Bank as low-income countries. While scalding is the predominant mechanism of injury in childhood, burns from fire or flames are the most common among adults. Contact and electrical burns, as well as explosion injuries, are much rarer causes of thermal injuries.

The basal pathomechanism of burn is the denaturation of proteins by heat. The depth of damage caused is therefore the result of the strength of the energy applied (temperature) and the duration of exposure. At the centre of the applied energy, there is tissue destruction, while in the surrounding area, the microcirculation is disturbed. This tissue is therefore potentially susceptible to becoming necrotic over time. A zone of reactive hyperaemia surrounds these two

zones, which also explains why specific measures, e.g. excessive cooling, can lead to 'afterburning', i.e. progressive tissue destruction.

From about 20% of burnt skin, there is a systemic involvement, the so-called burn sickness, in addition to the localised problems. This systemic involvement is characterised by the loss of integrity of the vessels, with fluid loss into the interstitium as well as microcirculation changes and a prothrombogenic and immunosuppressive state.

13.4 Preclinical care and admission to a burn centre

Analgesia and volume substitution are the most critical measures in preclinical care. Wound cleansing or blister removal should be avoided. Extensive, prolonged and intense cooling should also be prevented. Ideally, cooling should take place promptly and with lukewarm water (➤ Fig. 13.1). The temperature gradient is thus still sufficient to neutralise the thermal energy without further negatively influencing the microcirculation of the tissue.

All patients with severe burns should be treated in an appropriate centre. The admission criteria for such a centre include:
• Burns in complicated areas (face, hands, anogenital, large joints)
• Severe pre-existing conditions or accompanying injuries
• Inhalation traumas

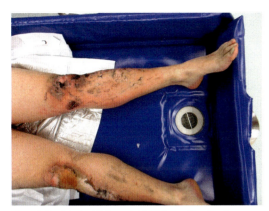

Fig. 13.1 Patient with burns to both lower legs in a burn treatment bath. [P578]

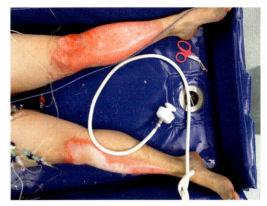

Fig. 13.2 Only after mechanical debridement of blisters and soot can the depth of the burn be estimated more accurately. The right lower leg is mostly indicative of a IIa-degree burn (reddish wound base); the left one, especially centrally, presents a IIb degree burn (also blistering, but with a white, avascular wound base). [P578]

- Circular burns with threatening perfusion disorder
- Electrical injuries
- > 15% second-degree burns
- > 10% third-degree burns
- < 8 and > 60 years

13.5 Treatment for a burn wound

The treatment for the burn wound depends first and foremost on its depth (see above).

As a rule, first-degree burns only require a symptomatic therapy.

In the case of second-degree burns, the blisters should first be removed in analgosedation. This step is essential for assessing the depth and thus determining any further therapy (➤ Fig. 13.2).

In the case of **IIa-degree burns,** spontaneous healing can be expected within approximately two weeks. There are a large number of wound dressings for this indication. This ranges from fatty gauze, to dressings made of silk, lactic acid or similar. Aims of topical therapy are to avoid infection, extend possible intervals between dressing changes as much as possible, low pain for the patient and rapid healing. According to our experience, fatty gauze can be used very well in combination with a topical antiseptic in gel form in many patients. In this case, a two-day

dressing change is recommended for renewed gel application and assessment of the wound surfaces. Alternatively, wound dressings can be used which, as described above, allow longer intervals between dressing changes. This is particularly recommended for secure IIa-degree burns and also for children to keep the periprocedural load as low as possible.

Due to the impairment of perfusion and the destruction of the basal cell layer, no spontaneous healing is to be expected in case of a **IIb-degree burn.** Therefore, the initial topical therapy serves to avoid infections in particular and in most cases, fatty gauze and topical antiseptics are used. Any further therapy of the IIb-degree burn usually takes place surgically.

The situation is similar for a **third-degree burn** (➤ Fig. 13.3). In the case of circular third-degree burns, it should also be noted that they contract strongly and can thus lead to perfusion disorders in the extremities, or to excursion problems in the thorax.

13.5.1 Debridement

With a IIb-degree burn and worse, necrotic tissue parts are present which must be removed to achieve healing. Until the 1970s, surgical debridement was often deferred in the hope that the patient would stabilise. Dr. Janzekovic began to do early excision of the necrosis and subsequent covering of the defect

13

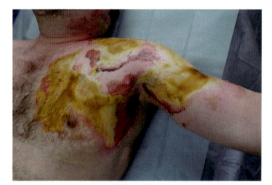

Fig. 13.3 Largely third-degree burn of the shoulder and arm. Note the leathery aspect of the lesion. [P578]

with autologous skin grafts. She was able to show that such a procedure was associated with significantly lower morbidity and mortality. Thus, early excision and grafting has become the standard therapy in burn care.

Debridement of the necrotic tissue parts can take place in different ways. In recent years, enzymatic debridement has become increasingly important and is done, for example, using pineapple enzymes (**NexoBrid**®) and has the advantage of a more selective removal of the eschar.

Surgical debridement distinguishes between two fundamentally different techniques. In tangential debridement, thin layers of tissue are removed tangentially until a vital wound bed – recognisable by punctual bleeding – emerges. The advantage of this technique is the potential preservation of dermal and subdermal structures, which in the long-term leads to better scarring. Disadvantages are the high expenditure of time and increased blood loss. The tangential technique is used in particular for IIb-degree burns because with intradermal damage, vital parts of the dermis remain and can be preserved in this way. A tangential debridement is usually performed with a special knife, the so-called Weck-Knife®. By preselecting a calibrated setting, a defined ablation depth can be set. For larger areas, the Humby-Knife® is ideal, with the help of which even large-area necroses can be quickly debrided. For tricky areas such as the hands or face, hydrosurgery systems can be particularly useful to achieve as fine and economical an ablation of the necrosis as possible.

The counterpart to tangential debridement is epifascial debridement. Here the complete skin,

including subcutaneous fatty tissue, is removed up to the muscle fascia. It is usually used for third-degree burns because of transdermal damage. Conventional instruments are used for this purpose. Monopolar cutting instruments are used primarily to minimise blood loss. An epifascial debridement offers the advantage of a fast and blood-saving procedure, but at the expense of the subcutaneous tissue and any existing dermis as a whole. The subsequent skin transplantation directly onto the fascia often leads to strongly adherent, painful and restricting scars due to the lack of a shifting layer. For this reason, the current practice for most patients is to debride only partially into the subcutaneous fatty tissue and not down to the fascia. Utilising various conditioning techniques, e.g. negative pressure therapy, the wound bed can be prepared to take a split skin graft. For extensive areas or unstable patients, it may be necessary to perform an epifascial debridement to save time and blood. Also, a longer time taken before definitive closure increases the risk of infection (➤ Fig. 13.4). Achieving a potentially better scar quality must, therefore, be carefully weighed up against the longer course of treatment and the associated risks.

Electrical and charring injuries often affect deeper structures, such as muscles, fascia and tendons. In these cases, radical resection of all avital tissue must be performed to prevent infections. Often, decompression of the muscle compartments is indicated in these patients.

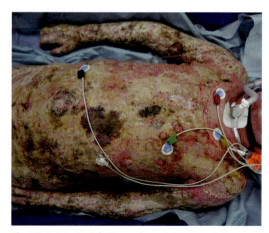

Fig. 13.4 Massive infection and remaining necrosis in a patient with 85% burnt body surface and temporary cover with xenografts. [P578]

13.5.2 Skin replacement

After debridement of the necrotic tissue, closure of the wound surface is of decisive importance to achieve prompt healing. In most cases, this is done through an autologous split skin graft. With a dermatome, the skin is harvested with a thickness of 0.2–0.3 mm. Classic donor sites are the thighs and, in children, the head. In the case of extensive burn injuries, the choice of available donor sites is often limited, so that less favourable sites must also be accepted.

In aesthetically and functionally relevant areas such as the face and hands, the skin to be transplanted is often only pricked to ensure drainage of the wound secretion. In other areas, expanding the skin is paramount, so that so-called mesh grafts are used here (➤ Fig. 13.5). For this purpose, the skin is expanded into a reticular shape using a roller. Depending on the roller used, surface enlargements of 1:1.5 to 1:9 can be achieved. The larger the mesh size, the poorer and slower the healing, which is why in most cases a ratio of 1:1.5 is chosen.

If there is not enough autologous skin available due to the extent of the burn, the debrided areas can also be covered with temporary skin replacement materials to wait until donor sites or IIa-degree burn areas have regenerated. For example, human donor skin or xenogeneic products are used.

13.5.3 Further procedures

A unique form of skin replacement is the Meek technique in which the harvested skin is transplanted as epithelial islands, using a complex system. This technique enables the efficient use of even the smallest donor sites and an even higher expansion ratio.

The preparation of autologous keratinocytes into spray suspensions and their subsequent application to the wound can also be used for burns. Autologous keratinocytes can be cultured for particularly extensive burns, where there are not enough autologous donor sites available. This requires a skin biopsy of just a few square centimetres, from which autologous keratinocytes can be cultured and propagated in specialised institutes. These are then applied as sheets to the burn wounds and can be combined with dermal matrices or donor skin (sandwich procedure), for example.

In addition to the restoration of the skin barrier, the subcutaneous tissue and the resulting scar quality is of particular importance. As already mentioned above, the subcutaneous fatty tissue can be conditioned to take a skin transplant. If this is not possible, e.g. due to thermal destruction, it is possible to use commercially available dermal replacement matrices. Depending on their thickness and texture, these can either be covered directly with a skin graft or take some time for vessels to sprout from the wound bed and vascularise the matrix.

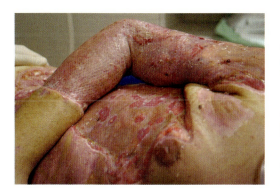

Fig. 13.5 Condition after surgical debridement and split skin transplantation. Note the mesh pattern on the arm after mesh grafting to a tangential debridement site. The distinct soft tissue stage on the ventral thorax after an epifascial debridement is also conspicuous. Amid the skin grafts that have mostly taken, pockets of hyperseptic granulation are visible. [P578]

13.6 Treatment of infected burn wounds

13.6.1 Prevention, diagnostics and bacterial spectrum

One of the main risks in patients with extensive burn injuries is wound infection. In addition to the large wound areas, this can also be explained by the reduced immune competence. Therefore, preventive measures are of decisive importance here. These begin with the corresponding nursing staffing ratio to guarantee 1:1 or 1:2 care for severely burnt patients. Also, burn patients should be accommodated individually with

13

a separate thermoregulation and laminar flow system. Bandages should be changed under sterile conditions to reduce the bacterial load as much as possible.

Despite all these measures, local and systemic infections can occur. The primary diagnosis of wound infection is performed clinically during dressing changes, when smears of the wound and the nasopharynx can also be obtained. Coagulase-negative staphylococci are most frequently detected in the local flora. However, gram-negative bacteria are particularly problematic. They are associated with a higher mortality rate and lead more regularly to transplant losses.

As in other areas, multi-resistant organisms (MRO) are gaining in importance in burn patients. In addition to MRSA, multi-resistant pseudomonads are significant. Even bacteria with high resilience, such as *Acinetobacter baumanii* in particular, are increasingly a problem for intensive burn wards. From this point of view, regular surveillance of the individual bacterial spectrum is an absolute necessity.

13.6.2 Topical and systemic therapy

Every topical and systemic antibiotic therapy is associated with the risk of generating resistant bacteria and should therefore be used with caution. As described above, many topical antiseptics may also be used in infected wounds. Currently, polihexanide preparations are most frequently used in these cases. However, these have, for example, a so-called *Pseudomonas* gap, so that preparations such as iodine can be used here. In addition to the low cytotoxicity of the preparations to be used, attention should also be paid to possible interactions with wound dressings and a possible protein error. Given the increase in MRO, reserve therapeutics may also be considered in individual cases for topical treatment.

Systemic anti-infective therapy should only be used in clinically relevant systemic infections. If the general condition is stable, a targeted therapy based on the results of the swabs taken should be initialised. In the case of severe infections, a calculated broad-spectrum antibiotic can be started. It should however be taken into account that gram-positive bacteria often dominate initially, while the bacterial spectrum shifts to the gram-negative range over the course of treatment.

13.6.3 Surgical therapy

Except for small, isolated areas of infections, an infected burn wound also requires surgical therapy in most cases. Such infections are mostly caused by remaining necroses that require surgical debridement.

13.7 Burn consequences

The most critical consequence of burns is the formation of large scars. Scar quality can be improved by maintaining or replacing subcutaneous tissue. Covering a defect quickly also contributes to a reduction of the scar load, since the time until healing correlates directly with the formation of scars. Often, follow-up interventions are necessary due to functionally and aesthetically disturbing scars. These range from using Z-plasties to break down a pronounced band of scar tissue, using full skin transplants or free flap reconstruction. Autologous fat grafting to improve scar quality is also becoming increasingly important. Percutaneous collagen induction (medical needling), dermabrasion or laser resurfacing can also be used to enhance the quality of the scar.

There is also always a risk of malignant development in the area of burn scars with the development of squamous cell carcinoma, the so-called Marjolin ulcer. In the case of chronic wounds in the field of scars or unstable skin areas, a biopsy should therefore be performed to clarify whether a neoplasia is present, whereby the risk correlates with how long the scar or ulcer have been present.

13.8 Conclusion

The correct estimation of depth and extent is essential for the adequate therapy of patients with burns and for determining a strategy. Today, when treated appropriately, even the most severe burns are injuries that can be survived. In addition to a multidisciplinary concept, this requires early surgical debridement and reconstruction of the skin surface. Improving the resulting scar quality, e.g. through the use of dermal substitutes and thus improving quality of life is highly desirable beyond pure survival. Despite extensive preventive measures, infections are a frequent problem and can be accompanied by the loss of split skin grafts and a higher mortality rate. Even beyond the acute phase, burn patients often still need follow-up interventions to correct scar induced problems.

REFERENCES

Hirsch T, Limoochi-Deli S, Lahmer A, et al. Antimicrobial activity of clinically used antiseptics and wound irrigating agents in combination with wound dressings. Plast Reconstr Surg 2011; 127: 1539–1545.

Kolbenschlag J, Goertz O, Behr B, et al. [Skin antiseptics in plastic surgery]. Handchir Mikrochir Plast Chir 2012; 44: 254–258.

Lehnhardt M, Hartmann B, Reichert B (Hrsg.). Verbrennungschirurgie. Heidelberg: Springer; 2016.

Pruit, BA Jr, McManus AT, Kim SH, et al. Wundinfektionen verbrennen: aktueller Status. Welt J Surg 1998; 22: 135–145.

Pruitt BA Jr, McManus AT. Die sich ändernde Epidemiologie der Infektion bei Verbrennungspatienten. Welt J Surg 1992; 16: 57–67.

Vogt PM, Mailänder P, Jostkleigrewe FRB, Hartmann B, Adams HA. Zentren für Schwerbrandverletzte in der Bundesrepublik Deutschland. GMS Verbrennungsmedizin 2008. GMSVerbrennungsmedizin 2008; 2: Doc03.

13

14

Joachim Dissemond, Knut Kröger

Rare causes of chronic wounds

─────────────── **Key notes** ───────────────

- For the successful treatment of patients with chronic wounds, it is important to diagnose all pathogenetically relevant factors to enable causal therapy.
- In addition to vasculitis and vasculopathy, there are, for example, neuropathic, metabolic, haematological and exogenous factors as well as neoplasia, infections, drugs, genetic defects

and different dermatoses that can cause chronic wounds.
- There may also be multiple causes as well as cofactors and comorbidities that lead to chronic wounds or inhibit their healing.
- Particularly in the case of atypical localisation or therapy-refractory process of wounds, clarification of otherwise rare causes is of decisive importance.

14.1 Introduction

In Europe, most chronic wounds can be attributed to venous leg ulcers, diabetic foot ulcers, pressure ulcers or arterial wounds. However, at least 10 to 20% of all wounds do not correspond to any of these more common causes. Several hundred of rarely diagnosed entities for chronic wounds have already been reported, of which a selection is given here (➤ Table 14.1).

After appropriate diagnostics, knowledge of the cause(s) is the basis for an adequate, mostly interdisciplinary and interprofessional therapy.

14.2 Clinical pictures

14.2.1 Vasculitis

Vasculitis comprises various clinical views that lead to inflammation of the vessel walls with subsequent damage. The classification is based on that of the Chapel-Hill consensus conference (➤ Table 14.2). Despite considerable differences between the various vasculitides, there are some similarities in the clinical appearance of the skin. For example, purpura often occurs, and necroses may happen in the further course

of the disease. When ulcerations arise, they are usually multiplied and more frequently localised at the lower extremities and surrounded by livid erythema. Typical is also a distinct painfulness.

The most frequently diagnosed vasculitis in patients with chronic wounds is cutaneous leucocytoclastic angiitis (➤ Fig. 14.1). It describes a relapsing inflammation of the cutaneous blood vessels caused by drugs, infections or neoplasia. Clinically it initially

Table 14.1 Causes of chronic wounds (a selection)

- Vascular diseases, e.g. chronic venous insufficiency, peripheral artery disease, lymphoedema
- Vasculitis/vasculopathy, e.g. cutaneous leukocytoclastic angiitis, polyarteritis nodosa, livedoid vasculopathy
- Dermatological diseases, e.g. pyoderma gangrenosum, necrobiosis lipoidica, epidermolysis bullosa
- Infectious diseases, e.g. ecthyma, leishmaniasis, mycobacteriosis
- Neoplasia, e.g. basal cell carcinoma, squamous cell carcinoma, lymphoma
- Metabolic disorders, e.g. calciphylaxis, oxalosis, diabetes mellitus
- Drugs, e.g. hydroxycarbamide, anagrelide, coumarin
- Exogenous factors, e.g. artefacial wounds, irradiation, trauma
- Haematological diseases, e.g. sickle cell anaemia, dysprotein anaemia, leukaemia
- Genetic disorders, e.g. Klinefelter syndrome, progeroid syndrome, factor V Leiden mutation

14

Table 14.2 Classification of vasculitis according to that of the Chapel-Hill Consensus Conference from 2012

Group	Disease
Large vessel vasculitis	• Takayasu arteritis • Giant cell arteritis
Medium vessel vasculitis	• Polyarteritis nodosa • Kawasaki disease

Small vessel vasculitis	• ANCA-associated vasculitis
	  – Microscopic polyangiitis
	  – Granulomatosis with polyangiitis (Wegener's)
	  – Eosinophilic granulomatosis with polyangiitis (Churg-Strauss)
	• Immune complex vasculitis
	  – Anti-glomerular basement membrane disease
	  – Cryoglobulinemic vasculitis
	  – LgA vasculitis (Henoch-Schönlein)
	  – Hypocomplementemic urticarial vasculitis

Variable vessel vasculitis	• Behçet's disease • Cogan's syndrome
Single-organ vasculitis	• Cutaneous leukocytoclastic angiitis • Cutaneous arteritis • Isolated aortitis • Primary central nervous system vasculitis • Other
Vasculitis associated with systemic disease	• Lupus vasculitis • Rheumatoid vasculitis • Sarcoid vasculitis • Other
Vasculitis associated with probable etiology	• Hepatitis C virus-associated cryoglobulinemic vasculitis • Hepatitis B virus-associated vasculitis • Syphilis-associated aortitis • Drug-associated immune complex vasculitis • Drug-associated ANCA-associated vasculitis • Cancer-associated vasculitis • Other

leads to palpable purpura and in the further course to painful ulcerations. Appropriate diagnostics should be carried out to rule out visceral manifestation, particularly with kidney involvement. In addition to conventional histopathological diagnostics, direct immunofluorescence (DIF) should also be performed.

The detection of IgA vasculitis (Henoch-Schönlein) in the DIF is often associated with systemic involvement.

Systemic immunosuppression with glucocorticoids, for example, is necessary for the therapy of pronounced vasculitis.

14.2.2 Thromboangiitis obliterans

Thromboangiitis obliterans is a rare non-arteriosclerotic inflammation of the small and medium-sized arteries and veins. It mainly affects young male smokers between the ages of 20 and 45. In Central Europe, an incidence of ten patients per 100,000/year has been described, but with a decreasing tendency in the last two decades. Histopathologically it is a vasculitis of unclear aetiology. In contrast to other vasculitides, the architecture of the vessel wall is preserved. Fibrinoid central necrosis is not observed, and the internal elastic lamina remains intact. Immunohistochemical analysis shows infiltration of cytotoxic T-lymphocytes as well as T-helper lymphocytes.

The diagnostic criteria of thromboangiitis obliterans are not yet standardised. The clinical criteria, according to Shionoya, are the most widespread. These include smoking, disease onset before the age of 50, segmental arterial occlusions of the lower or upper extremities, phlebitis migrans and the absence of other arteriosclerotic risk factors. A reliable clinical diagnosis requires the fulfilment of all five criteria. The duplex sonographic or angiographic detection of so-called corkscrew collaterals also supports the diagnosis. There are no specific laboratory changes, and even a biopsy only helps if the typical early changes can be detected. Typical but not specific symptoms are often described as an initial one-sided intermittent claudication, pain at rest or Raynaud's syndrome. Clinically, acral livid erythema, plaques and nodi occur until finally, necrosis and ulceration develop, which can lead to spontaneous stimulation (➤ Fig. 14.2). The course of the disease is usually chronic in relapses. The predilection sites are the forefoot areas and toes.

The most important therapeutic measure is strict nicotine intolerance. A rheological treatment with prostaglandins can be initiated with medication. Vascular surgery or endovascular therapy only makes sense in individual cases.

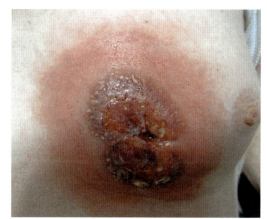

Fig. 14.3 Pyoderma gangrenosum on the chest. [P580]

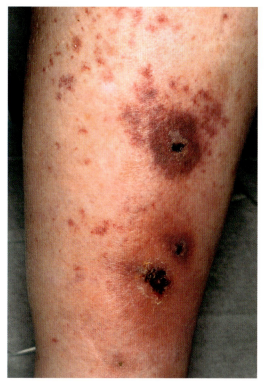

Fig. 14.1 Cutaneous leucocytoclastic angiitis with palpable purpura and several ulcerations of the lower leg. [P580]

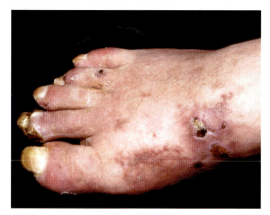

Fig. 14.2 Painful wounds in thrombangiitis obliterans. [P580]

14.2.3 Pyoderma gangrenosum

Pyoderma gangrenosum is a rare destructive ulcerous neutrophilic dermatosis of unclear aetiology. There is a frequent association with chronic inflammatory (intestinal) diseases, neoplasias or metabolic syn-

drome. Following minimal injuries or surgical interventions, the occurrence is described as a pathergy phenomenon. Typical are initially pressure-sensitive, erythematous nodi or sterile pustules, which are often misinterpreted as 'insect bites' and quickly ulcerate. Polycyclic ulcerations usually have a dark, livid, partly undermined, extremely painful rim (➤ Fig. 14.3). The course of the disease is self-limiting after several weeks to years. A diagnostic aid is the PARACELSUS score, which summarises the most important diagnostic criteria (➤ Table 14.3).

Table 14.3 PARACELSUS score for the diagnosis of a pyoderma gangrenosum; ≥ 10 points = Pyoderma gangrenosum highly probable, < 10 points = Pyoderma gangrenosum highly unlikely

Major criteria (3 points)	• **P**rogressing disease (defined as a clinically evident ulcer developing within less than six weeks) • **A**ssessment of relevant differential diagnoses • **R**eddish-violaceous wound border
Minor criteria (2 points)	• **A**melioration by immunosuppressant drugs • **C**haracteristically irregular ulcer shape • **E**xtreme pain (VAS > 4) • **L**ocalisation of lesion at the site of trauma (pathergy phenomenon)
Additional criteria (1 point)	• **S**uppurative inflammation in histopathology • **U**ndermined wound borders • **S**ystemic diseases associated

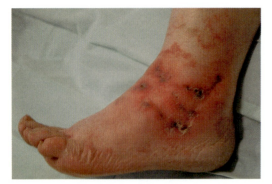

Fig. 14.4 Acute phase of a recurrent livedoid vasculopathy. [P580]

Glucocorticoids are the first choice for systemic therapy. The best evidence from RCTs otherwise exists for ciclosporin and the TNFα inhibitor infliximab.

14.2.4 Livedoid vasculopathy

Livedoid vasculopathy is a rare thrombotic vasculopathy of cutaneous vessels, which leads secondarily to very refractory ulcerations. The first manifestation is often a young adult without a family predisposition. Women are affected approx. three times more frequently than men. Predilection sites are the distal lower legs and especially the malleolar regions. Nonspecific cardinal symptoms of livedoid vasculopathy (➤ Fig. 14.4):
• Livedo racemosa
• Ulcers
• Atrophie blanche
The most painful ulcerations are bizarrely shaped and surrounded by an inflammatory hemorrhagic periwound area. The clinical course of the disease is chronic and recurrent. A biopsy should be taken for diagnosis.

For systemic therapy, rheologically effective drugs such as low molecular weight heparin or direct oral anticoagulation (DOAK), such as rivaroxaban and compression therapy are used.

14.2.5 Calciphylaxis

Calciphylaxis is a rare, potentially lethal disease of unclear etiopathogenesis. Of central importance in this disease are disorders of the calcium-phosphate metabolism. The disease mainly affects patients with (terminal) renal insufficiency. A reduced vitamin D3 synthesis and a compensatory increase in parathyroid hormone occur. The result is an increase in the calcium phosphate product. If the solubility threshold is exceeded, calcium salts are deposited in vascular walls and subcutaneous fat tissue, which leads to tissue ischaemia. Clinically, livid erythema is impressive, leading to extremely painful and very refractory ulcerations, especially on the distal lower legs (➤ Fig. 14.5). Calciphylaxis is a disease which should be histopathologically confirmed and which leads to a high mortality rate.

In therapy, forced dialysis may be essential in combination with the systemic administration of sodium thiosulfate. Vitamin K antagonists should be discontinued.

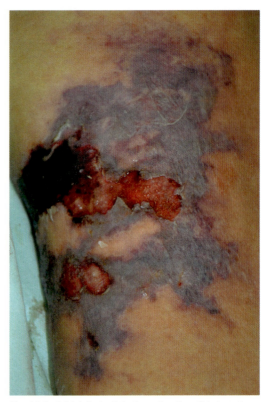

Fig. 14.5 Calciphylaxis of the lower legs in a dialysis patient. [P580]

14.2.6 Hypertensive ischaemic leg ulcer (Martorell's ulcer)

Hypertensive ischaemic leg ulcers are the occurrence of rare, ischaemic, very painful necrosis and ulcerations in patients with arterial hypertension. Women are affected more often than men, with a peak between the ages of 50 and 75. Besides the insufficiently adjusted arterial hypertension, more than half of the patients have diabetes mellitus type 2. Due to stenosing arteriosclerosis of the dermal and subcutaneous arterioles caused by subendothelial intimal fibrosis, reactive hyalinosis of the media occurs. The extremely painful ulcerations have a polycyclic, violet-black wound margin, are mostly found on the dorsolateral distal lower legs and occur on both sides in half of the patients (➤ Fig. 14.6). The diagnosis should be confirmed histopathologically by a large biopsy.

Excision with surgical coverage is described as the therapy of choice.

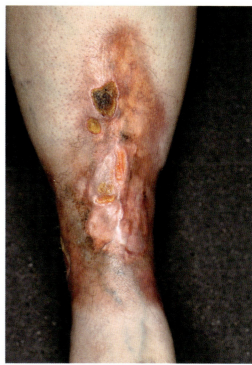

Fig. 14.7 Ulcerative necrobiosis lipoidica diabeticorum. [P580]

14.2.7 Necrobiosis lipoidica

Necrobiosis lipoidica is a rare inflammatory granulomatous skin disease. At least half of the patients are linked with diabetes mellitus; women are affected two to three times more frequently. The disease usually begins with a brownish-red papule with a livid rim, which later develops into a coarse plaque with a yellowish centre and telangiectasias. If the centre then becomes increasingly atrophic, very painful ulcerations can occur (➤ Fig. 14.7). The predilection sites are the extensor sides of the lower legs and the backs of the feet. A biopsy should be taken for diagnostics.

There is no approved or well-evaluated therapy. In addition to glucocorticoids and UV therapies, there are a few studies on successful systemic therapy, for example with fumaric esters, ciclosporin or TNFα inhibitors.

14.2.8 Infectious diseases

Numerous infectious diseases can lead to chronic wounds. In many parts of the world such wounds

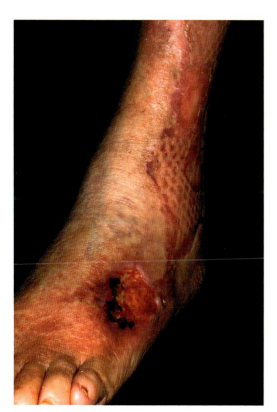

Fig. 14.6 Hypertensive ischaemic leg ulcer (Martorell's ulcer). [P580]

are very common. Predisposing factors include poor hygiene, malnutrition, obesity, diabetes mellitus, immunosuppression or eczema.

Ecthyma (simplex) is the name for an ulcerating purulent inflammation of the skin caused by a bacterial superinfection of pre-existing injuries. Clinically, the primary symptom is a pustule with surrounding erythema. Secondarily, sharply defined, less painful ulcerations develop, which are rarely larger than 3–5 cm. Typical is the erythematous border, which appears punched out (➤ Fig. 14.8). The occurrence of ulcers, which are very refractory to therapy and usually occur in multiple cases, is preferentially observed on the legs and gluteal. The clinical findings and anamnesis are so typical that mostly no further diagnostic is necessary after clinical inspection. Therapy is usually performed exclusively topically, for example, with antiseptics.

Obligate intracellular protozoan Leishmania parasites cause leishmaniasis. They are found in the tropics, Asia, East Africa and increasingly in the Mediterranean. Rodents and dogs are the pathogen reservoir. The pathogens enter the skin of the affected

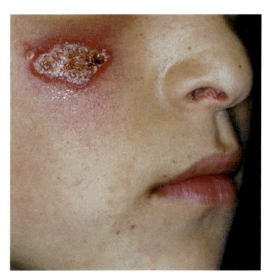

Fig. 14.9 Cutaneous leishmaniasis on the cheek. [P580]

person via the saliva of sand flies. The predilection sites are all areas that are not covered by clothing. In addition to cutaneous leishmaniasis, there are visceral (kala-azar) and mucocutaneous (espundia) forms. In cutaneous leishmaniasis, erythema develops at the puncture site. After an incubation period of two weeks to one year, an erythematous papule with a livid rim is visible, which often ulcerates (➤ Fig. 14.9). The most painless ulcerations are 1–5 cm in size. For diagnostic purposes, several biopsies should be taken for both conventional histopathology and cultural detection.

Without therapy, cutaneous leishmaniasis usually heals spontaneously after one to two years. In the case of findings of a growth in size, or mucocutaneous and visceral progression, systemic therapy should always be performed. Therapies with N-methylglucamine antimonate, miltefosine, pentamidine or amphotericin B are recommended.

14.2.9 Neoplasms

Primary cutaneous neoplasms that can lead to wounds include malignant melanomas, basal cell carcinomas, cutaneous lymphomas and spinocellular carcinomas (SCC).

An SCC is a locally destructively-growing, primarily epithelial malignant tumour. The average age at first manifestation is 70 years; men are affected two times

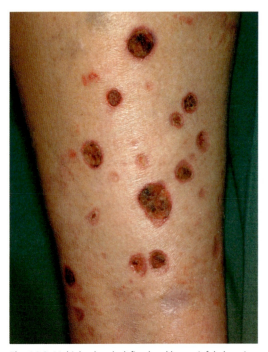

Fig. 14.8 Multiple, sharply defined and less painful ulcers in ecthyma. [P580]

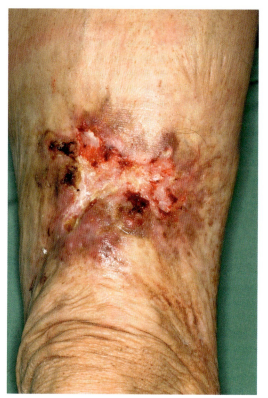

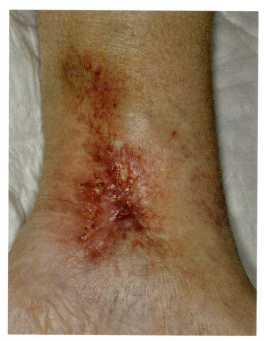

Fig. 14.11 Ulcerations after long-term ingestion of hydroxy-carbamide. [P580]

Fig. 14.10 Spinocellular carcinoma (Marjolin ulcer) of the tigh on a longterm burn scar. [P580]

more frequently than women. Clinically, SCC often begins with an erythematous macula on which hyperkeratosis develops. In the further course of the disease, an indolent tumour develops, which can ulcerate (➤ Fig. 14.10). A unique form of SCC is the so-called Marjolin ulcer. After several years or decades, carcinomatous transformation occurs, particularly in the scars of burns.

If a neoplasm is suspected, one or rather more biopsies should be taken. The therapy of choice is usually a complete excision.

14.2.10 Drugs

Chronic wounds can also be caused by taking various drugs, such as hydroxycarbamide. Hydroxycarbamide is a drug taken by patients with myeloproliferative diseases such as chronic myelogenous leukaemia (CML), polycythaemia vera or essential thrombo-

cythaemia. When taken for a period of time, usually several years, atrophie blanche and very painful ulcerations can occur. These skin changes are often located symmetrically on the distal lower legs and especially around the malleoli (➤ Fig. 14.11). The diagnosis is based on a review of the anamnesis, the clinical findings and the histopathological result.

There is no specific therapy for these wounds other than discontinuation of the causative drug.

14.2.11 Dermatitis artefacta

Dermatitis artefacta is a self-damaging skin condition that occurs in almost all areas of medicine. It is an autoaggressive action with damage to the body without a direct intention of suicide. A dermatitis artefacta can frequently be found in women between the ages of 20 and 40, especially in patients with medical knowledge. In some patients, cutaneous artefacts serve as a secondary gain illness, e.g. in the context of gaining a pension or attention. Chemical substances, needles, razor blades or constricting bands are often used for self-injury in areas that are easily accessible.

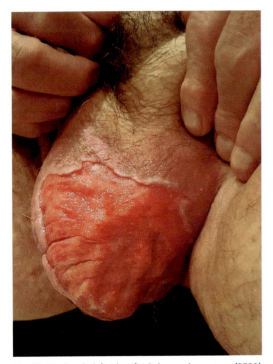

Fig. 14.12 Sharply defined artificial ulcer on the scrotum. [P580]

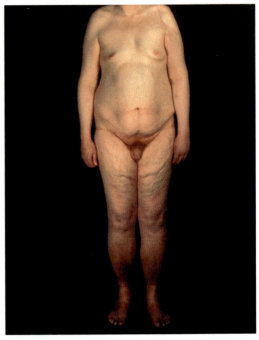

Fig. 14.13 Patient with Klinefelter syndrome and post-thrombotic leg ulcer. [P580]

The clinical picture is very heterogeneous. Dermatitis artefacta are mostly clearly circumscribed, often striate and well distinguishable from the surrounding skin (➤ Fig. 14.12). The anamnesis of the patients gives a regular occurrence of 'overnight'.

Psychiatric treatment would be useful but is often rejected by patients. Without the acknowledgement of the affected person and the wish for therapy, no meaningful treatment is possible. It may be possible to establish readiness for therapy by talking to their relatives.

14.2.12 Genetic diseases

There are numerous genetic diseases potentially associated with the occurrence of chronic wounds. Klinefelter syndrome is the most frequently described genetic defect with a prevalence of 1:590 male neonates. In most cases, a numerical chromosomal aberration in the form of a trisomy (47,XXY) is the basis. The patients show gynaecomastia, testicular hypoplasia, azoospermia, elevated serum follicle-stimulating

hormone (FSH) levels, excessive tallness, obesity, osteoporosis and adaptation disorders. The incidence of phlebothrombosis is up to 20 times higher than in the average population due to various thrombogenic factors. The chronic wounds usually correspond to a postthrombotic leg ulcer (➤ Fig. 14.13).

Progeroid syndromes are genetic diseases that lead to premature ageing symptoms. Examples of these sporadic diseases are Werner syndrome, Xeroderma pigmentosum and Rothmund-Thomson syndrome. A faulty DNA repair results in oxidative stress and altered transcription control. In addition to wound-healing disorders, others such as neurodegenerative diseases, arteriosclerosis and neoplasia are also common. Rothmund-Thomson syndrome type II is an autosomal recessive genodermatosis based on a mutation of the RECQL4 gene-coding for a helicase. Clinical symptoms include facial poikiloderma, delayed growth, low body hair, cataracts and skeletal abnormalities (➤ Fig. 14.14). Often chronic wounds can occur after microtrauma, and genetic analysis is necessary for the diagnosis of genetic defects. In all patients with progeroid syndromes, it is crucial

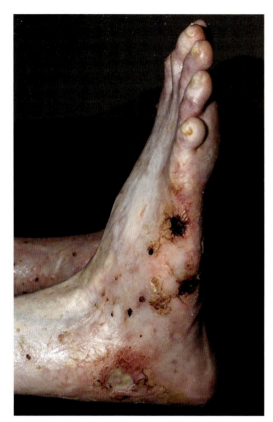

Fig. 14.14 Chronic wounds of the feet of a patient with Rothmund-Thomson syndrome type II. [P580]

to exclude neoplasia as the cause of wound-healing disorders.

Therapeutically, only symptomatic therapy is possible for most genetic diseases.

14.3 Conclusion

Even if CVI, PAD, pressure or diabetes mellitus is the main pathophysiological factors in most patients with chronic wounds, the relevant differential diagnoses should be known and possibly excluded, especially in the case of atypical localisation or therapy refractory courses. It should also be noted that there is increasing knowledge about relevant cofactors and comorbidities, such as obesity, diabetes mellitus, haematological diseases, eczema or (lymphatic) oedema, which rarely cause chronic wounds but can be of decisive importance for the refractory course of treatment.

REFERENCES

Dissemond J. Blickdiagnose chronischer Wunden – Über die klinische Inspektion zur Diagnose. 4th edition, Köln: Viavital-Verlag; 2020.

Dissemond J, Körber A, Grabbe S. Differential diagnoses in leg ulcers. J Dtsch Dermatol Ges 2006; 4: 627–634.

Jockenhöfer F, Gollnick H, Herberger K, et al. Aetiology, comorbidities and cofactors of chronic leg ulcers – Retrospective evaluation of 1,000 patients from 10 specialised dermatological wound care centres in Germany. Int Wound J 2016; 13: 821–828.

Körber A, Klode J, Al-Benna S, et al. Etiology of chronic leg ulcers in 31,619 patients in Germany analyzed by an expert survey. J Dtsch Dermatol Ges 2011; 9: 116–121.

Mekkes JR, Loots MA, Van Der Wal AC, Bos JD. Causes, investigation and treatment of leg ulceration. Br J Dermatol 2003; 148: 388–401.

14

15

Joachim Dissemond, Knut Kröger, Jan Kottner

Pathological skin changes

15.1 Wound or no wound?

Joachim Dissemond, Knut Kröger

─────────────────── **Key notes** ───────────────────

- Disease patterns that are associated with blisters or erosions, for example, should be clarified pathophysiologically. An interdisciplinary treatment of the partly autoimmunological or infectiological diseases is often necessary.
- Eczema is not a wound. Therefore the use of wound dressings is not appropriate here.

- There are clinical pictures such as intertrigo or gram-negative bacterial toe web infection which are associated with severe exudation and for which moist wound treatment is contraindicated.
- Modern moist wound treatment is contraindicated for dry necroses.

15.1.1 Introduction

Not everything that looks like a wound will need regular chronic wound care. Some syndromes show certain changes to the skin, but the rules of modern moist wound treatment do not always lead to success and are sometimes even contraindicated. It is therefore important for nurses and medical wound experts to know what would be appropriate in modern moist wound care. The following are examples of some diseases for which localised moist wound treatment is not appropriate.

15.1.2 Gram-negative bacterial toe web infection

Gram-negative bacterial toe web infection is a very exudative inflammation caused by gram-negative bacteria, but often also by a mix of infections, which usually begins in the interdigital areas and spreads proximally (➤ Fig. 15.1a). Patients often have a tinea pedis of the interdigital area which has been treated with antimycotics for a long period. These antimycotics are also effective against some gram-positive bacteria. The growth of gram-negative bacteria, especially *Pseudomonas aeruginosa* or *Klebsiella-*, *Enterobacter-*, or *Proteus* species, is promoted by

skin maceration in the course of mycosis and the eradication of gram-positive bacteria. Other local factors are the wearing of less breathable footwear or plantar hyperhidrosis. Also, diabetes mellitus and atopic diathesis, peripheral artery disease (PAD) or chronic venous insufficiency (CVI) appear to be more frequent in patients.

In addition to the physical examination with very typical symptoms, it is necessary to take a bacteriological swab, establish a mycological culture and determine the inflammatory serological parameters such as the blood count, erythrocyte sedimentation rate (ESR), and C-reactive protein (CRP). The clinical findings are usually characterised by the intense, sweet, foul odour of the gram-negative bacteria. In addition to the possibly distinctive oedema, there are strongly exudative, painful erosions, which can also develop into ulcerations in the further course of the disease ➤ Fig. 15.1b). The symptoms are often found in varying degrees on both sides. Chronic ulcerations or distinctive local infections can develop into sepsis.

In contrast to the otherwise propagated modern moist wound care, it is crucial here to eliminate the moist wound environment. Localised treatment is based on creating a dry environment, and antiseptic topical therapies. Systemic antibiotics can be useful for very severe cases or a soft tissue infection. Also, it is necessary to diagnose and adequately treat the

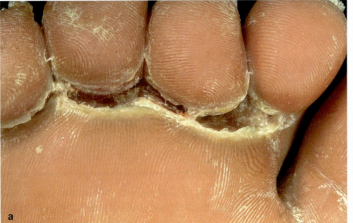
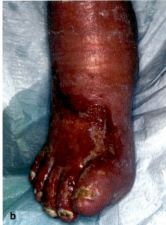

Fig. 15.1 a Initial gram-negative bacterial toe web infection with distinctive fungal foot infection; **b** gram-negative bacterial toe web infection with noticeable soft tissue infection. [P580]

favourable factors that led to the development of the gram-negative bacterial toe web infection, as a chronic recurrent course may otherwise occur.

15.1.3 Hidradenitis suppurativa

Hidradenitis suppurativa, synonymously called acne inversa, is a chronic recurrent disease caused by an inflammation of the follicular epithelium of the sebaceous glands and the terminal hair follicles. Secondarily, the apocrine sweat glands are also involved in the inflammatory process. An initial manifestation can occur at any age after puberty; mostly younger adults between the ages of 20 and 30 are affected for the first time. The exact prevalence of hidradenitis suppurativa is not known, but it is believed to affect at least 1% of the adult population in western countries. The incidence has risen over the past four decades, particularly among women. The ratio of affected women to men is about 2–5:1. A family history is positive in 40% of patients.

The exact aetiology of hidradenitis suppurativa is unknown. A causal connection with cigarette consumption is under discussion, because up to 97% of all those affected were found to be smokers in various clinical studies,. There is also a high incidence of obesity. These clinically often very pronounced and recurrent bacterial infections are seen as a secondary problem to the actual disease process. A local factor is tight-fitting clothing. A very noticeable course can

also be associated with immunosuppression or diabetes mellitus.

The predilection sites of hidradenitis suppurativa are the intertriginous areas (➤ Fig. 15.2). In men,

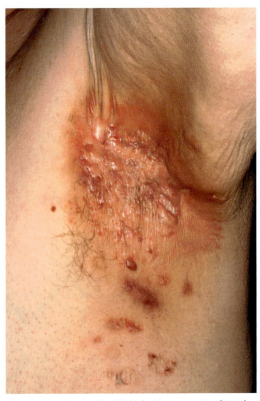

Fig. 15.2 Axillary localised hidradenitis suppurativa. [P580]

hidradenitis suppurativa frequently occurs at the perineum or perianal area and is often more severe than in women who are more frequently affected in axillary or submammary areas. Clinically, the patients show cutaneous inflammation with multiple nodi, pustules or abscesses. In case of a longer persistent course, the occurrence of bumpy scar tissue and fistulating tracts, from which pus can often be expressed, is typical. Also, erosions, ulcerations, macerations and eczema may occur in the wound environment.

Classification of hidradenitis suppurativa according to Hurley:

- Stage I – one or more distinct abscesses; no fistulae
- Stage II – one or more abscesses with fistulae and scarring which lie far apart from each other
- Stage III – extensive infestation with abscesses, fistulas and scarring

In addition to the physical changes, the patients – who often have limited mobility – feel considerably stigmatised and psychologically burdened due to the disease, which can lead to social isolation. Rare but dreaded late complications may be secondary amyloidosis or squamous cell carcinoma.

Many guidelines recommend the long-term systemic administration of clindamycin (and rifampicin) or doxycycline. Since 2015, the tumour necrosis factor (TNF)-α inhibitor adalimumab has been approved for systemic treatment. A radical excision should be performed, especially in the case of scars or fistulas. A local concomitant treatment, for example with antiseptics, is recommended. The risk factors, especially cigarette use and obesity, should be eliminated.

15.1.4 Intertrigo

Pathological erythematous skin changes in the intertriginous areas are summarised as intertrigo. Intertriginous are all areas of the body where skin surfaces touch each other directly. Aetiologically, skin friction causes physical irritation and secretion congestion. An increased sweat production, which macerates the skin surface, and thus weakening the skin barrier function, has a locally favourable effect. Additionally, those affected often suffer from obesity or diabetes mellitus.

The clinical picture is usually so typical that no further diagnosis is necessary. However, relevant microorganisms that lead to superinfection of the disorder should be searched. Infections with *Candida albicans* are particularly frequent here. In addition to bacteriological swabs, mycological examinations are therefore also useful. In the intertrigo, there is sharply limited erythema, which often shows central macerations. In this erythema, erosions or even ulcerations can develop over time (➤ Fig. 15.3a). Patients often describe an unpleasant feeling of warmth with itching and burning pain. In the case of candidal intertrigo caused by yeasts, additional pustules are typically seen at the edges and in the surroundings of the erythema ➤ Fig. 15.3b). The predilection sites of intertrigo are inguinal, submammary, in the abdominal folds and the intergluteal cleft. In the differential diagnosis incontinence-associated dermatitis (IAD) (➤ Chap. 15.2) should be excluded.

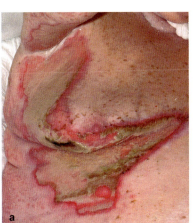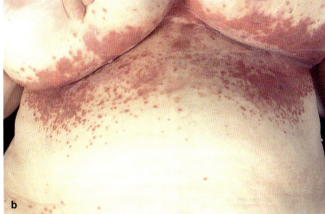

Fig. 15.3 a Very pronounced erosive, partly ulcerating intertrigo; **b** candidal intertrigo. [P580]

Specific treatment is based on the pathogens that may have been detected. In contrast to the basic principles of moist wound treatment, the aim is to achieve a dry environment for the affected patients. After cleansing, for example, the wound is cushioned with dry, non-irritating compresses. Adjuvant measures should eliminate favourable factors. For example, weight reduction and the avoidance of tight-fitting clothing and friction should be targeted, as otherwise a chronic relapse may occur.

15.1.5 Dry necrosis, dry gangrene

According to the current definitions of the Initiative Chronische Wunden (ICW) e. V., necrosis is defined as dead, previously vital tissue (➤ Fig. 15.4a). Gangrene is a dead body part, for example, a toe or a forefoot (➤ Fig. 15.4b). When describing dead tissue in wounds, we therefore speak of necrosis and not of gangrene.

Dry necroses and gangrene are usually not infected and do not release decaying tissue products to the underlying wound. They adhere firmly to the underlying wound and form a clean, germ-free wound-covering. Since the wound is already bacteria-free and firmly covered, moist wound treatment is counterproductive in such a situation. It only leads to dry necrosis becoming moist and being infected by bacteria. A wound dressing cannot penetrate dry necrosis to positively influence wound-healing. The therapeutic goal in the case of dry necrosis is to keep it dry and to use it as a wound cover until it dissolves spontaneously or has to

be removed for further wound treatment. Dry necrosis or gangrene which comes loose and detaches from the wound edges does not form a firm wound-covering. Covered by this loose necrosis, the wound cannot be assessed and cleaned, and the necrosis should be removed promptly.

If necrosis or gangrene is moist, this usually indicates a bacterial infection. Moist necrosis has a negative effect on wound-healing because it releases decaying tissue products (➤ Fig. 15.4c). They also provide a breeding ground for bacteria, which can survive in that environment despite the local application of antiseptics or systemic use of antibiotics. Moist necrosis must not be preserved by moist wound treatment. It must be removed promptly and entirely from the wound by adequate, surgical debridement. Moist gangrene should be surgically amputated. The debridement should be carried out as soon as possible, but until then, moist necrosis should be covered with a bandage which is firmly strapped over the exudate of the wound, so that the moisture is extracted from the bacterial tissue decay. Superabsorbers are suitable for this purpose, for example.

15.1.6 Blisters on skin

There are numerous pathophysiological reasons why blisters appear on the skin (➤ Table 15.1). Often it is causal (localised) oedema in inflammatory changes.

For adequate treatment, it is necessary to find out the cause of the blister formation and, if possible, to treat the cause. In localised blister treatment, it is vital

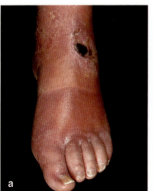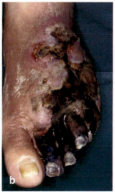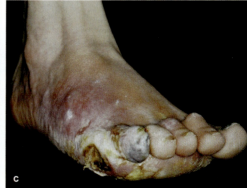

Fig. 15.4 a Dry necrosis; **b** dry gangrene; **c** foot with wet necrosis and gangrene. [P580]

Table 15.1 Disease patterns in which blisters may occur on the skin

- Physical/mechanical damage, e.g. dermatitis solaris, frostbite
- Adverse drug reactions, e.g. Steven-Johnson syndrome, toxic epidermal necrolysis (➤ Fig. 15.5a)
- Bullous autoimmune dermatoses, e.g. bullous pemphigoid (➤ Fig. 15.5d), pemphigus vulgaris (➤ Fig. 15.5e)
- Insect bite reactions, e.g. mosquito bite, bullous arthropod bite
- Internal diseases, e.g. porphyria cutanea tarda, bullosis diabeticorum
- Infectious diseases:
  - Viruses, e.g. herpes simplex, zoster (➤ Fig. 15.5b)
  - Bacteria, e.g. erysipelas (➤ Fig. 15.5c), impetigo contagiosa
  - Fungi, e.g. candidiasis, cryptococcosis

to prevent bacterial superinfection as well as pain caused by adhesive bandages. There is no fundamental need to open blisters which are primarily sterile, or even to remove the top of the blister. Pustules need a differential diagnosis. In pustules, the content of the blister consists of pus. If blisters cause pressure pain or, for example, prevent getting dressed, they can be punctured in a sterile manner and covered with dry, sterile bandages.

Bullous pemphigoid

Bullous pemphigoid (BP) is the most common form of subepidermal bullous autoimmune dermatosis. Women are more frequently affected than men. Most patients are older than 60 years at first manifestation.

The binding of autoantibodies causes subepidermal cleavage to the basement membrane zone. The antibodies are directed against hemidesmosomes, which ensure a connection between the basal keratinocytes and the basal membrane zone. Various drugs or ionising radiation have been discussed as triggers for flare-ups. Also, patients with BP have a potential association with neoplasms. A tentative diagnosis can usually be made just after the anamnesis and clinical examination. The specific IgG antibodies against BP230 or BP180 should be determined serologically by indirect immunofluorescence (IIF). Also, biopsies should be taken to perform both conventional his-

tology with HE staining and direct immunofluorescence (DIF).

Initially, patients described reticular erythema and pronounced itching. In most cases, bulging blisters which are initially clear, later haemorrhagic, occur in phases. When these blisters burst, sharply delineated erosions or sores occur (➤ Fig. 15.5d). The mucous membranes are rarely affected.

The treatment is primarily based on systemic therapy with immunosuppressive drugs with systemic glucocorticoids as the first choice. Further therapy is often supplemented with other substances such as azathioprine or mycophenolate mofetil. In therapy-refractory courses, successful treatment was reported with the anti-CD20 antibody rituximab. With localised findings, exclusively topical treatment with highly potent glucocorticoids (mostly clobetasol) can also be attempted.

Pemphigus vulgaris

Pemphigus vulgaris (PV) is the most common form of intraepidermal bullous autoimmune dermatosis. It occurs in men and women in a comparable frequency. The first manifestation usually occurs in the third to sixth decade of life.

The formation of autoantibodies against desmosomal proteins causes acantholysis with cleft formation within the epidermis. The autoantibodies are directed against desmoglein 1 or 3, which as cadherins are responsible for keratinocytes adhesion. There may be an association with various other diseases such as myasthenia gravis, lupus erythematosus, neoplasms or even drugs. After anamnesis and clinical examination, a tentative diagnosis can usually be made. A typical, but not proven, clinical test procedure is the positive Nikolsky sign. The upper skin layers on apparently unaffected skin can be shifted or 'dislodged' with the tangential pressure of a finger. Serologically, antibodies against desmoglein 1 or 3 can be detected. Also, the collection of biopsies is useful for conventional and DIF staining. In about half of the patients, the disease begins with therapy-refractory erosions of the mucous membranes. As the disease progresses, additional flaccid blisters may develop on the entire integument. Due to the fragile 'roof' of the blisters, they burst very quickly,

15

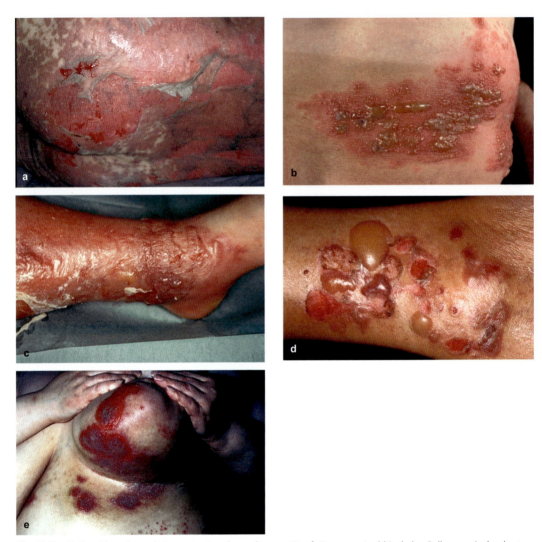

Fig. 15.5 a Toxic epidermal necrolysis as a severe adverse drug reaction; **b** Herpes zoster (shingles); **c** Bullous erysipelas due to streptococcus infection; **d** Bullous pemphigoid; **e** Pemphigus vulgaris. [P580]

so that clinically erosions often occur exclusively (➤ Fig. 15.5e).

Without treatment, a lethal process can occur. The treatment is comparable to that of BP, but often much more protracted.

15.1.7 Eczema

Eczema, synonymously known as dermatitis, is a symptom of various diseases (➤ Table 15.2).

Concerning the symptomatic description, a distinction must be made between acute and chronic eczema. Acute eczema usually occurs in different stages. Clinically, light erythema with itchy blisters occurs initially. If the blisters burst, weeping results. After drying, yellowish crusts form. When healing begins, scaling can be observed (➤ Fig. 15.6). Finally, postinflammatory hyperpigmention results. These stages do not always have to be passed through successively. In many patients, different aspects can be seen at the same time.

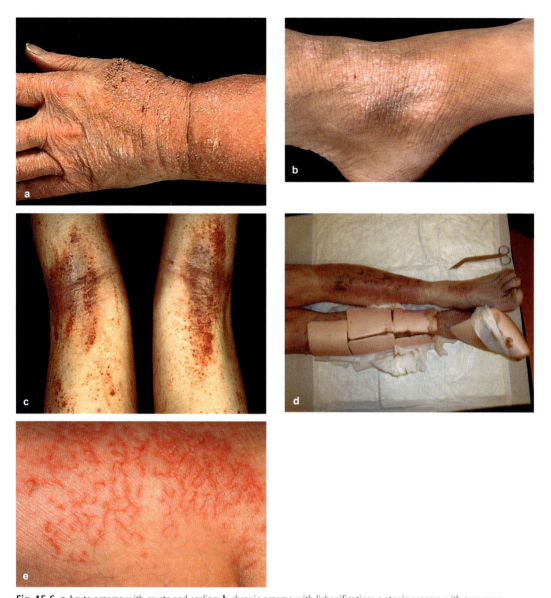

Fig. 15.6 **a** Acute eczema with crusts and scaling; **b** chronic eczema with lichenification; **c** atopic eczema with numerous excoriations; **d** wound dressings are used for the treatment of eczema. This procedure is wrong! **e** Eczema craquelé in a patient with asteatotic eczema. [P580]

In chronic eczema, lichenification occurs, which describes a coarsening and thickening of the skin structure (➤ Fig. 15.6b). Papules can also occur.

Due to itching, acute and chronic eczema often show excoriations of varying depth caused by scratching the skin (➤ Fig. 15.6c).

For successful treatment, a diagnosis should be made. A dermatological assessment is usually useful for this purpose. 'Sore/erosive skin' or 'superficial wounds' are often considered to be symptoms of eczema and then incorrectly treated with wound dressings or so-called wound-healing ointments (➤ Fig. 15.6d). As this is a cutaneous, non-infectious inflammation, at least in the case of more notable findings, external agents with glucocorticoids should be used for a limited time (➤ Chap. 37). With long-

Table 15.2 Diseases indicated by eczema symptoms

- Atopic eczema
- Asteatotic eczema
- Stasis dermatitis
- Seborrheic eczema
- Scabies and post-scabial eczema
- Cutaneous T-cell lymphoma, e.g. mycosis fungoides
- Contact eczema:
  - Allergic contact dermatitis
  - Toxic contact eczema
  - Photo-toxic/allergic contact eczema

term therapy of chronic diseases, other external agents can often be used as alternatives, such as calcineurin inhibitors. To prevent recurrence, consistent skin-care (➤ Chap. 41) is usually sufficient. Contact with potential allergens should be avoided (➤ Chap. 42). Excessive washing and bathing or the excessive use of soaps or shower products contribute to drying out the skin and thus lead to an increase in itching.

Asteatotic eczema

Asteatotic eczema from dry skin is also referred to as eczema craquelé. It is an eczema caused by re-duced sebum production of the skin (sebostasis). Asteatotic eczema is a type of itchy dermatitis that occurs particularly frequently in older adults and atopic patients.

Rare causes are malnutrition, ichthyosis or system-ically taken drugs such as retinoids. Dry skin (or xerosis cutis) often does not cause any symptoms in the first decades of life. From mid-life onwards, increasing dehydration leads to an unpleasant feeling

of skin tightness. Typically, the drying process is more frequently aggravated in winter (heating period). The symptoms often begin in the lower legs. Morphologic-ally, eczema is accompanied by typical net-like tears in the skin, which are reminiscent of a dried-out river bed (➤ Fig. 15.6e).

15.1.8 Conclusion

There are always patients showing symptoms which cannot be treated 1:1 with the basic principles of modern moist wound care. Here it is important to diagnose and treat the underlying factors as inter-disciplinarily and interprofessionally as possible. The use of modern wound products is usually not recommended and is sometimes even con-traindicated.

REFERENCES

Dissemond J, Augustin M, Eming SA, et al. Modern wound care – practical aspects of non-interventional topical treatment of patients with chronic wounds. J Dtsch Dermatol Ges 2014; 12: 541–554.

Has C, He Y. Focal adhesions in the skin: lessons learned from skin fragility disorders. Eur J Dermatol 2017; 27: 8–11.

Ingram JR, Woo PN, Chua SL, et al. Interventions for hidra-denitis suppurativa. Cochrane Database Syst Rev 2015; 10: CD010081.

Lichterfeld-Kottner A, El Genedy M, Lahmann N, Blume-Peytavi U, Büscher A, Kottner J. Maintaining skin integrity in the aged: a systematic review. Int J Nurs Stud 2020; 103: 103509.

von Kobyletzki LB, Beckman L, Smirnova J, et al. Eczema and educational attainment: a systematic review. Br J Dermatol 2017; 177: 47–49.

Weidner T, Tittelbach J, Illing T, Elsner P. Gram-negative bac-terial toe web infection – a systematic review. J Eur Acad Dermatol Venereol 2018; 32: 39–47.

15.2 Incontinence-associated dermatitis

Jan Kottner

─────────────────────────── **Key notes** ───────────────────────────

- Direct and repeated contact of the skin with urine or faeces can cause incontinence-associated dermatitis (IAD).
- Clinical signs of IAD are erythema, erosions, excoriations and pain.

- Prevention and therapy of IAD consists of conti-nence promotion, adequate use of absorbent or draining products and structured skin protec-tion.

15.2.1 Etiology and pathogenesis

The so-called incontinence-associated dermatitis (IAD) is caused by the repeated and prolonged contact of urine or faeces with the skin. It is therefore a toxic contact dermatitis (L24.-). Exposure to faeces, in particular liquid faeces, represent a particularly high risk for the skin. Occlusive conditions due to inadequate incontinence material or prolonged lying down on a non-ventilated surface or mattress and repeated skin cleansing also contribute to the development of IAD.

This phenomenon occurs in all age groups. The diagnosis 'nappy rash' (L22) is established in newborns and infants. In young people and adults, however, the term 'IAD' should be used, since the term 'nappy' is not considered appropriate in this age group and the IAD can develop regardless of the type of continence material used.

Comparable to other forms of contact dermatitis, contact with urine or faeces leads to direct damage of the skin barrier and subsequent inflammatory reaction. Specifically, the following pathogenetic mechanisms are discussed:

1. The increased **moisture** on the skin surface leads to hyperhydration of the stratum corneum (SC). The SC and the entire epidermis lose their structural integrity and resistance to mechanical loads. At the same time, the permeability of the SC is increased; irritating substances on the skin surface (e. g. surfactants from skin cleansing products) can penetrate more quickly into the epidermal and dermal layers and cause irritations there. Repeated changes of moisture on the skin surface and drying (e. g. air exposure during or after changing incontinence pad) lead to a loss of natural moisturising factors in the corneocytes, causing the SC to dry out.
2. Urine contains urea, which is split into ammonia and carbon dioxide by urease. Ammonia dissolves in water and produces a basic solution, which increases the **pH** of the skin surface. As a result, the cohesion of the SC is further weakened, and the skin flora changes.
3. **Digestive enzymes** – lipases and proteases – are found in the faeces. These directly attack the lipids and proteins of the SC. Since the passing of faeces is particularly fast in liquid faeces, the enzymes are still active, which explains why the IAD risk in diarrhoea is particularly high.

4. The faeces on the skin surface cause a high load of bacteria and fungi. A **secondary infection** often occurs, especially on previously damaged skin. Infections with *Candida albicans* are most common. It has also been shown that bacteria penetrate deep epidermal and dermal layers due to the disturbed skin barrier, where they cause inflammatory reactions.
5. Occlusion by incontinence material or prolonged lying down on occlusive mattresses lead to an increase of humidity and temperature on the skin surface **(microclimate of the skin)**. This temperature increases the hyperhydration of the SC (see point 1) and increases permeability. In particular, the increased skin temperature contributes to the increased tendency for inflammation.
6. Repeated skin cleansing procedures also increase the moisture on the already damaged skin. Active **cleansing agents** (surfactants) in the skin cleansing products have an irritating effect. Some skin cleansers have an alkaline pH, which increases the pH of the skin surface. The repeated friction on the skin surface with washcloths and during the drying process causes a **mechanical irritation.** Due to the increased SC hydration, the friction coefficient is higher than in dry skin, and therefore the resulting shear forces within the epidermal and dermal layers are particularly high.

Although each of the six pathogenetic mechanisms contributes to the development of IAD, the factors coincide in clinical reality. These interact and reinforce each other.

Causes for the development of incontinence-associated dermatitis (IAD)

- Stratum corneum overhydration
- Increased pH on the skin surface
- Digestive enzymes
- Bacteria and fungi
- Occlusion and friction
- Skin cleansing procedures

15.2.2 Symptoms and classification

The IAD shows the classic signs of an inflammatory reaction of the skin. Early forms of IAD are characterised by erythema, but the epidermis is still intact. Another characteristic symptom is the disappearance of the skin profile and a 'shiny' aspect (➤ Fig. 15.7).

15

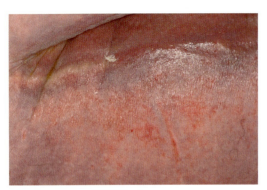

Fig. 15.7 Early form of IAD with oedema and 'shiny' skin. [P580]

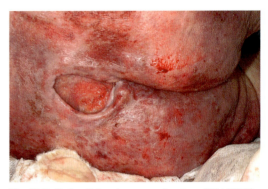

Fig. 15.8 Distinct IAD and pressure ulcer stage III/IV. [P580]

Macerated skin has a whitish appearance. In its progression, typical clinical signs of contact eczema, erosions and excoriations, some of which may be extensive, develop. Every type of IAD is excruciating, especially during manipulations or changing position. Abnormal sensations such as burning, tingling or itching also occur frequently.

The IAD typically occurs perianally, perineally or at the inside of the thighs. It should be noted that IAD only occurs where urine or faeces come into direct contact with the skin. Depending on the body position, the convex body areas are most frequently affected.

Pronounced erythema or other pathological skin signs that are visible in areas that have not come into direct contact with urine or faeces (e. g. in skin folds in obese patients) are not IAD. Typical differential diagnoses are intertrigo or other forms of contact dermatitis, which must be distinguished from IAD. There may also be a possibility of confusion with pressure ulcers in stage 1 and 2. Differential diagnostic information can be found in ➤ Table 15.3. In practice, IAD and pressure ulcers very frequently occur simultaneously (➤ Fig. 15.8).

Secondary infections are common due to the disturbed skin barrier. *Candida albicans* is the most common fungal infection associated with IAD. Satellite lesions in the form of pustules are typical. The diagnosis should always be based on a microbiological sample.

Internationally there are at least ten standardised instruments for the assessment of the IAD risk or the IAD severity. A very simplified classification is the 'Ghent Global IAD Categorisation Instrument (GLOBIAD)' (www.skintghent.be). It is available in over 15 languages and thus allows comparable international communication. Category 1 is reddened skin, but there is still no skin loss. Category 2 is characterised by skin loss (➤ Fig. 15.9). In both cases, there may be additional clinical signs of infection.

15.2.3 Prevention and therapy

All incontinent patients are at risk of developing an IAD. Prophylactic measures are therefore necessary. If an IAD has developed, it must be treated. The transition between prevention and therapy is blurred. The

Table 15.3 Comparison of clinical characteristics of pressure ulcers and IAD

	Pressure ulcers	Incontinence-associated dermatitis
Localisation	Over a bony prominence or a medical device (e.g. cannula, catheter, splint)	Perineal, perianal, inside of thighs, buttocks
Aetiology	Immobility, limited sensory perception	Urine or faecal incontinence
Depth	At the beginning, category I or deep tissue injury, at the end, category III/IV as a rule	Partial loss of skin (erosion, excoriation)
Shape	Round, oval, clearly defined edges	Uneven shape and blurred edges
Other features	Necrosis and undermining may occur	Surrounding skin typically macerated

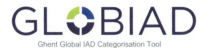

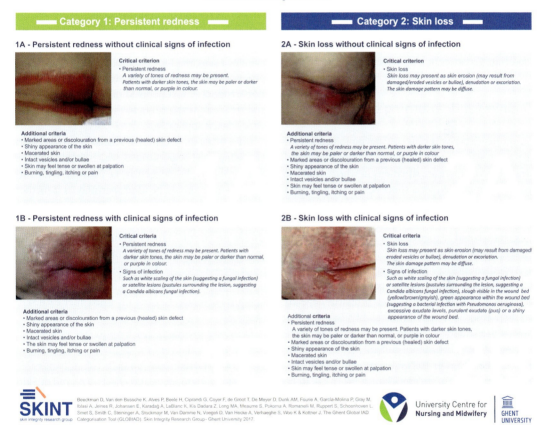

The categories do not necessarily relate to the natural history of IAD and are not intended to suggest how IAD may develop or progress. This categorisation tool may prove useful in the monitoring of IAD prevalence and incidence, and for research purposes.

Fig. 15.9 Ghent Global IAD categorisation instrument (GLOBIAD). [T1052]

evidence for or against certain measures is weak, but there are three basic principles.

Promoting continence

Whenever possible, continence should be promoted, restored or maintained. A range of conservative (e. g. pelvic muscle floor training, bladder training) and surgical procedures can be considered. This form of causal therapy is the most effective in terms of IAD prevention and therapy. Nevertheless, this therapeutic goal is not realistic in many areas, e. g. intensive care medicine, geriatrics or long-term care.

Draining and absorbing devices

Incontinence per se is generally not an indication for the use of systems such as bladder indwelling catheters. However, there are situations in which drainage systems can be used for a short period with either a heavy, large IAD area or if a high amount of thin faeces is flowing uncontrollably. Then, for example, faecal collectors should be used to promote IAD healing and protect the skin.

Absorbent devices play a much more significant role in the care of incontinent patients. The quality and effectiveness of these products primarily depends on their absorbency and breathability. In principle, preference should be given to products that have efficient absorbent material and are soft and breathable. Especially after faecal incontinence episodes, absorbent devices must be changed immediately. Devices that create occlusive conditions promote the development of IAD.

Side effects of absorbent devices can be allergic contact dermatitis. Numerous chemical compounds in the absorbent material can cause sensitisation, especially when the absorptive capacity is exhausted, and there is a reflux of fluid from the absorbent core back to the skin, which must be prevented by frequent changes.

Structured skincare

Skin protection products can help to prevent or reduce the direct contact of the skin with urine or faeces. Typical active components of these topical formulations are lipophilic viscous (e. g. vaseline, paraffin) or film-forming substances and polymers (e. g. dimethicone, acrylates). In so-called 'barrier products', mixtures of these components are often present, together with other auxiliary substances such as emulsifiers or preservatives and fragrances. The presence or concentration of a particular ingredient does not indicate the efficacy of the overall formulation. Due to the heterogeneity of the products on the market and the available studies, it is currently not possible to say whether one skin protection product is better than another. However, available evidence suggests that the use of a skin protection product is better than using nothing. Skin protection products must be used in sufficient quantity and frequency (according to the manufacturer's instructions, if applicable).

Once urine or faeces are on the skin surface, **skin cleansing** must be performed, which should be done as thoroughly, but as gently, as possible with soft cloths. Water should be used sparingly as it further damages the pre-damaged skin. Washing solutions with mild surfactants can be used to remove faeces. Under no circumstances should normal alkaline soaps be used. For damaged and vulnerable skin, appropriate wet wipes or disposable washing systems can be an alternative to water and skin cleansing products. The surface should be carefully dried after each skin cleansing.

Skincare products can help to strengthen and restore the skin barrier. The distinction between skin protection and skincare products is hardly possible because the ingredients and effects are similar. Skin protection products help to regenerate irritated skin, and many skincare products have a concomitant skin-protecting effect.

An existing IAD must be treated. IAD healing can be significantly accelerated if exposure to irritants is reduced to a minimum. The topical treatment depends on the clinical picture. Acutely weeping IAD can be treated with drying preparations or with soft zinc-containing products (e. g. soft zinc paste) for a short time. Reepithelialisation can be promoted with skin protection or lipophilic skincare products. If an infection is present, antimicrobial or antifungal treatment must be applied.

Measures for the prevention and therapy of incontinence-associated dermatitis

- Promotion of continence
- Absorbent (or drainage) devices
- Structured skincare: skin protection, skin cleansing, skincare

15.2.4 Conclusion

Repeated and prolonged exposure to urine or faeces leads to irritative contact dermatitis of exposed skin areas. Excessive moisture on the skin surface, increased pH, occlusion, faecal digestive enzymes and repeated skin cleansing procedures are the causes of IAD. Effective strategies for the prevention and therapy of IAD are continence management, the use of efficient, absorbent aids and structured skin protection and care.

REFERENCES

Beeckman D, Van Damme N, Schoonhoven L, et al. Interventions for preventing and treating incontinence-associated dermatitis in adults. Cochrane Database Syst Rev 2016; 11: CD011627.

Kottner J, Kolbig N, Bültemann A, Dissemond J. [Incontinence-associated dermatitis: a position paper]. Hautarzt 2020; 71: 46–52.

15

16 Pathological scars

Joachim Dissemond

Key notes

- Hypertrophic scars are limited to the original area of injury and occur particularly frequently after burns.
- Keloid scars or keloids extend beyond the original injured area.
- There seems to be a genetic predisposition for the likelihood of developing keloids.

- Exogenous factors that increase the risk of developing pathological scars include traction and compression.
- There are many different interventional and non-interventional treatment options, often to be used in combination, for patients with pathological scars.

16.1 Introduction

A central goal of wound treatment is complete wound closure. All chronic wounds heal with the formation of a scar. Scar-free wound-healing (restitutio ad integrum) has so far only been possible as a foetus in humans. Scars consist of replacement tissue rich in fibres, mainly formed by fibroblasts. After this wound closure, tissue degradation and remodelling continues in the scar area for several months and in some cases for years, and is mainly regulated by matrix metalloproteinases (MMPs). Over time, a contraction of the myofibroblasts causes scar shrinkage; the density of the blood vessels decreases and leads to the scar tissue becoming paler. In the case of disturbance in the process of physiological scar formation, pathological scars in the form of hypertrophic or keloid scars may also develop.

16.2 Pathological scars

Pathological scars often represent a considerable burden for those affected, which a treating physician can only detect if this factor is also determined. The Vancouver Scar Scale (VSS) (➤ Table 16.1) is somewhat more time-consuming for everyday clinical practice but can support a line of treatment

for patients and health care professionals alike, especially in connection with photo documentation if therapy is desired.

Table 16.1 Assessment of pathological scars according to the Vancouver Scar Scale (VSS)

Characteristic	Property	Point value
Vascularity	Normal	0
	Pink	1
	Red	2
	Purple	3
Pigmentation	Normal	0
	Hypopigmentation	1
	Hyperpigmentation	2
Pliability	Normal	0
	Supple	1
	Yielding	2
	Firm	3
	Ropes	4
	Contracted	5
High	Flat	0
	< 2 mm	1
	2–5 mm	2
	> 5 mm	3
Total		max. 13

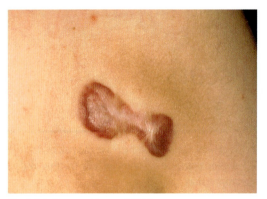

Fig. 16.1 Hypertrophic scar. [P580]

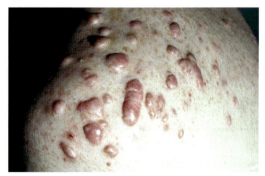

Fig. 16.2 Keloids. [P580]

16.3 Pathophysiology

16.2.1 Hypertrophic scars

Hypertrophic scars are limited to the original area of injury and often appear only a few weeks after wound closure. They are higher than the surrounding skin level and can disturb patients cosmetically or functionally (➤ Fig. 16.1). So far, no genetic predisposition has been described in those affected, and the scars can recede over time, either spontaneously or through therapy; the risk of those affected in the case of renewed injuries in other areas is not higher than in the average population. The incidence of hypertrophic scars after burns is particularly high, at 67%.

16.2.2 Keloids

The term keloid goes back to the French dermatologist Jean Louis Alibert, who in 1816 derived the term 'cheloid' from the Greek term 'chele' for crab pincers. Keloids extend beyond the initially injured area (➤ Fig. 16.2). Although they occur exclusively in previously injured tissue, the injuries can also be minimal traumas, such as folliculitis, excoriations or insect bites. They usually form several months, sometimes even years, after the wound has closed. Keloids can occur anywhere on the body. However, typical predilection sites are ears, sternum, shoulders and neck. Here, a potential correlation with increased skin tension has been discussed. The age of initial manifestation is usually between 10 and 30 years for both sexes, or 23 years on average; there is no sexual predisposition.

A pathophysiologically central aspect of disturbed scar formation seems to lie in the disordered regulation of myofibroblasts, which leads to a prolonged and intensified activation of the cells with an unphysiological increase in collagen synthesis. In hypertrophic scars and keloids, the activity of MMP-1 is decreased, and the activity of other MMPs such as MMP-2 is increased, which promotes catabolism in the extracellular matrix (ECM). Structural proteins such as fibrin, fibronectin, glycosaminoglycans and type III collagen are replaced by collagen, predominantly type I.

Various factors influence the stimulation of myofibroblasts. In the case of exogenous influence, these are physical factors such as tensile and compressive force. It is known from burn treatment that wound-healing periods can also influence scar formation. If wounds persist for longer than three weeks, the cytokine-mediated control of the complex interaction between epidermal keratinocytes and wound fibroblasts slips away; fibroblast activity becomes autonomous and overproduction of collagen results. Endogenous factors include cytokines, of which the effects of overexpressed Transforming Growth Factor (TGF)-β isoforms and Platelet-Derived Growth Factor (PDGF) are best studied.

Also, various genetic factors are discussed, although more than one gene locus seems to be involved. For many years now, a connection with a positive family and own anamnesis, as well as dark skin types, has been reported here. Under discussion are autosomal

Table 16.2 Controllable factors in surgical procedures with a potential influence on the course of scar
formation

Align incision lines with Langer's cleavage lines
Vertical section guide
Atraumatic wound edge treatment
Minimisation of centripetal drag during the operation
Minimisation of the centripetal drag by sufficient under-mining or tension-free plastic and a stratified suture for strain relief
Select suitable suture material
Reduced compression bandages, e.g. strips or bandages on extremities
Adequate dressings and changes of dressings, e.g. with elastic plasters or silicone films
Avoidance of postoperative infections

dominant modes of inheritance with incomplete penetration as well as more frequent autosomal recessive modes of inheritance.

16.4 Prevention of pathological scars

Scars are the final stage of wound-healing. In this respect, scar formation in humans is inevitable after a relatively deep wound. However, there are numerous factors which can influence both the extent and the probability of pathological scarring. For example, surgical procedures on patients at increased risk of pathological scarring should be planned to be as atraumatic as possible. The occurrence of scarring often cannot be prevented, especially during interventional procedures. However, several factors can be taken into account to reduce the risk of pathological scars (➤ Table 16.2). It is also crucial in this context to inform patients about possible risks in advance.

16.5 Scar therapy

Since hypertrophic scars, as well as keloids, are benign skin changes, medical treatment is only necessary when symptoms, perceived as distressing by those affected, occur. These include, in particular, the occurrence of itching or pain. Functional impairments are also very problematic, e.g. movement restrictions in scars over joints with resulting contractures. Very rarely, squamous cell carcinomas can also develop in scars. Often, however, it is aesthetic or cosmetic impairments that tend to require therapy.

16.5.1 Wait-and-see

In the case of hypertrophic scars, there should first be a wait-and-see approach for a spontaneous regression within the first 12–24 months. Especially in the case of so-called immature scars, which are clinically red, itchy and usually only discreetly raised, no invasive therapies should be carried out.

16.5.2 Cryotherapy

Cryotherapies are a well-established therapeutic procedure for the treatment of pathological scars. Liquid nitrogen is mostly used, reaching temperatures of up to minus 190 °C. Tissue necrosis is achieved by direct cell and vessel damage with ischaemic cell death. The application can be carried out as a spray or contact procedure and is also suitable for outpatient use. In practical application, the freezing is usually applied twice for 10–30 seconds. Treatment can be repeated every 4–6 weeks in the case of insufficient success. Generally, at least three treatments are necessary. The effectiveness of cryotherapy can be increased by using intralesional procedures.

Frequently observed side effects of cryotherapy are pain during therapy but, mostly, partially reversible depigmentation. Since postinterventional blisters and subsequent weeping erosions often occur, attention should be paid to antiseptic follow-up treatment. Response rates are about 40–80% and recurrence rates 0–45%. Several studies have shown that the effectiveness of cryotherapy can be increased by combining it with triamcinolone injections.

16.5.3 Glucocorticoids

Intralesionally applied glucocorticoids, and especially triamcinolone acetonide, have been successfully used for many decades to treat pathological scars. They have anti-inflammatory and vasoconstrictive effects, inhibit fibroblast proliferation and inhibit collagen synthesis. Practical application is carried out with 10–40 mg triamcinolone acetonide pure or diluted 1:1–1:4 in combination with lidocaine. Strictly intralesional injections are performed with syringes or high-pressure injectors (Dermojet). A blanching effect of the injected tissue indicates the endpoint of the infiltration. Usually, several more injections follow at intervals of 2–6 weeks. Freezing immediately before the intralesional glucocorticosteroid injection facilitates the subsequent injection by the formation of oedema and reduces pain. Response rates after therapy with intralesional glucocorticosteroids are about 50–100% in various studies, and recurrence rates are 9–50%.

The intralesional glucocorticoid injection is easy to perform, inexpensive and shows high effectiveness with low side effects. However, it should be noted that too deep an injection can lead to irreversible atrophy of the subcutaneous fat tissue. Glucocorticoids are often used as a combination procedure, especially for the prevention of recurrence after excision with excellent results.

16.5.4 Pressure treatment

Pressure treatment causes local hypoxia, which, among other things, leads to an acceleration of collagen maturation through reduced wound tension. For the pressure treatment of pathological scars, for example, individually adapted stockings, gloves, magnetic buttons or ear clips can be used. Vacuum therapy can also be used, especially postoperatively. However, it is often useful to plan treatments in cooperation with specialists in orthopaedic technology or epithetics.

In general, pressure treatments should be started as early as possible and carried out over the entire day for at least six, or preferably 24 months. To use the materials effectively, they should provide pressure values of around 20–30 mmHg. However, the consistent implementation of the therapeutic recommendations by the patients in these therapeutic procedures is stated to be < 40%. The response rates are about 60%.

Potential side effects of pressure treatments may include pruritus, heat accumulation, contact eczema, swelling, erosion and even skeletal deformation.

16.5.5 Silicone

Silicone is used as gel, cream, ointment, spray, pad or foil in scar therapy. The effects are improved skin hydration, temperature increase and cytokine-mediated signaling of keratinocytes on fibroblasts. It is recommended to use the pad for 12–24 h/day for 12–24 weeks. The response rates are 60–100%.

The advantage of treatment with silicone is the painless and uncomplicated application. Only the occurrence of folliculitis has been described as a frequently observed side effect.

16.5.6 Radiotherapy

Radiotherapy of hypertrophic scars or keloids can be performed with x-ray radiation, electron radiation or as brachytherapy. The propagated antiproliferative effects are mediated by inhibition of cell regeneration and ECM formation as well as induction of fibroblast apoptosis. An anti-inflammatory effect is also under discussion. Keloids are often irradiated in a fractionated manner in 6–10 sessions every one to two days with a total dose of 10–12 Gy, since the expected side effects are then significantly lower than with higher doses. If postoperative irradiation is to be performed, it is recommended to start within the first 24 hours after surgery. The response rates are 10–94%, and the recurrence rates 50–100%.

Side effects occur in the form of erythema, depigmentation and possibly erosion and increased carcinogenicity. In most cases, radiotherapy is only recommended in combination with other procedures.

16.5.7 Onion extract

The onion extract *extractum cepae* has a bactericidal effect and inhibits both inflammation and fibroblast proliferation. Among the underlying mechanisms of action discussed were the induction of MMP-1 and the inhibition of the TGF-β signalling pathway. After re-epithelialisation, the application should be performed several times a day with massage of the scar tissue for several weeks to months. For older scars, an application under occlusion is also possible. Scar massage can be seen as a separate suppurative therapy measure when using scar gels.

Apart from the rarely described allergic contact dermatitis, there are hardly any side effects from the application of external agents containing onion extract.

16.5.8 Laser therapy

Ablative systems use, for example, erbium-yttrium-aluminium-garnet lasers (Er:YAG laser) or carbon dioxide (CO_2) lasers. The goal of ablative laser treatment of scars is primarily the levelling of exophytic parts. Utilising short pulse emissions, successively defined cell layers are vaporised (CO_2) or explosively ablated (Er:YAG) in water with minimal bleeding. However, the Er:YAG laser can also be used purely thermally for scar treatment. The thermal effect mediates a heat-shock reaction, which can have a modulating influence on the activity of the keloid fibroblasts and TGF-β by inducing various heat shock proteins (HSP). Even though response rates of up to 100% have been reported, keloid ablation with ablative lasers alone is contraindicated today, as up to 90% of those affected experience recurrences. These recurrence rates can be significantly reduced when ablative lasers are used in combination with intralesional glucocorticosteroid injections, cryotherapy, radiotherapy or compression therapy.

Side effects of ablative laser treatment are often weeping erosions, crusts, erythema, and de- and hyperpigmentation.

16.5.9 Surgical methods

The excision of keloids alone is contraindicated due to recurrence rates of up to 100%. Only the tangential excision of keloids at the earlobes is described here as an exception. An excision should, therefore, always be used in combination with other therapies. Especially in the case of hypertrophic scars or functional limitations, surgical interventions can provide relief. Here, Z-, W- and Y-V-plasty, rotational flaps, free flaps, tissue expanders or transplants are used. These plastics shift the direction of scar traction by up to 90° and extend the scar. The resulting relief in tightness can result in an absence of recurrence. It is debatable whether an intramarginal scar excision, which leaves a narrow hem of the scar tissue, reduces the recurrence rate.

16.6 Conclusion

There are numerous different treatment options for patients with pathological scars. There is no single optimal therapy for all patients, but there are several good options that can be discussed. Subsequently, it is possible to choose between different alternatives and, above all, combined, multimodal procedures to create an individually adapted treatment process.

REFERENCES
Dissemond J. Pathologische Narben. Dtsch Dermatologe 2016; 64: 34–41.
Lingzhi Z, Meirong L, Xiaobing F. Biological approaches for hypertrophic scars. Int Wound J 2020; 17: 405–418.
Nast A, Eming S, Fluhr J, et al. German S2k guidelines for the therapy of pathological scars (hypertrophic scars and keloids). J Dtsch Dermatol Ges 2012; 10: 747–762.
Sidgwick GP, McGeorge D, Bayat A. A comprehensive evidence-based review on the role of topicals and dressings in the management of skin scarring. Arch Dermatol Res 2015; 307: 461–477.
Wagner JA. Therapy of pathological scars. J Dtsch Dermatol Ges 2013; 11: 1139–1157.

16

17

Knut Kröger, Joachim Dissemond

Cooling down and wound-healing

Key notes

- Lowering the temperature can be useful for acute injuries and prolonged operations, as hypothermia slows down the metabolic processes in healthy tissue.
- In chronic wounds, however, lowering the temperature leads to an additional disturbance of the metabolic processes and is, therefore, a factor that potentially further delays wound-healing.
- As biological processes, such as blood flow, enzyme activity and cell division are temperature-dependent, all situations that disturb the healing process should be avoided in the treatment of chronic wounds.

17.1 Introduction

Lowering the body temperature can be useful in acute injuries and prolonged operations, as hypothermia slows down the metabolic processes in healthy tissue and reduces energy consumption, thus protecting the tissue to a certain extent from the consequences of hypoxia. In the case of chronic wounds, precisely the opposite is the case. These wounds are chronic because the normal healing process and the associated metabolic processes are disturbed and are already delayed. This delay is likely due to underlying diseases, such as diabetes mellitus, peripheral artery disease (PAD) and chronic venous insufficiency (CVI), or due to repeated disturbances such as pressure loads and oedema formation. An additional lowering of the temperature delays the metabolic processes even further and thus presents potential further delays in wound-healing. Metabolic processes come to a standstill and take several hours before they resume their regular activity.

Cooling down can have various causes. Primary ischaemic cooling rarely has any significance for the healing of chronic wounds, as acute ischaemia at the base of an embolism or bypass occlusion must be revascularised within a few hours. Also, these patients generally do not (yet) have chronic wounds. In chronic ischaemia, as is the case in patients with closure situations that cannot be revascularised in a meaningful way, cooling would more significant-ly be due to insufficient blood circulation. In these patients, for example, cottonwool dressings or fur boots can prevent the inadequately perfused extremity from cooling. Chronic wounds often cool down unintentionally by leaving the wound open too long during dressing changes or by cleaning it with a cold irrigation solution.

17.2 Blood circulation

Blood is a complex fluid consisting of plasma and blood cells as corpuscular components. Cooling of the extremity or exposed parts of the wound reduces blood flow properties. A distinction is made between plasma and whole blood viscosity. Plasma viscosity is determined by the water content and the proportion of macromolecular components. Plasma is a highly concentrated protein solution in which protein-protein interactions play a role. In the literature, the normal values for plasma viscosity at 37 °C are 1.2 ± 0.1 mPas/s depending on age and sex. At 22 °C, it increases to 1.6 ± 0.2 mPas/s.

Whole blood viscosity depends on the shear forces present and is determined by temperature, haematocrit, plasma viscosity, aggregation tendency and deformability of the erythrocytes. For blood, therefore, not only a viscosity value can be given, but also the measurement conditions must always be specified. For example, the whole blood viscosity is 4.7 ± 0.9 mPas/s at slow flow velocity and 3.3 ± 0.6 mPas/s at high flow velocity. At 22 °C, these values increase to 7.6 ± 1.6 mPas/s and 5.0 ± 0.8 mPas/s, respectively.

Erythrocytes are highly deformable at normal temperatures but become stiffer at a temperature below 18 °C. This physical property is of great importance in the microcurrent path. The tendency of erythrocytes to aggregate reversibly is another crucial determinant of the apparent viscosity of the blood. The size of the erythrocyte aggregates is inversely proportional to the size of the shear forces. Cooling down of the limb reduces the flow properties of the blood, which suddenly becomes very viscous at a critical temperature and lack of perfusion pressure. This stationary blood is not clotted, but it requires increased shear forces to return it to a liquid state. Also, the risk of thrombocyte aggregation increases with decreasing temperature.

17.3 Enzyme activity

The rule for temperature dependence of rate of reaction, or the van't-Hoff equation, which was first described in 1884, is a rule of thumb which states that chemical reactions run two to three times faster at a temperature increased by 10 K. In this way, an increase in temperature causes an acceleration of enzymatic and non-enzymatic reactions.

In biological systems, reactions at 0 °C hardly take place at all. If the temperature is raised to above 0 °C, the response is slowly accelerated until it reaches a maximum at 37 °C. For many enzymes, temperatures above 37 °C change the spatial structure (tertiary structure), which is essential for their function, and the reaction speed is thus reduced. For most enzymes, the optimal effective temperature is between 30 and 45 °C; at temperatures < 10 °C or > 60 °C, most enzymes no longer work. At physiologically low temperatures in the acral area or on cooled wound surfaces, the body must increase the regional excess blood flow to conduct warmer blood from the inside of the body to the acral area or wound surface. This mechanism is only possible to a limited extent in chronic wounds due to the disturbed microcirculation

present in diabetic foot syndrome (DFS), PAD and CVI. In the wound itself, the granulation tissue is well supplied with vessels and can transport warm blood to the wound. Enzymes that are released in the wound and serve autolysis or other signalling substances can only be reached indirectly by heat conduction.

17.4 Cell division

Like all biological processes in our body, cell division is temperature-dependent. In cell culture, human fibroblasts multiply exponentially. Their proliferation decreases with temperature reduction and finally ends at incubation temperatures of 30 °C and below. The cells that are in the synthesis (S) phase of the cell cycle at the time of switching to the low temperature complete their DNA synthesis and are locked into the G1 phase of the cell cycle. The locked cells can be stimulated to proliferate by restoring the optimal growth temperature (37 °C).

Cooling the cells below 25 °C is accompanied by a passive dehydration process, while the rehydration process during heating reflects an active energy-consuming process. During this phase, oxygen consumption is increased. It is therefore easier to inhibit the division of a cell by cooling it below 30 °C than to reactivate cell division by heating it above 30 °C.

17.5 Conclusion

Since biological processes such as blood circulation, enzyme activity and cell division are temperature-dependent, all situations that lead to cooling and thereby disruption of the healing process should be avoided during wound treatment.

REFERENCES
Baskurt OK. In vivo correlates of altered blood rheology. Biorheol 2008; 45: 629–638.
Chien S, Usami S, Dellenback RJ, Gregersen MI, Nanninga LB, Guest MM. Blood viscosity: influence of erythrocyte aggregation. Science 1967; 157: 829–831.

Christmann J, Azer L, Dörr D, Fuhr GR, Bastiaens PI, Wehner F. Adaptive responses of cell hydration to a low temperature arrest. J Physiol 2016; 594: 1663–1676.

Enninga IC, Groenendijk RT, van Zeeland AA, Simons JW. Use of low temperature for growth arrest and synchronization of human diploid fibroblasts. Mutat Res 1984; 130: 343–352.

Késmárky G, Kenyeres P, Rábai M, Tóth K. Plasma viscosity: a forgotten variable. Clin Hemorheol Microcirc 2008; 39: 243–246.

Schmid-Schönbein H, Gallasch G, Volger E, Klose HJ. Microrheology and protein chemistry of pathological red cell aggregation (blood sludge) studied in vitro. Biorheol 1973; 10: 213–227.

17

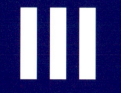

III

Factors which inhibit wound-healing

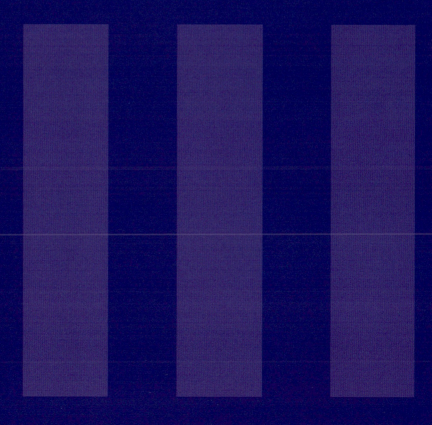

18 Nutrition for patients with chronic wounds

Madeleine Gerber

Key notes

- Malnutrition can be an important reason why a wound is not healing.
- If the energy supply via oral food is insufficient, it should be supplemented or entirely covered by enteral and parenteral nutrition.
- Wound-healing requires a fully balanced diet; the administration of additional proteins must fit into the overall nutrition concept; maximum limits must be taken into account.
- Individual evidence-based recommendations on patient nutrition have been developed for surgical departments to prevent the postoperative risk of malnutrition.

18.1 Introduction

Wound-healing and nutrition are closely related since cell proliferation requires macro- and micronutrients. These must be supplied to the body from the outside, at best through natural food. If this does not happen with sufficient quality and quantity, it can lead to disturbances in the entire metabolism. The consequences include wound-healing disorders. It is therefore important to detect malnutrition at an early stage to counteract the corresponding disorders as preventively as possible. The frequently used term 'nutrition management' has to be used meaningfully.

18.2 What is malnutrition?

Malnutrition is generally understood to be a deficit between demand and supply of essential nutrients.

The term disease-associated malnutrition covers clinically relevant deficiencies caused either by reduced food intake, malabsorption and maldigestion or by increased protein catabolism or inflammation. According to the guidelines of the German Society for Nutritional Medicine (DGEM) on 'terminology in clinical nutrition', disease-associated malnutrition is defined by three criteria:

1. Body Mass Index (BMI) less than $18.5 \, kg/m^2$ **or**
2. unintentional weight loss of more than 10% in the last 3–6 months; **or**
3. BMI below $20 \, kg/m^2$ and accidental weight loss of more than 5% in the last three to six months.

18.3 Causes of malnutrition

Malnutrition is a common diagnosis in older adults. A meta-analysis summarising the results of 18 studies showed that up to 83% of older adults in institutions and up to 31% of older adults still living in their own homes have subnormal nutritional parameters. Multimorbidity and/or loneliness due to the loss of one's partner reduce appetite and thereby the amount of necessary food intake. Dementia also often leads to malnutrition. An excess in activity can also demand a high energy supply which cannot be dealt with orally, or the sense of taste has changed, or food is no longer recognised as such. Also, some drugs are suspected of causing malnutrition. Gegenbacher et al. showed that on the day of ingestion of these drugs in patients with severe pressure ulcer, there was pronounced zinc deficiency at 78%, albumin deficiency at 79% and vitamin B_{12} deficiency at 33%.

18.4 Diagnostics of malnutrition

➤ Table 18.1 summarised parameters for acquisition, aetiology and therapy. The recommendations are based on the current German guidelines for enteral nutrition.

In the geriatric sector and nursing in general, the use of screening and assessment tools is recommended to help detect malnutrition at an early stage. Examples include the **M**ini **N**utritional **A**ssessment (MNA) and **N**utritional **R**isk **S**creening (NRS), or the **M**alnutrition **U**niversal **S**creening **T**ool (MUST) in inpatient long-term/elderly care. These instruments should not only be used for the initial application, but also monitoring and control.

18.5 Energy demand assessment

There are various approaches to determining the energy demand. All standard formulas are based on the basal metabolic rate for further calculation. The basal metabolic rate, the working metabolic rate and individual factors such as growth rate and/or illness in relation to each other form the performance metabolic rate of a person.

For the level of physical work, a multiplier is used, called the Physical Activity Level (PAL). Various formulas are available to determine the basal metabolic rate (➤ Table 18.2, ➤ Table 18.3, ➤ Table 18.4).

The Harris-Benedict formula was first published in 1918 for the calculation of the basal metabolic rate. This formula rigidly takes into account size, age and influencing factors. The method presumes strict resting conditions and shows the basal metabolic rate for the post-absorptive state after waking up, at complete physical rest and under thermoneutral conditions. The basal metabolic rate is usually calculated using multipliers assigned to illnesses to determine the increased need. Once the total amount of energy required has been determined, it can be distributed among the macro- and micronutrients.

Experts recommend the PAL values ➤ Table 18.5 to determine power conversion.

Regular weight checks can only determine the actual energy demand or consumption. The individual factors which, apart from BMI and PAL, are influential

Table 18.2 Harris-Benedict equation for determining basal metabolic rate

Men	Women
Basal metabolic rate (kcal/24 h) = 66.47 + (13.7 × weight in kg) + (5 × height in cm) – (6.8 × age in years)	Basal metabolic rate (kcal/24 h) = 655.1 + (9.6 × weight in kg) + (1.8 × height in cm) – (4.7 × age in years)

Table 18.1 Recording, aetiology and therapy of malnutrition

Summarising the problem	Clarification of the causes	Consequences
Determine BMI. Fat mass is a primary indicator for malnutrition. Fat mass can be determined in a bio-impedance analysis; indirectly, the BMI gives information about the fat mass of the body.	Nutrition protocol. Check for malassimilation. Determine the necessary energy consumption.	Increase of the energy supply. Treatment of possible malassimilation.
Measurement of triceps skinfold thickness (malnutrition = triceps skinfold thickness < 10 mm).	Unwanted weight loss. Nutrition protocol.	Increase of the energy supply.
Determine protein deficiency. Muscle mass and plasma protein concentration are assessment criteria for malnutrition.	Nutrition protocol. Composition of the diet.	Possible substitution of missing protein via oral or enteral food. Recommended protein amounts: 1–15 g/kg body weight.
Specific nutrient deficiency may lead to skin changes, neurological changes and physical symptoms, such as fatigue or diarrhoea.		Targeted supply.

18

Table 18.3 Basal Metabolic Rate (BMR) according to WHO

Age group	Women	Men
≤ 3 years	BMR = 0.244 × BW (kg) − 0,130	BMR = 0.249 × BW (kg) − 0.127
3–10	BMR = 0.085 × BW (kg) + 2.033	BMR = 0.095 × BW (kg) + 2.110
11–18	BMR = 0.056 × BW (kg) + 2.898	BMR = 0.074 × BW (kg) + 2.754
19–30	BMR = 0.062 × BW (kg) + 2.036	BMR = 0.063 × BW (kg) + 2.869
31–60	BMR = 0.034 × BW (kg) + 3.538	BMR = 0.048 × BW (kg) + 3.653
≥ 60	BMR = 0.038 × BW (kg) + 2.755	BMR = 0.049 × BW (kg) + 2.459
BMR = Basal metabolic rate; BW = Body weight		

Table 18.4 Mifflin St. Jeor calculator

Men	Women
BMR = (10 × weight in kg) + (6.25 × height in cm) − (5 × age in years) + 5	BMR = (10 × weight in kg) + (6.25 × height in cm) − (5 × age in years) − 161
BMR = Basal metabolic rate	

Table 18.5 PAL value as a function of level of work load

Workload	PAL	Example
Sedentary/lying down lifestyle (partial mobility)	1.2	Bedridden, frail
Sedentary	1.4–1.5	Office worker
Sedentary, both standing and walking	1.8–1.9	Craftsman, seller
Heavy labour	2.0–2.4	Construction workers, competitive athletes, hyperactive dementia-altered people

Table modified according to DGEM reference values (2008) in MDS statement of principle (2014)

must be considered in such a differentiated way that there can be no uniform formula for them. The basal metabolic rate correlates with the fat-free body mass. With increasing age, the body fat mass increases, the metabolism slows down, and activity decreases overall. Those with mobile restlessness due to dementia can however have a calorie requirement of 3,500 kcal or more in 24 hours.

18.6 Food composition

The German Nutrition Society (DGE) recommends a diet consisting of 55% carbohydrates, 30% fat and 15% protein.

The D-A-CH (an abbreviation for the countries Germany, Austria and Switzerland, whose professional societies jointly publish these reference values) has published reference values for protein, fat and carbohydrate intake. It is based on the calculated average adult requirement for high-quality protein. A recommended intake of 0.8 g protein/kg BW/day in a mixed diet is considered sufficient for a healthy adult.

With existing wounds and other conditions which require nutrition, the protein intake must be increased to counteract the degradation of body protein. The current NPUAP guidelines recommend a protein intake of 1.25–1.5 g/kg BW/day for existing pressure ulcers. However, this protein input should always be checked in relation to the kidney function. A protein input of more than 2 g/kg BW/day – corresponding to about 120 g for women and 140 g for men – is not considered sensible in the literature, as this can lead to kidney or liver dysfunction and, above all, dehydration in older patients. If renal insufficiency is present, protein intake may be limited. In the diet, particular attention must be paid to the biological value of the proteins in the composition of the food. If the body better utilises food than egg protein, its value is more than 100%. The most favourable combination consists of potato and egg; here, the biological value is 135%.

In addition, renal insufficiency leads to increased calcium excretion, which in turn increases the risk of osteoporosis.

18

What should also be considered is the fact that wound exudate contains protein. The composition of exudate is similar to blood serum. One litre of wound exudate contains about 30 g albumin. In strongly exuding wounds, this protein loss has to be replaced.

18.7 Oral food – enteral nutrition – parenteral nutrition

Natural food taken orally undoubtedly has the highest value. If, however, a patient cannot consume any or only insufficient food, enteral and parenteral nutrition must be used. Enteral nutrition does not necessarily have to be administered via a percutaneous endoscopic gastrostomy (PEG) tube, but can also be ingested in the form of liquid. Here, fully balanced products are available. Balanced in this context means that the nutrient composition corresponds to that of a normal healthy diet. Statutory health insurers usually reimburse fully balanced dietary supplements on the condition that the patient is already malnourished or is showing signs of imminent malnourishment. A diagnosis is required for the prescription. A disadvantage is that there is no uniform diagnostics analysis for outpatient. Moreover, liquid food is not a drug but is legally regarded as a drug, and is included in the budget of general practitioners in Germany.

In cooperation with other professional associations, the DGE has developed guidelines on clinical nutrition in surgery. This guideline concludes that supplemental perioperative nutrition is also indicated for patients without obvious malnutrition, if the patient cannot foreseeably consume sufficient energy postoperatively. Catabolism and malnutrition should be prevented preemptively.

Recommendations:
- Patients without aspiration risk may eat solid food up to six hours before anaesthesia.
- Glucose may be infused into non-diabetics up to two hours before surgery if enteral nutrition is not possible.
- After uncomplicated surgeries, food intake should not be interrupted (with individual tolerance taken into account). Even after colorectal surgery, food intake can begin a few hours after surgery.

- Patients without malnutrition who are however unable to eat oral food for more than seven days after surgery, should preferably be fed enterally. The same applies to patients who can only consume about 60–75% of the recommended amount of energy orally over ten days postoperatively.
- If the energy requirement cannot be covered orally/enterally, a combination with additional parenteral nutrition should be made if the expected period is longer than four days.
- A central venous catheter (CVC) is only recommended if the parenteral diet lasts 7–10 days.
- Total parenteral nutrition should be started if enteral artificial feeding is not feasible or contraindicated.
- Patients with a severe metabolic risk should receive nutritional therapy before surgery, even if the operation has to be postponed.

18.8 Conclusion

Proper wound healing requires a functional nutritional status. People affected by wounds require an increase in absolute energy intake. With formulas and tables, this requirement can be determined accordingly.

The status or risk of malnutrition must be assessed at an early stage to ensure sufficient nutrition in good time, preferably as a preventive measure. Only in this way can wound healing be adequately supported by nutrition.

Requirements can be calculated; however, requirement and habits, as well as availability, play an equally important role in the implementation of the recommended diet.

Individual specifics must be taken into account. The involvement of a dietician can be of decisive importance for the success of the treatment.

REFERENCES
Bialski HK, Bischoff SC, Puchstein C. Ernährungsmedizin, Curriculum der Bundesärztekammer. 4th ed, Stuttgart: Thieme; 2010.
Deutsche Gesellschaft für Ernährung e.V. D-A-CH Referenzwerte für die Nährstoffzufuhr. www.dge.de/wissenschaft/referenzwerte (last acessed 12 October 2020).

Deutsches Netzwerk für Qualitätsentwicklung in der Pflege (DNQP). Expertenstandard „Ernährungsmanagement zur Sicherstellung und Förderung der oralen Ernährung in der Pflege". Osnabrück, 2008.

ESPEN (European Society for Clinical Nutrition and Metabolism). Guidelines on enteral nutrition, clinical nutrition. 2006. www.clinicalnutritionjournal.com/article/S0261-5614%2806%2900051-3/abstract?cc=y (last acessed 12 October 2020).

Leitzmann C, Müller C, Michel P, et al. Ernährung in Prävention und Therapie. Stuttgart: Hippokrates; 2009.

Weimann A, Breitenstein S, Breuer JP, et al. S3-Leitlinie der Deutschen Gesellschaft für Ernährungsmedizin (DGEM) in Zusammenarbeit mit Geskes, AKE, DGCH, DGAI und DGAV – Klinische Ernährung in der Chirurgie. Akt Ernährungsmed 2013; 38: 155–197.

18

19

Knut Kröger, Joachim Dissemond, Anya Miller

Disease patterns in oedema, lymphoedema, and lipoedema

19.1 Systematics of oedema

Knut Kröger, Joachim Dissemond

Key notes

- A reduction in interstitial pressure often causes acute oedema as a result of local mechanisms that induce rapid fluid influx from the capillaries into the loose connective tissue.
- The driving force for chronic oedema is increased intracapillary pressure which affects both arteriovenous and lymphatic capillaries.

- Oedema formation is always a pathological condition. It is accompanied by a change in the composition of loose connective tissue that disrupts the microcirculation and regeneration of the tissue.
- Oedemas hinder undisturbed wound-healing and should therefore always be considered within the course of wound treatment.

19.1.1 Introduction

There are a multitude of causes for oedema (> Table 19.1). In the end, however, the result is always the same. There is a pathological accumulation of more or less protein-rich or cell-rich fluid in the tissue. This fluid is located between the cells in the so-called loose connective tissue. The loose connective tissue is an integral part of all organs. It contains the vast majority of the interstitial fluid volume and surrounds the peripheral blood and lymph vessels. For a long time, it was assumed that the amount of interstitial fluid was regulated within narrow limits and that it was only a compensation space for the fluid filtered through the capillary wall. It is now known that the connective tissue is not only a loose link between the tissues but also actively influences the transcapillary fluid exchange via the interstitial fluid pressure. This interstitial fluid pressure is the pressure that can be measured in the tissue fluid when a catheter is inserted into the tissue. This pressure works to fill the initial lymphatic system when no other external forces such as muscle contractions support the filling of the initial lymphatic system.

Interstitial fluid pressure is an essential factor in determining transcapillary fluid flow. It can be changed dynamically and actively. Thus, the pressure on the outside of the capillary can be increased or decreased by controlling cellular tension on extracellular collagen and microfibrillar networks mediated by collagen-binding β1 integrins. The term interstitial compliance describes these altered properties of loose connective tissue. Such a change in the loose connective tissue can lead to increased transcapillary fluid flow, which must be understood as an apparent altered capillary permeability and which increases the transport of convective dissolved substances via the capillary wall. Through these mechanisms, the loose connective tissue actively influences the transcapillary exchange of fluid and proteins and the cellular exchange of information.

19.1.2 Composition of the extracellular matrix

The extracellular matrix (ECM) of the loose connective tissue consists of four main components. First, there is a fibrous collagen network that forms a scaffold. It provides a three-dimensional structure where the blood vessels of the organ are embedded, as are the basement membranes, to which the parenchyma cells

Table 19.1 Various causes of oedema

Oedema	Pathophysiology
Organ-related oedema	Heart, kidney, or liver failure
Venous oedema	Acute thrombosis of the deep or superficial veins; chronic venous insufficiency due to a post-thrombotic syndrome or primary varicosis
Lymphatic oedema	Primary or secondary lymphatic tissue damage
Lipoedema	Chronic and mostly progressive disease in women characterised by a fat distribution disorder.
Protein deficiency oedema	Oedema with a reduction of serum protein below approx. 5 g/dl or albumin below 3 g/dl
Traumatic oedema	Passages of swelling after fractures, operations, bruises, sprains etc., which disappear spontaneously after days to weeks; cause: tearing of small lymphatic and blood vessels
Inactivity oedemas	Paraplegic oedema predominantly in flaccid paresis due to neurological diseases such as paraplegia, multiple sclerosis or apoplexy; cause: lack of muscle pump function
Orthostatic oedema	Oedema due to prolonged standing or sitting stress, e.g. during a typical working day
Obesity-associated oedema	Functional venous or lymphatic drainage disorders caused by obesity
Toxic oedema	The toxic effect, e.g. wasp or bee sting, snake bite
Acute allergic oedema	Localised, acute, often volatile oedema after allergen contact
Angioedema/angioneurotic oedema/Quincke oedema	Oedema occurring in seizures, especially in intestinal mucosa, larynx and extremities; mostly histamine-mediated angioedema in the sense of urticaria; cause: e.g. mastocytosis, paraneoplastic, parainfectious, medications
Drug-induced oedema	Triggering drugs, e.g. calcium channel blocker, beta-blockers, clonidine, hydralazine, minoxidil, methyldopa, corticosteroids, estrogens, NSAID, pioglitazone, rosiglitazone, monoamine oxidase (MAO) inhibitors Three causes have been described: • Sodium retention, e.g. antibiotics, • Disturbance of kidney function, e.g. NSAID, antihypertensive, cytostatic drugs, • Induction of hyperpermeability of blood vessels, e.g. calcium antagonists.

19

are attached. The ECM also contains the microfibre elastin system and the primary substance formed by proteoglycans. These proteoglycans consist of glycosaminoglycans covalently bound to a core protein and the free glycosaminoglycan hyaluronan. Glycosaminoglycans are long, unbranched amino sugar polymers that can interact with the fibrous components of ECM, but also occur freely and unbound in the interstitial fluid.

The ECM is the transport medium for nutrients and waste products and determines the physical transport properties of the tissue, such as hydraulic conductivity and compliance. Finally, the ECM contains the interstitial fluid, an ultrafiltrate of the plasma with a total protein concentration of about 50–60% of the plasma content, but with a similar electrolyte composition. The composition of the interstitial fluid concerning the plasma proteins is the result of the fluid flow through the capillary, the size and charge of the molecules and the permeability of the capillary wall.

Some of the structural components of the ECM can be washed out of the interstitium by increasing fluid flow. The regular exchange via the capillaries is determined by the transcapillary hydrostatic and colloid osmotic pressure. The skin and skeletal muscle together contain about two-thirds of the extracellular fluid. In someone with an extracellular fluid volume of 15 l, the plasma volume is about 3 l, and the total lymphatic return is 3–5 l/day. The most significant contribution to the total lymphatic return is made by the intestine, followed by the skin and skeletal muscles. The interstitial fluid in the skin and skeletal muscles are exchanged once every 24–48 hours.

19.1.3 Control of the extracellular fluid volume

The interstitial volume is physiologically controlled by the kidney and the central nervous system (CNS). These regulate the interstitial volume via transcapillary microvascular exchange in the sense of a control loop. However, there is evidence that independent regulation of the interstitial fluid volume via tissue macrophages in the skin takes place through a shift in sodium salts. The mechanisms involved include the activation of so-called enhancer-binding proteins in the mononuclear phagocytes of the loose connective tissue that reacts to tonicity. These proteins bind to the promoter of the gene-coding for vascular endothelial growth factor (VEGF)-C and induce VEGF-C secretion by macrophages. Exhaustion of mononuclear phagocytes or accumulation of VEGF-C leads to interstitial hypertension with increased volume retention and decreased endothelial nitric oxide synthase expression. VEGF-C controls the regulation of blood pressure via osmosensitive influences. The necessary amount of sodium should be localised to glycosaminoglycans or intracellularly. This regulation would require either an increased amount of negative charge on the glycosaminoglycans or an altered electrolyte composition of the interstitial fluid and the plasma. One explanation under discussion is that the intracellular sodium content in connective tissue cells is increased. These local mechanisms ensure that the control of the sodium balance is at least partially decoupled from the renal regulation of the extracellular fluid volume.

19.1.4 Acute oedema

Acute inflammatory reactions are often associated with rapid and significant changes in the transcapillary exchange of fluid and protein flows. When oedema is associated with acute inflammation, it often occurs within less than ten minutes. The interstitial volume must at least double during this period to do this. It usually takes one to two days to filter this amount of fluid out of the capillary via the fluid flow. In severe cases, such as large-scale combustion, the fluid flow is maybe 200 to 300 times higher than normal. The capillary filtration coefficient must be two to three times higher than the normal value and leave the filtration pressure in the vessel system unchanged to explain most of the liquid inflow. The increase in net filtration pressure is calculated at 250–300 mmHg and is higher than the blood pressure of the circulatory system.

Surprisingly, a decrease in pressure in the interstitial fluid is also associated with oedema. In experimental studies, a reduction of the pressure in the interstitial fluid to 150 mmHg was associated with a physical denaturation of collagens. Various inflammation inhibitors, cytokines and chemokines have the same effect on the pressure in the interstitial fluid. The most pronounced reduction of the pressure in the interstitial fluid is observed in frostbite and burns. It is based on the release of local inflammation mediators as a pathophysiological reaction in addition to direct tissue injury. The same reaction patterns are found in anaphylaxis, acute allergic asthma or neurogenic inflammation due to stimulation of the vagus nerve. Overall, there is a broad range of conditions leading to a reduction of pressure in the interstitial fluid. In all cases, the loose connective tissue can actively enhance capillary filtration. This process ends as soon as a new balance has been established between the tension in the fibre networks, swelling of the basic substance, interstitial fluid pressure and increased capillary filtration.

The reduction of pressure in interstitial fluid leads to oedema formation during the initial phase of inflammation due to the rapid inflow of fluid. The simultaneous initial discharge of large protein molecules then shifts the balance of the colloid osmotic pressure gradient across the capillary. Once oedema has occurred, and the mechanisms that triggered the initial fluid inflow have subsided, increased pressure values remain in the interstitial fluid. The maintenance of oedema then depends on the capillary pressure and the colloid osmotic pressure of the loose connective tissue.

19.1.5 Chronic oedema

Chronic oedema usually develops more slowly than acute oedema. The driving force for oedema formation here is not an acute pressure reduction in the interstitial fluid, but the increased intracapillary pressure.

19

This increase affects both the arteriovenous and lymphatic capillaries and leads on the one hand to an increased occurrence of interstitial fluid and on the other hand to reduced reuptake of the fluid into the venous and lymphatic capillaries.

This chronically increased intracapillary pressure leads to a permanent increase in the filtration coefficient of the arteriovenous capillaries with an increase in interstitial fluid. At the same time, the increased intracapillary pressure causes chronic damage and dysfunction of the microcirculation. The skin capillaries are progressively enlarged and twisted, forming bulges and loops reminiscent of glomerular capillaries. Also, there is swelling of endothelial cells with enlarged interendothelial spaces and a resulting increase in macromolecular permeability with plasma, erythrocyte and fibrinogen leakage. This results in a chronic inflammatory process of the capillary bed and surrounding tissue. The diagnosis of dermatolipofasciosclerosis is histologically associated with septal fibrosis, lipomembrane necrosis, erythrocyte extravasation and iron deposition.

In contrast to chronic oedema with increased venous pressure, lymphoedema has larger lobules of fatty tissue surrounded by thick collagen fibres and interstitial lymphatic fluid. Adipocytes from lymphoedema show hypertrophic changes and increased collagen fibre deposition. The number of capillary lymph channels in the dermis is increased. Crown-like structures of dead adipocytes surrounded by M1 macrophages have been less frequently seen in biopsies of lymphoedema tissue. Flow cytometric studies show that less cellular fat-typical stem cells and M2 macrophages occur in the oedematous fat tissue of patients with lymphoedema than in healthy controls. Overall, the tissue appears less mature. Mechanical stimulation of lymphatic endothelial cells of people with secondary lymphoedema can stimulate the differentiation of these cells again. Experimental studies have shown that mechanical stretching of such lymphatic endothelial cells leads to increased expression of a mature lymphatic phenotype. It promotes lymphangiogenesis and reduces collagen deposition and cytokine secretion.

19.1.6 Conclusion

In the normal state, the loose connective tissue in the skin, subcutis and fascia is rather underhydrated. This condition is actively maintained by the fibre network in the loose connective tissue. Oedema formation is always a pathological condition associated with a change in the composition of the loose connective tissue and disrupts the microcirculation of the tissue. If this process lasts longer and becomes chronic, it leads to a disturbance of cell maturation in the ECM and accompanying inflammatory processes. A chronic oedematous tissue is therefore not only a normal tissue with increased fluid but a tissue whose function and structure are disturbed, which among other things inhibits physiological wound-healing.

REFERENCES

Chao CY, Zheng YP, Cheing GL. The association between skin blood flow and oedema on epidermal thickness in the diabetic foot. Diabetes Technol Ther 2012; 14: 602–609.

Choonhakarn C, Chaowattanapanit S, Julanon N. Lipo-dermatosclerosis: a clinicopathologic correlation. Int J Dermatol 2016; 55: 303–308.

Lund-Johansen P, Stranden E, Helberg S, et al. Quantification of leg oedema in postmenopausal hypertensive patients treated with lercanidipine or amlodipine. J Hypertens 2003; 21: 1003–1010.

O'Hearn DJ, Gold AR, Gold MS, Diggs P, Scharf SM. Lower extremity oedema and pulmonary hypertension in morbidly obese patients with obstructive sleep apnea. Sleep Breath 2009; 13: 25–34.

Reed RK, Lidén A, Rubin K. Oedema and fluid dynamics in connective tissue remodelling. J Mol Cell Cardiol 2010; 48: 518–523.

Reed RK, Rubin K. Transcapillary exchange: role and importance of the interstitial fluid pressure and the extracellular matrix. Cardiovasc Res 2010; 87: 211–217.

Tashiro K, Feng J, Wu SH, et al. Pathological changes of adipose tissue in secondary lymphoedema. Br J Dermatol 2017; 177: 158–167.

Virgini-Magalhães CE, Porto CL, Fernandes FF, Dorigo DM, Bottino DA, Bouskela E. Use of microcirculatory parameters to evaluate chronic venous insufficiency. J Vasc Surg 2006; 43: 1037–1044.

Wang S, Nie D, Rubin JP, Kokai L. Lymphatic endothelial cells under mechanical stress: Altered expression of inflammatory cytokines and fibrosis. Lymphat Res Biol 2017; 15: 130–135.

19

19.2 Lymphoedema
Anya Miller

Key notes

- The lymphatic vasculature plays a vital role in the uptake of interstitial fluid from the tissues and in immunological interaction.
- The treatment of lymphoedema is an integral part of the therapy of patients with chronic wounds.

- Lymphoedema therapy is divided into two phases: decongestion and maintenance therapy.
- Successful therapy requires a team consisting of physician, lymph therapist/physiotherapist, medical supply store with the patient at the centre.

19.2.1 Introduction

In the lymph vessel system, the microfiltration is absorbed from the tissue, concentrated in the lymph nodes and returned to the bloodstream along the left venous angle. Substances such as proteins, fats, cell detritus and bacteria can only be absorbed and transported lymphatically. An important immunological examination takes place, especially in the lymph nodes. Lymphoedema develops either primarily, as a result of faulty development of the lymph vessel system with limited transport, or secondarily, as a result of various causes such as operations and inflammations (➤ Table 19.2; ➤ Fig. 19.1). Neuropathic disorders and internal causes also lead to reduced performance of the drainage system. Here, too, the cause is an increase in the lymph load, which exceeds the transport capacity. In chronic wounds, inflammation leads to a rise in this lymph load and the often accompanying fibrosis leads to a disturbance in transport. Typical clinical changes of the resulting chronic lymphocytosis on the skin are pachydermia, papillomatosis cutis lymphostatica, cysts and fistulas (➤ Fig. 19.2; ➤ Fig. 19.3; ➤ Fig. 19.4; ➤ Fig. 19.5; ➤ Fig. 19.6).

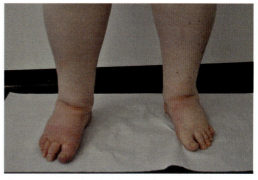

Fig. 19.1 Primary lymphoedema with aggravation by recurrent erysipelas and obesity. [P579]

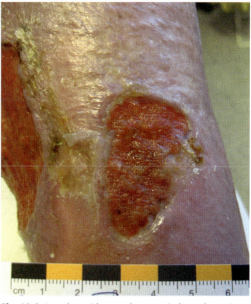

Fig. 19.2 Leg ulcer with an oedematous indurated margin. [P579]

Table 19.2 Primary and secondary causes of lymphoedema

Primary	Secondary
• Aplasia/atresia	• Surgical interventions
• Hypoplasia	• Lymphonodectomy
• Hyperplasia/dysplasia	• Radiation
• Lymph node fibrosis	• Neoplasms
• Lymph node agenesia	• Traumatic/post-traumatic
	• Post-/infectious
	• Obesity
	• Advanced stages of CVI
	• Artificial

19

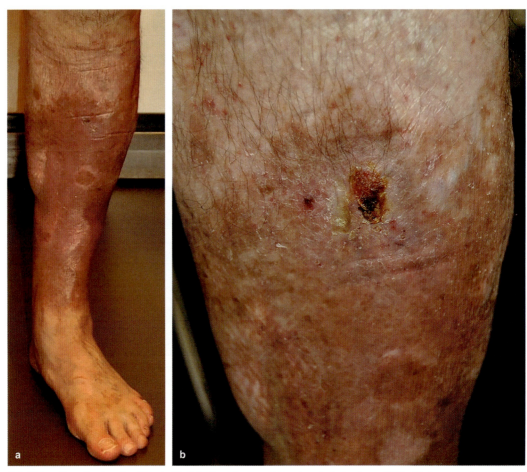

Fig. 19.3 a Secondary lymphoedema in Klinefelter's syndrome and postthrombotic syndrome (PTS) with recurrent ulcers; **b** ulcer of the patient in **a** [P579]

19.2.2 Definition

Lymphoedema is a chronic, inflammatory disease of the interstitium resulting from primary (hereditary) or secondary (acquired) damage to the lymphatic drainage system, i. e. the initial lymph vessels, pre-collectors, lymph collectors, lymphatic strains and lymph nodes.

19.2.3 Epidemiology

Exact figures on the frequency of lymphoedema are not available. Worldwide, the figures vary between 0.0115‰ and 0.3‰ for primary lymphoedema. The incidence in women is higher (m:w = 1:6–10).

19.2.4 Clinical signs of lymphoedema

• Indentable and non-indentable oedema
• Swelling of the foot/back of the hand (➤ Fig. 19.7)
• Sunken malleolus setting (Bisgaard area)/wrist joints
• Box toe (positive Stemmer's sign)
• Column-like deformity of the arm/leg
• Lichenification of the skin

19.2.5 Skin changes in lymphoedema

Lymph cysts   Dilated initial lymphatic vessels (lymph sinus); lined with endothelium (➤ Fig. 19.8). The cause is an intravascular increase in pressure due

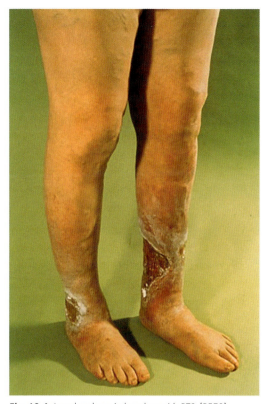

Fig. 19.4 Lymphoedema in leg ulcer with PTS. [P579]

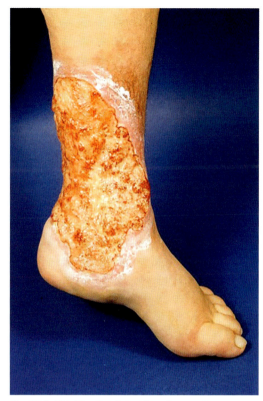

Fig. 19.5 Distal lymphoedema of pyoderma gangrenosum. [P579]

to a central flow disorder. Congenital lymphatic cysts are rare.

Lymph fistula   Bulging of lymph due to a defect in the lymph vessel, e. g. ruptured lymphatic system or iatrogenic due to injury during surgery.

Pachydermia   Fibrosclerosis of the skin due to stasis of the lymph load in the skin. The cause of the activation of fibroblasts which increase collagen synthesis is not known. Inflammatory processes lead to an increase in matrix metalloproteinases (MMP) and to the formation of reactive oxygen species (ROS) and thus to tissue remodelling. The thickening of the skin is the pathophysiological basis for the Stemmer sign in distal lymphoedema, which describes the inability to lift up a fold of skin on the second toe (thickened skin fold).

Papillomatosis cutis lymphostatica   Verrucous changes caused by acanthosis and hyperkeratosis

(➤ Fig. 19.6). It develops late in the course of the disease and is therefore a clinical sign of a longstanding lymphoedema. If papillomatosis is pronounced, fissuring produces a micro milieu which significantly increases the risk of infection.

Yellow nail syndrome   Typical medical triad of thickening and yellowing of the nails, scleronychia, lymphoedema and lung disease. The pathophysiological connection is unknown.

19.2.6 Diagnostics

The diagnosis of lymphoedema is usually clinically possible. A detailed history with inspection and palpation of the skin reveals the typical clinical signs of lymphoedema. The affected region shows oedema and changes of the skin depending on the stage (➤ Table 19.3).

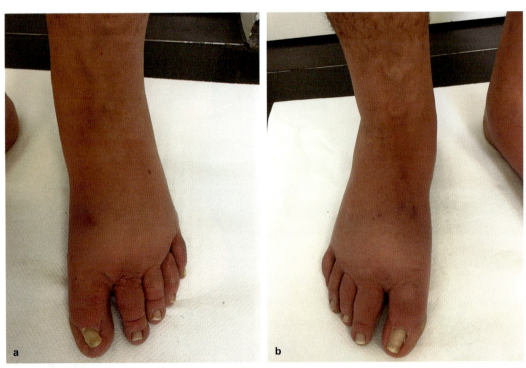

Fig. 19.6 a, b Hereditary lymphoedema with papillomatosis cutis lymphostatica, pachydermia and nail growth disturbances. [P579]

Table 19.3 Classification of the lymphoedema stages

Stage	Clinical
Latency stage	Disturbed lymph transport, no clinically measurable swelling, but e.g. pathological lymph scintigram
Stage I	Oedema of soft consistency; elevation reduces swelling
Stage II	Oedema with secondary tissue changes; elevation remains without effect
Stage III	Massively disfiguring hard swelling; often lobular form with typical tissue changes

History

- Start of oedema
- Spreading of oedema
- Other diseases/operations
- Drugs
- Previous therapy
- Family anamnesis

Apparative diagnostics   In the case of unclear cases and expert opinions, further diagnosis is necessary.

Sonography   It is not possible to differentiate a lymphoedema of the skin reliably from oedema of another genesis. Duplex sonography is primarily used to exclude differential diagnoses such as phleboedema due to CVI and changes in lymph nodes, e.g. metastases.

Functional lymph scintigraphy   Injection of a radioactively labelled carrier (^{99m}Tc nanocolloid) into the subcutis with the subsequent defined movement of the limb. The transport time (uptake) in the groin/axilla is measured with the gamma camera. The weakening due to individual depth of the lymph nodes is then corrected. Lymph flow scintigraphy provides information about the function of the lymph vessel system. In the case of a lymphatic flow disorder or insufficient movement, the uptake is reduced.

Static lymph scintigraphy   Following the functional lymph scintigraphy, ventral whole-body scintigraphy or partial body scintigraphy is performed. The lymphatic collectors are band-shaped radioactivity

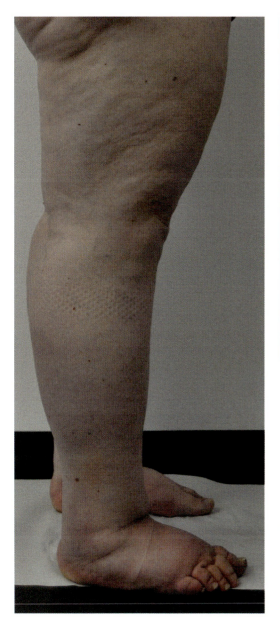

Fig. 19.7 Primary lymphoedema with swelling on back of the foot. [P579]

deposits. Indirect lymphangiography can show pathological localised radioactivity accumulations in the case of damage to the lymph vessel system or lymphocytes.

Indirect lymphangiography Intracutaneous injection of non-ionic dimeric contrast agents. Epifas-

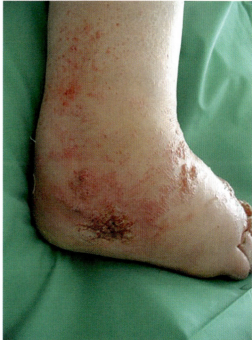

Fig. 19.8 Ulceration in lymphoedema with expanding lymph cysts. [P579]

19

cial lymph vessels with a length of 30 cm can be visualised from the resulting contrast medium depot. The procedure is used, for example, preoperatively for planning plastic operations on the lymph vessel system.

Magnetic resonance imaging (MRI) After the application of a water-soluble contrast medium containing gadolinium, the lymph collectors, lymph strains and lymph nodes can be displayed in MRI. The contrast medium is currently not approved for interstitial MRI. Indications are mainly diagnostics for lymphoedema in the context of malignancies and malformations.

Indocyanine green Indocyanine green is absorbed by the lymphatic system and fluoresces after illumination with a special camera which allows *in vivo* imaging of lymph channels after injection.

19.2.7 Therapy

Basic therapy is the complete or complex decongestive therapy (CDT):
- Manual lymphatic drainage
- Compression
- Movement in compression
- Skincare
- Instructions for self-management

Manual lymphatic drainage   Manual lymphatic drainage is a massage technique using special hand movements that stimulate lymphangiomotor activity, among other things, which leads to an increase in lymphatic volume and a decongestive effect. In the case of anatomical interruptions of the lymphatic system – e. g. due to scars – bypass circuits are activated. Manual lymphatic drainage always begins centrally above the venous angle and at the neck. Subsequently, treatment continues according to the oedema localisation.

Compression therapy
- **Decongestion phase:** Multilayer lymphological compression bandaging, starting with fingers or toes. The padding of sensitive regions and balancing of concave areas with foam and pads, followed by bandaging with short- and long-stretch bandages. The bandage is applied after lymph drainage and left until the next therapy.
- **Maintenance phase:** Adaptation of mostly flat-knitted compression stockings of compression classes 1–4 according to individual oedema localisation and characteristics. Combinations can be useful in individual cases. Special ulcer compression stockings are available for chronic wounds.

Movement in compression   Muscle activity causes further compression of the tissue and the absorption of interstitial fluid into the lymph vessel system. When moving in water (upright position) with leg oedema, the water pressure causes compression up to compression class 4 with simultaneous relief of the joints and muscle activity.

Breathing exercises   Special breathing techniques create a suction that increases lymph drainage.

Skincare   Unctuous and moisturising external preparations to support the epidermis. Skincare products with urea, glycerin or ceramides are used. Individual sensitivities, e. g. to fragrances or preservatives, should be taken into consideration. If there is a tendency to interdigital foot infections, regular prophylactic antifungal therapy is recommended. In the case of acute wounds, disinfection should be carried out as quickly as possible to prevent infections. In the case of chronic wounds, care should be taken to protect the wound edges.

Instructions for self-management   A detailed explanation of the clinical picture by the doctor, as far as possible, and instructions for independent central decongestion, application of compression bandages and exercise treatments. Self-management is an integral part of Phase 1 treatment (➤ Chap. 35). Further information is also well provided by self-help groups.

Further conservative therapies

Apparative compression therapy   Adjuvant therapy with multi-chamber devices that produce a wave-like dosed compression, which results in a central shift of fluid. Treatment is also possible for patients with chronic wounds and peripheral artery disease (PAD).

Nutrition   Protein-containing diets and a reduction of long-chain triglycerides are indicated for lymph vessel abnormalities of the intestine and chylous effusions.

Obesity   Causes a deterioration of lymph vessel function and should be prevented or treated.

Surgical therapy

There is no standard surgical therapy for lymphoedema. Different procedures are used depending on the cause of oedema:
- Reconstructive microsurgical procedures
- Microsurgical autogenous lymph vessel transplants
- The interposition of autogenous veins
- Flap plastic surgery with the incorporation of lymph vessels

19

- Separation methods:
  - Lymphovenous, lymphonodulovenous anastomoses
  - Autogenous lymph node transplants
- Resection procedures:
  - Liposuction
  - Tissue resection

19.2.8 Conclusion

The lymph vessel system is an essential component of the homeostasis of the tissue and thus also of wound-healing. The treatment for lymphoedema is therefore a primary component of the therapy of chronic wounds. The focus is on complete decongestive therapy (CDT) as an essential treatment.

REFERENCES

AWMF. S2k-Leitlinie Diagnostik und Therapie der Lymph-ödeme. AWMF Reg. 058–001. 2017. www.awmf.org/uploads/tx_szleitlinien/058-001l_S2k_Diagnostik_und_Therapie_der_Lymphoedeme_2017-05.pdf (last accessed 12 October 2020).

Földi M, Földi E, Kubik S. Lehrbuch der Lymphologie für Ärzte Phyiotherapeuten und Masseure/medizinische Bademeister. München: Elsevier; 2010.

Gültig O, Miller A, Zöltzer H. Leitfaden Lymphologie. München: Elsevier; 2016.

International Society of Lymphology. The diagnosis and treatment of peripheral lymphoedema: 2013 Consensus Document of the International Society of Lymphology. Lymphology 2013; 46: 1–11.

Levick JR, Michel CC. Microvascular fluid exchange and the revised Starling principle. Cardiovasc Res 2010; 87: 198–210.

Moffatt CJ, Franks PJ, Doherty D, et al. Lymphoedema: an underestimated health problem. QJM 2003; 96: 731–738.

Weissleder H, Schuchhardt C. Erkrankungen des Lymphgefäßsystems. Köln: Viavital Publisher; 2015.

19.3 Lipoedema

Knut Kröger

───────── **Key notes** ─────────

- Lipoedema is not primarily an oedema, but a hereditary fat distribution and reproduction disorder.
- There are no reliable criteria and no medical devices which prove or exclude the diagnosis of lipoedema. The diagnosis is based on anamnesis and clinical appearance.

- There is no causal therapy for lipoedema. With oedema, complete decongestive therapy is increasingly of great importance.
- Lipoedema *per se* does not cause wounds. Wounds that occur in patients with lipoedema are usually primarily caused by local infection or trauma and are delayed in their healing by the microcirculation disorders associated with the vast masses of fatty tissue.

19

19.3.1 Introduction

An important differential diagnosis of lipoedema is lymphoedema. The term 'oedema' is currently misleading, as it is primarily not oedema, but a fat tissue disorder. In the case of a narrow trunk and waist, an excessive and symmetrical accumulation of fatty tissue in the gluteal and hip region as well as on the legs (approx. 97%) or arms (approx. 30%) usually occurs after puberty. Typically, the foot and hand regions are omitted.

The cause of local fat tissue proliferation has not been clarified. An X-chromosomal dominant or autosomal dominant inheritance with gender-specific li-

mitation is under discussion. Activated adipogenesis is suspected in the lipoedema tissue leading to hypoxia and consecutive adipocyte necrosis and macrophage recruitment.

19.3.2 Definition

Lipoedema is a fat distribution and reproduction disorder, usually caused by a predisposition, which occurs predominantly in women. The tissue is painful under pressure and has a high tendency to haematoma due to capillary fragility. Since this is not primarily a liquid-induced increase in volume, there is no reduction in the size of the limb overnight or during elevation.

In the course of the disease, spontaneous pain often occurs additionally, which can lead to limited mobility. However, painfulness alone is not a sufficient differential diagnostic criterion, as the pain is difficult to objectify. As a result of the disproportionate increase in fat tissue in the legs, an altered gait and a malposition of the joints can also occur in advanced cases. The skin colour is not changed in uncomplicated lipoedema. Erythema and hyperpigmentation only happen as a result of complications, such as congestive dermatitis or functional chronic venous insufficiency accompanied by obesity (➤ Fig. 19.9).

Pure lipoedema is not a form of obesity and is not associated with the typical secondary diseases of obesity such as arterial hypertension, lipid metabolism disorders or diabetes mellitus. Therefore, lipoedematous fat tissue is assumed to have a different metabolism of fat cells with altered receptors. However, in about 50% of patients, there is concomitant obesity.

19.3.3 Diagnostic

There are no specific criteria which prove or exclude the diagnosis of lipoedema. Despite studies on histology, lymph scintigraphy, phlebography, MRI and lymphangiography, no examination procedure can determine specific signs of lipoedema. Therefore, the diagnosis is usually based only on the clinical assessment and experience of the examiner, which makes the handling of this clinical picture difficult, both for questions of a scientific nature and in discussions with cost bearers.

The anamnesis usually shows a slow increase of the leg or arm circumferences from puberty or early adulthood. Patients complain of pain with light touching or pressure and a tendency for seemingly spontaneous haematomas.

The clinical examination shows only a slight increase in fat tissue in the early stages, and regarding it as diseased is controversial (➤ Fig. 19.10). In the advanced stages, there is an altered skin aspect similar to orange peel, with a formation of dents and subcutaneous pasty knots. As long as there are no signs of oedema with denting under pressure, the Stemmer sign is negative, and the back of the foot/hand is not affected. In the area of the joints, mostly at the ankles, but also at the knees, elbows and wrists, a typical band formation can be found as a decisive morphological criterion (➤ Table 19.4).

The oedema component is only added in the course of the disease. In some cases, signs of secondary lymphoedema (so-called lipolymphoedema) form, not

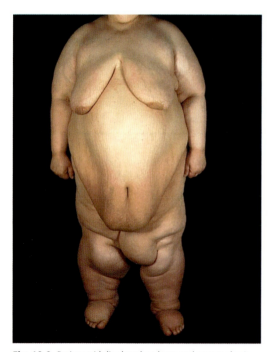

Fig. 19.9 Patient with lipolymphoedema and severe obesity. [O1089]

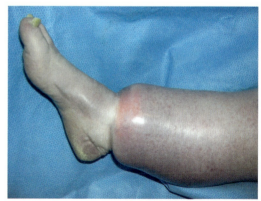

Fig. 19.10 Lipoedema with the typical picture of the fat reproduction on the lower leg (band formation), which is delimited at the foot. [O1089]

Table 19.4 Stages of lipoedema based on skin changes and amount of fatty tissue. There is no differentiation concerning the amount of oedema or the symptoms

Stage	Clinical findings
Stage I	Smooth skin surface, increased subcutaneous fat tissue
Stage II	Uneven skin surface, nodular structure of subcutaneous fatty tissue
Stage III	Severe contour deformities, large knots and dewlaps
Stage IV	Combination with secondary lymphoedema

always with a positive Stemmer's sign. The cause of the lymphatic system being affected in patients with lipoedema is unclear. Primarily lipoedema seems to have an increased supply of extracellular fluid, and the initially intact lymph vessel system of the body reacts with an increased lymph transport. It is hypothetical whether the permanent loading of the lymph vessels leads to degenerative changes of the vessel wall with a consequent reduction of the transport capacity (high-volume transport insufficiency). Other hypotheses assume that in the course of the disease, the increase in the number of crammed fat tissue cells also has a direct effect on lymph drainage. If the tissue fluid, which mainly accumulates in the dependent parts of the body, can no longer be sufficiently eliminated, oedema can occur. Also, patients with lipoedema in orthostasis showed a delayed and reduced veno-arterial reflex. The disorder of this reflex favours orthostatic oedema.

The body mass index (BMI) in patients with lipoedema can be misleading in determining a new onset of obesity, as it takes into account the total weight but not the disproportionate distribution of fatty tissue in the extremities. Therefore, in many patients with lipoedema, there is apparent obesity (BMI > 25). The Waist-to-Hip-Ratio (WHR) is better suited for the assessment of obesity in these women. This is < 0.8 for normal-weight women and < 0.9 for normal-weight men. Values > 0.85 for women and > 1.0 for men are considered obese – even in patients with lipoedema.

Important differential diagnoses

➤ Table 19.5

Normal variants of the leg shape

Normal variants of the leg must be differentiated from lipoedema. Measurements of the leg are wide-ranging and partly ethnically justified. The clinical signs of painfulness, haematoma tendency and band formation above the ankle are helpful in the differential diagnosis.

Lipohypertrophy in obesity

The most critical delineation from lipoedema is lipohypertrophy in obesity. Here, there is an increase in fat tissue, which affects the trunk as well as the appearance on the extremities. The BMI should be significantly increased, and the WHR should also show pathological values.

In extreme obesity, the lower leg oedema is the result of functional chronic venous insufficiency, with all associated characteristics and complications, or even lymphoedema.

Lipomatosis dolorosa

Lipomatosis dolorosa, also called adiposis dolorosa or Dercum's disease, is a rare disease characterised by obesity and chronic, therapy-resistant pain. Typical are severe pains in the area of fatty tissue deposits. Further symptoms can be fatigue, depression and other psychiatric and psychological abnormalities. Especially the juxta-articular form shows partial overlaps with lipoedema.

19.3.4 Therapy

Since the cause of lipoedema is unknown, there is no causal therapy. The aim of the treatment is therefore an improvement of the subjective symptoms, prevention of lipoedema progression concerning further fat tissue increase, as well as prevention of lipolymphoedema development. The early stages of lipoedema therefore focus on weight regulation and physical activity. This therapy does not alter the fat tissue distribution disorder, but slows down the progression of fat tissue proliferation and alleviates subjective symptoms. Since lipoedema is not watery, or protein-rich oedema and lymphatic reflux are even increased in the early

19

Table 19.5 Differential diagnoses of lipoedema according to Shavit et al.

Specialities	Lipoedema	Lymphoedema	Obesity	Dercum's disease
Pathophysiology	Multifactorial, lipohyper-trophy, primary	Disorders of the lymphatic vessels, primary or secondary	Multifactorial	Genetic
Disproportion	+	–	–	+
Onset	Puberty	Any age	Any age	Postmenopausal
Gender	Female	Both genders	Both genders	Female
Skin consistency	Firm	Soft to sclerotic	Firm	Firm
Skin colour	Normal, ecchymoses	Brown	Normal	Normal, sometimes ecchymoses
Expansiveness	Bilateral, mainly legs	Unilateral or bilat-eral, most commonly arms and legs	Bilateral, centrally emphasised	Bilateral, trunk, arms, legs
Symmetry	Symmetrical	Can be asymmetrical	Symmetrical	Symmetrical
Clinic	'Cuff sign' or band forma-tion, missing definition of the Achilles tendon	Papillomatosis, po-sitive Stemmer sign	Central obesity	Painful lipomas, the involvement of ex-tremities and trunk
Participation of the feet/hands	–	+	–	+
Response to compression therapy	–	+	–	+
Frequent associations	Depression, chronic venous insufficiency, hypermobility	Recurrent erysipelas	Metabolic syn-drome	Mood swings, dia-betes

19

stages of the disease, manual lymphatic drainage is not indicated. With increasing oedematisation of the tissue in the sense of lipolymphoedema, patients need a decongestive therapy which then resembles the therapy of lymphoedema (➤ Chap. 19.2.7).

A reduction of the pathologically increased fat tissue cannot be achieved with conservative means. Liposuc-tion can be helpful here. Liposuction of lipoedema usually requires the removal of significantly larger amounts of fat than cosmetic surgery. The scientific data on the questions of when and according to which criteria liposuction is indicated and how good the long-term results are concerning symptom relief and weight reduction is insufficient.

19.3.5 Lipoedema and wounds

Lipoedema doesn't cause wounds per se. Wounds that occur in patients with lipoedema are usually primarily caused by a local infection (➤ Fig. 19.11) or trauma (➤ Fig. 19.12) and delayed in their healing due to the microcirculation disorders associated with the vast masses of fatty tissue. In contrast to lymphoedema, erysipelas plays a minor role in soft tissue infections in patients with lipoedema. The infections are often caused by staphylococci and tend to form an abscess. After infection remediation, compression therapy is at the centre of the therapy, along with all other aspects of wound care.

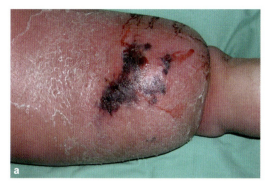

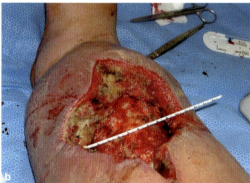

Fig. 19.11 Anamnestic infection of fat tissue resulting from an insect bite in a patient with lipoedema. **a** Pain due to pressure, necrotising soft tissue infection at first presentation; **b** after surgical evisceration, the thick subcutaneous fatty tissue layer and the exposed muscle fascia are visible. [O1089]

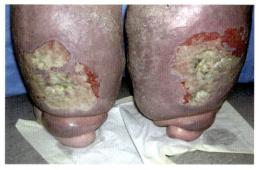

Fig. 19.12 Superficial wounds in a patient with lipoedema. This is due to recurrent trauma while lying down and getting up from bed or chair. Due to the large circumference and the weight, high shear forces occur. Therapeutically, in addition to adequate wound care (exudate management) and complete decongestive therapy (reducing weight and improving microcirculation), avoiding further trauma is important as a cause. [O1089]

REFERENCES

Bellini E, Grieco MP, Raposio E. A journey through liposuction and liposculture: Review. Ann Med Surg 2017; 24: 53–60.

Caruana M. Lipoedema: A commonly misdiagnosed fat disorder. Plast Surg Nurs 2018; 38: 149–152.

Reich-Schupke S, Schmeller W, Brauer WJ, et al. S1 guidelines: Lipedema. J Dtsch Dermatol Ges 2017; 15: 758–767.

Shavit E, Wollina U, Alavi A. Lipoedema is not lymphoedema: A review of current literature. Int Wound J 2018; 15: 921–928.

Wollina U, Heinig B. [Differential diagnostics of lipedema and lymphedema : A practical guideline]. Hautarzt 2018; 69: 1039–1047.

19

20

Wolfgang Tigges, Eike Tigges

Obesity-associated wound treatment

Key notes

- Obesity and being overweight is a disease with an increasing prevalence in Western countries.
- Obesity is a disease that can lead to chronic wounds.
- The specific treatment options for people with chronic wounds, in particular adjuvant wound treatment measures, must be regularly reviewed for their effectiveness.

- Weight reduction with a balanced diet should be included as a secondary treatment objective in the planning of treatment at an early stage.
- Treatment planning adapted to obesity in an interprofessional and interdisciplinary team can support the healing of chronic wounds and reduce the tendency to relapse.

20.1 Introduction

According to the WHO, obesity is defined as a chronic disease with excessive weight development and increased body fat.

Being overweight and obesity are defined by the Body Mass Index (BMI) (➤ Table 20.1), which however has only limited significance concerning disease-related weight development, since neither the absolute nor the relative fat content is taken into account.

The distribution of fat also determines the pathological value. Visceral fat is associated here with the highest health risk and shows a positive correlation with the waist to hip ratio. The 'waist-to-hip ratio' (WHR), which should not exceed 0.85 for women and 1.0 for men, has been shown to be a worthwhile assessment of the risk of being overweight and obesity. Among other things, it could be presented as a risk factor for the development of diabetes mellitus type 2, myocardial infarction and increased mortality.

According to the study on adult health in Germany (health monitoring by the Robert Koch Institute in 2013), the number of obese patients in the total population is 67.1% of men and 53.0% of women.

20.2 Influence of obesity on chronic wounds

Even if obesity has not been described as an independent risk factor for the development of chronic wounds, multimodal pathogenesis suggests an association. Wound complications after surgery have already been observed. Recently, an increased rate of postoperative wound complications after kidney transplantation in obese patients was demonstrated.

Table 20.1 Bodyweight classification

BMI (kg/m^2)	Classification	Waist-to-hip ratio
< 18.5	Underweight	
18.5 < 25	Normal weight	< 0.85; < 1.0
25.0 < 30.0	Overweight	
30.0 < 35.0	Grade I obesity	
35.0 < 40.0	Grade II obesity	
> 40.0	Grade III obesity	

Obesity-associated mechanisms of chronic venous insufficiency

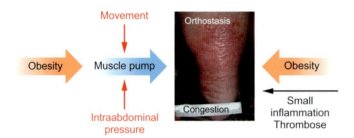

Fig. 20.1 Obesity-associated mechanisms of chronic venous insufficiency. [P581/L231]

Various pathophysiological patterns may explain the development of chronic wounds in obese patients.

20.2.1 Venous leg ulcers

There is an increased intra-abdominal pressure in obese patients as well as a limited pumping function of the musculature due to the limited mobility with atherogenic congestion syndrome. Due to degenerative joint changes in the context of an increased static load, the venous return is also counteracted, which leads to increased hydrostatic pressure in the venous vascular system. In this context, one speaks of the obesity-associated dependency syndrome.

The BMI as a measure of obesity has been described as an independent risk factor for the degree of reflux of the epifascial veins in terms of chronic venous insufficiency (CVI) (➤ Fig. 20.1).

Also, a linear relationship has been described between the BMI, the degree of obesity, and the development of deep vein thrombosis. In extremely obese patients, the same study showed a 3.4-fold increased risk compared to normal-weight patients.

The natural course of the disease in the context of a chronic venous leg ulcer is well known.

20.2.2 Diabetic metabolic disorder and arteriosclerosis

Besides storing energy, fatty tissue also has endocrine functions.

Visceral fatty tissue, in particular, can form and express multiple hormones. These are described in their entirety as adipokines. They include inflammation-specific proteins such as TNF-α and IL-6. For this reason, obesity is referred to as a so-called small bowel inflammatory disease. The blockade of insulin receptors by TNF-α explains, among other things, insulin resistance, on whose pathophysiological effect the diabetic metabolic state of diabetes mellitus type II in obese patients is based, which is an independent risk factor for the occurrence of a diabetic foot ulcer (DFU).

Furthermore, a diabetic metabolic state correlates with a raised cardiovascular risk. Due to a high triglyceride content, small, dense low-density lipoproteins (LDLs) as well as a low high-density lipoprotein (HDL) content, direct, intimal damage may occur in the further course of the disease. Also, the risk of developing arterial hypertension in obese patients is six times higher than in normal-weight patients. Consecutive arteriosclerotic deposits can, depending on their severity, lead to peripheral artery disease (PAD) and, in advanced stages, lead to chronic ulcers and prevent their healing. A presentation of diabetes mellitus increases the risk of PAD by a factor of 3–4.

20.2.3 Intertriginous skin changes and pressure ulcers

Excess fatty tissue resulting from pronounced obesity can lead to the occlusion of intertriginous skin areas. A progressive milieu change in the corresponding areas leads to skin irritations, mycoses and superficial dermatitis. The inguinal and axillary areas are considered as predilection sites for this. In pronounced cases, abscesses may also form in the gluteal area (➤ Fig. 20.2).

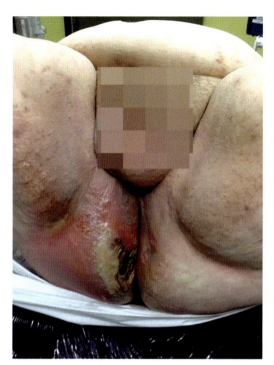

Fig. 20.2 Abscess infection with necrosis formation in obesity-related pressure ulcer. [P579]

In extreme obesity, the obesity-associated lack of exercise promotes the development of pressure ulcers. Social isolation with reactive depression, often observed in these cases, can lead to becoming bedridden.

Furthermore, lymphoedema of the lower leg is more likely in the context of pronounced obesity (➤ Fig. 20.3), which can promote the development

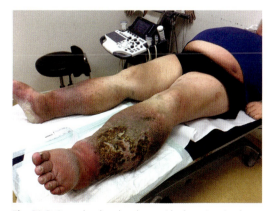

Fig. 20.3 Secondary lymphoedema with ulcerations in obesity. [P579]

of a chronic wound via dermatitis, erosion and ulceration. Lipoedema must be distinguished from this as an independent disorder without a direct connection to obesity.

20.3 Algorithm of wound treatment in obese patients

The complexity of the disorder makes a treatment algorithm useful, although the particular way in which wounds develop in obese patients and their specific treatment must not be neglected. If one first attempts to look at the various determinants and effects of obesity, it is possible to make a diagnosis as to which had an influence or a part to play in the development or lack of healing of a chronic wound (➤ Fig. 20.4).

For medical or non-medical wound therapists, the treatment of the underlying disease and the localised treatment of the chronic wound are in the foreground. It is rarely taken into account that obesity itself is the consequence of the underlying disease or is at least a factor in its development that should not be neglected. Insufficient knowledge about the treatment for obesity coupled with inadequate interdisciplinary networking giving specific information make it very difficult to give the necessary consideration for the treatment of obesity in combination with the treatment of the underlying chronic wound.

Local treatment of the chronic wound, improvement of arterial perfusion, compression and adjuvant metabolic adjustments can therefore promote healing. Still, only an accompanying obesity therapy will permanently prevent a recurrence.

Experienced wound therapists therefore need to include early considerations as to how obesity as an independent disorder can be clearly and permanently influenced concerning longterm weight reduction (➤ Fig. 20.5).

This algorithm cannot stand on its own because particular aspects are very specifically at the forefront. Nevertheless, it provides a guideline for initiating weight reduction and addressing the particular implications for the overweight patient during treatment. This guideline requires the patient to be dealt with in an understanding manner, to form a personal bond

20

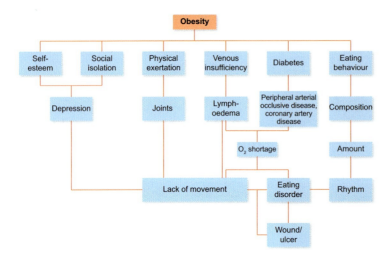

Fig. 20.4 Determinants of wound formation as caused by obesity. [P581/L231]

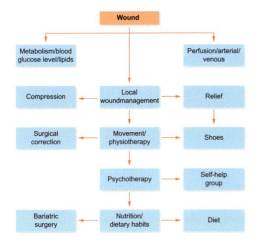

Fig. 20.5 Algorithm in the treatment process of patients with chronic wounds. [P581/L231]

and to be introduced to a network similar to the wound care centres available in some obesity centres.

20.4 Special features of wound management in obese patients

The unique features of wound treatment in obese patients result both from the local conditions, which pose particular challenges for the application of a dress-

ing, and from the adjuvant measures associated with each wound treatment, which must be differentiated according to the specific cause of the wound.

Aspects of specific wound treatment of the most common entities of chronic wounds of obese patients will be discussed below.

20.4.1 Venous leg ulcers

It is essential that wound treatment is always based on debridement, dressing techniques with exudate management, and compression therapy. The particularities in obese patients result from the anatomical and morphological changes of the limb with their pathophysiological effects. Obesity always causes an increase in body fat in the extremities, so that a venous leg ulcer can be associated with a combined oedema of phleboedema, lymphoedema and lipoedema. Leg ulcers with lipoedema are generally excruciating, which makes the use of analgesics particularly necessary for manipulation during wound treatment and debridement. Special wound dressings with analgesic ingredients have been developed to influence and reduce the intensity of pain in patients.

One of the main effects in the treatment of venous leg ulcers is compression therapy. Particularly in obese wound patients, the morphology of the lower extremity is associated with considerable restrictions for adequate compression therapy due to the distribution of fatty tissue. In the decongestion phase, multi-layer dressing systems which can compensate for disharmonious contours of the lower extremity have proved their worth. It must be clarified in each case whether a limited compression effect will be compensated for by a relatively pain-free effect. Besides, it must also always be considered that obese patients with chronic wounds have limitations in the formation of a venous return due to limited mobility. Thus adequate support of the muscle pump with compression therapy is limited. In extremely obese patients, therefore, a successful decongestion phase can be supplemented by intermittent pneumatic compression therapy, especially under inpatient conditions when surgical local wound therapy or surgical/interventional interventions on the epifascial venous system are necessary.

With the indication that the surgical procedure will influence congestion-related effects of the venous system (epifascial, rarely on the deep venous system), the risk of infection for postoperative wound infections must be considered, which is significantly increased by the patient's own risk of obesity. Also, the surgical procedure is sometimes performed in densely populated skin areas of the intertriginous area, so that an increased risk of infection must be expected.

Weight loss should be included in longterm treatment to avoid a recurrence of the leg ulcer in obese patients. Associated changes in body weight and anatomical and morphological changes in the lower extremity require necessary adjustments to the individually prescribed compression systems in the so-called maintenance phase of treatment.

20.4.2 Diabetic foot ulcers

Not every obese patient develops type 2 diabetes mellitus, but the probability of developing it increases with the duration of obesity. A peripheral insulin resistance develops, which is pronounced in the metabolic syndrome. The metabolic syndrome is characterised by:

- Obesity (pathological waist circumference in correlation to visceral fat)
- Arterial hypertension (> 135/85 mmHg)
- Hypertriglyceridaemia (> 150 mg/dl)
- Lowered high-density lipoprotein (HDL) levels

- Fasting glucose > 100 mg/dl

From this pattern of symptoms, obese patients who come for treatment with a presumed diabetic foot ulcer must first of all be checked for the metabolic syndrome, to then be referred to an accompanying internal medical treatment with a positive influence on the parameters as mentioned above.

In addition to the optimised adjustment of metabolism and blood pressure values, the treatment of the patient with a diabetic foot ulcer is determined by their local wound treatment as well as by the pathophysiological triad of peripheral neuropathy, infection and PAD. Managing the diabetic foot by wearing appropriate shoes, orthopaedic insoles or orthoses is an essential part of the treatment planning. These measures are complicated to achieve in obese patients. Peripheral neuropathy causes a restriction of sensitivity, which limits the safety of the patient's movements. At the same time, however, obesity means that many times the normal weight must be transferred to the feet and shoes, which in turn leads to a restriction of harmonious movement sequences. Patients who are overweight and obese often use a gait pattern that lessens the coordination of stability and sequence and restricts the adaptation of all joints to a natural series of movements. As a result, large body weights are often transferred abruptly via stretched knee joints and slightly abducted hip joints to the foot region, which is unable to counteract this weight with a springy and mobile action. A diabetic shoe or orthotic fitting can therefore only provide limited support, leading to insufficient relief. A close observation of the patient's gait pattern with appropriate support shoes, bandage shoes, interim shoes or orthoses should therefore be carried out after every local wound treatment. If the effect is insufficient or the gait is unsafe, further measures such as wheelchair care up to and including inpatient admission may have to be considered.

The diabetic foot ulcer may be accompanied by interstitial oedema, particularly with the involvement of infections and PAD, and is intensified in obese patients by reduced interstitial tissue pressure, which must be counteracted with adapted compression therapy. Compression therapy can also be included in the treatment of PAD. However, compression therapy is not permitted with an ankle brachial index (ABI) < 0.5, which describes the quotient of the blood pressure at the lower leg and of the arm; absolute values with an ankle artery pressure of 80 mmHg must not be undercut.

20.5 Nutrition and possibilities of weight reduction contribute to the healing of chronic wounds

A nutritional disorder can also exist in patients with obesity, leading to malnutrition over an extended period, if the diet is rich in carbohydrates and fats with a low proportion of fruit and vegetables.

Obese patients often have a protein deficit. However, an energy and protein intake covering the requirements is essential for the healing of chronic wounds, which means that obese patients, most of all, need a targeted change in diet and eating habits. An experienced nutritional therapist should make these two changes to the diet. Exercise therapy complements these measures and can be applied by exercise therapists as part of a conservatively oriented nutrition programme.

There is a variety of conservative nutrition programmes, in which three mainstays are taken into account, some of which are financially supported by health insurance companies: accompanying psychotherapy with progressive changes in eating habits, correction of the nutritional composition and exercise therapy.

Moderate hypocaloric diets require an average of 3–6 months before a weight reduction of 5–10% in those who are overweight is made possible; moreover, the longterm effect of further weight reduction is limited with this therapy despite strenuous support and shows high relapse rates. Two years after starting a low-calorie diet, only about one third of the patients benefit from a weight loss averaging 5%.

In addition to these conservative measures of weight reduction, surgical or so-called bariatric measures are available in specialised centres. Implementing such surgical measures requires stabilisation of the wound treatment and careful consultation with the patient as well as an unreserved willingness and self-discipline to have such a procedure performed.

In individual psychological/psychiatric consultations, the possibility of implementing such measures can be considered in addition to a bariatric surgeon. By reducing the size of the stomach as a special measure, or in combination with a gastric bypass, which shortens the absorption distance of the small intestine, significant weight reduction is achieved. The effects of a restriction of food intake and a malabsorption result lead to weight loss, which after two years is between 40 and 60% in those who are overweight. However, interventions involving a permanent change in diet to small portions usually require the supplementation of protein, trace elements and vitamins. After such operations, an improvement of obesity-related effects can be expected in up to 80% of cases. These changes are not necessarily accompanied by weight loss, but can sometimes be noticed after just a few weeks, e. g. by normalisation or improvement of the diabetic metabolic situation. This effect is attributed to a change in gastrointestinal hormone production. The term metabolic surgery is also used in this sense.

20.6 Networks

Networking means to complete the overall concept of a treatment procedure in an interprofessional, interdisciplinary team at the right time. This requires that everyone in this network recognises their limits, takes note of excellent disciplines or professions in a critical and necessary analysis and can promptly refer their patients to this cooperative community.

One of the prerequisites for this is to accept the patient as part of the network and to show understanding for them in their exceptional situation. This includes not always turning to supposedly necessary measures and steps that could lead to excessive demands and insufficient adherence and compliance of the patient.

Given the complexity of the patient's illness as a whole, an understanding conversation with the patient is an essential element in binding them to their treatment team.

Step by step, they should be included in the treatment process as a whole and positively supported. Educating the patient is complex and must be perceived in the context of the particular issue from the perspective of different disciplines and professions so that the patient's caregiver is not forgotten or neglected. Most obese patients bear the burden of their condition for years if not decades because they have never experienced an effective therapy or have been ignored. The development of an obesity-related chronic wound then leads to a new attempt to heal themselves, in order to heal or improve the wound itself. In addition to all the measures of modern wound management, this includes the consistent implementation of weight-reducing measures in the long term.

It is preferable to refer patients to obesity centres which have not committed themselves to only one of the measures. In this way, according to the individual assessment of the health care professionals, a longterm concept can be worked out for the patient without any pressure, initiating weight reduction and ensuring its success for many years. Obesity centres have specialised experience in the treatment of obese patients, in which various disciplines and professions are involved: psychology, psychiatry, nutritional counselling, endocrinology, and including very experienced surgeons in bariatric surgery as well as movement therapists. These centres also have specialised equipment with spacious facilities, ranging from the seating to the means of transport with a higher load capacity, for inpatient and outpatient treatment. Likewise, this adaptation must be consistent, with the use of special operating tables, and special operative-technical conditions must be fulfilled.

Obese patients are chronically ill patients who require lifelong contact with competent and understanding health care professionals.

REFERENCES

Danielsson G, Eklof B, Grandinetti A, Kistner RL. The influence of obesity on chronic venous disease. Vasc Endovasc Surg 2002; 36: 271–276.

Gößwald A, Lange M, Kamtsiuris P, Kurth BM. DEGS: Studie zur Gesundheit Erwachsener in Deutschland. Bundesgesundheitsblatt Gesundheitsforsch Gesundheitsschutz 2012; 55: 775–780.

Klovaite J, Benn M, Nordestgaard BG. Obesity as a causal risk factor for deep venous thrombosis: A Mendelian randomization study. J Intern Med 2015; 277: 573–584.

Lawall H, Huppert P, Rümenapf G. Deutsche Gesellschaft für Angiologie – Gesellschaft für Gefäßmedizin. S3-Leitlinie zur Diagnostik, Therapie und Nachsorge der peripheren arteriellen Verschlusskrankheit. 2015. www.awmf.org/uploads/tx_szleitlinien/065-003l_S3_PAVK_periphere_arterielle_Verschlusskrankheitfinal-2016-04.pdf (last accessed 12 October 2020).

Schwarz NT, Tigges W, Tigges H. Allgemein- und Viszeralchirurgie. Stuttgart: Thieme; 2017.

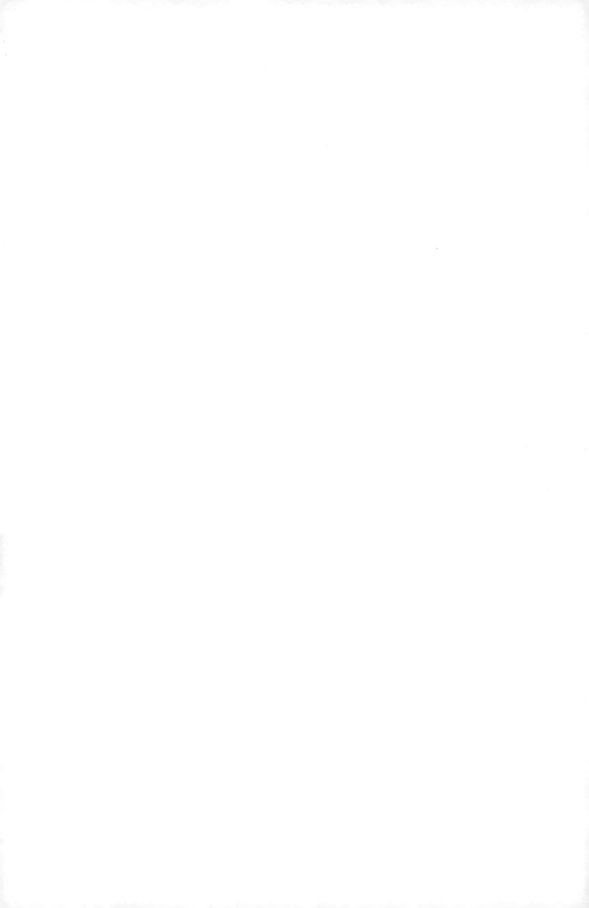

21

Richard Dodel, Frank Assmus

Wound care for patients with dementia

Key notes

- Wound care requires a high degree of patient cooperation, which is often limited in patients with dementia.
- Dementia is an established risk factor for the development and chronification of pressure

ulcers in particular, and leads to increased morbidity and mortality.
- Patients with dementia must be given a validating approach.
- A multi-professional team should provide care.

21.1 Introduction

Chronic wounds are common in the elderly and lead to impairment of everyday activities as well as the quality of life of those affected, and result in a need for increased care. For example, about 70% of pressure ulcers occur in people over 70 years of age. Significant factors leading to the development of these wounds are an advanced age and the risk factors associated with old age, such as reduced mobility, an increasingly sedentary lifestyle and poor nutritional status. The occurrence of dementia is another established risk factor that is responsible for both the development and chronicity of wounds. Memory and concentration problems of the patients make it difficult to take a medical history, and to prepare and provide care. An interview with a third party must involve a family member or a guardian to obtain an accurate medical history. The care must always be coordinated with the person who predominantly cares for the patient.

21.2 Dementia

Dementia is defined as the acquired impairment of higher cognitive functions and everyday skills. With most of the chronically progressive courses, there are impairments of many cortical functions including memory, thinking, orientation, perception, arithmetic,

learning ability, language, speaking and judgement. Usually, changes in emotional control, social behaviour or motivation accompany the cognitive impairments. Dementia is currently classified according to ICD-10 (➤ Table 21.1). In recent years, however, a large number of new diagnostic (research) criteria has been proposed.

In Germany around 1.7 million people currently live with dementia. The prevalence rates increase with age. In the 65–69 age group, about 1% are affected, and about 40% among those over 90 years of age. Dementia is comparatively rare in middle age. More women than men have dementia. Dementias are usually irreversible and last until death ➤ Fig. 21.1). They shorten the remaining normal life expectancy; however, the duration of the disease cannot be reliably predicted in individual cases. In general, the later in life the condition occurs, the more severe the symptoms are; the more accompanying physical illnesses there are,

Table 21.1 Dementia criteria according to ICD-10

Dementia is a syndrome due to disease of the brain, usually of a chronic or progressive nature, in which there is a disturbance of multiple higher cortical functions, including memory, thinking, orientation, comprehension, calculation, learning capacity, language, and judgement. Consciousness is not clouded.
The impairments of cognitive function are commonly accompanied and occasionally preceded by deterioration in emotional control, social behaviour, or motivation. This syndrome occurs in Alzheimer's disease, in cerebrovascular disease, and other conditions primarily or secondarily affecting the brain.

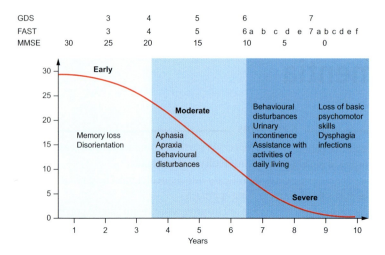

GDS			3	4	5	6					7						
FAST			3	4	5	6a	b	c	d	e	7 a b c d e f						
MMSE		30	25	20	15	10		5			0						

Fig. 21.1 Typical course of Alzheimer's disease over time, with accompanying scores on the Global Deterioration Scale (GDS) for assessment of primary degenerative dementia, Functional Assessment Staging Tool (FAST) and Mini-Mental State Examination (MMSE). (Adapted from Voisin and Vellas 2009) [F1023-001]

the shorter the survival time. A mean duration of the disease is 3–6 years as given in the literature, but the length of the disease varies greatly between patients; in some cases, survival times of 20 years and more have been reported.

Social behaviour or motivation, in addition to cognitive disorders and disorders of emotional control, can be found early on in the course. All these symptoms are included under the term 'behavioural and psychological symptoms of dementia'. The term 'challenging behaviour' refers to repetitive behaviour that is perceived by the social environment as unadapted or not appropriate to the situation. These include the following aspects:

- Agitation and aggression
- Irritability
- Apathy
- Depression
- Anxiety
- Delusions and hallucinations
- Tendency to run away
- Disinhibition
- Euphoria
- Constant shouting

These stressful non-cognitive symptoms can occur in the course of the disease in up to 90% of affected dementia patients. People with dementia who show these symptoms have a worse prognosis, need more care than others and are sent to nursing homes earlier.

Alzheimer's dementia is considered the most common form of dementia, accounting for about 60–70% of dementia cases. Other common diseases associated with dementia are vascular dementia (about 10–15%), dementia with Lewy bodies (5%), dementia with Parkinson's syndrome (3–5%) and frontotemporal dementia (5–10%). Secondary forms of dementia are listed with about 6%.

For diagnostic classification, the procedure according to the German S3-guideline for dementia (www.dgn.org/leitlinien/3176-leitlinie-diagnose-und-therapie-von-demenzen-2016) is suggested, which first proposes a syndrome diagnosis and then a subsequent etiological classification. For syndrome diagnosis, the use of short tests is recommended. For an orientation assessment of a cognitive disorder, the Mini Mental Status Test (MMST), the DemTect, the Test for the Early Diagnosis of Dementia with Differentiation from Depression (TFDD) and the Montreal Cognitive Assessment Test (MoCA) are mentioned. The clock-drawing test, in combination with the other short test procedures discussed above, can increase the diagnostic significance but is not suitable as the sole cognitive test. It should be noted, however, that the sensitivity of these procedures is limited for mild and questionable dementia, and the test procedures mentioned are not suitable for the differential diagnosis of various dementias. An in-depth neuropsychological examination with an established series of tests, such as CERAD, should be carried out to determine the individual pattern and extent of impairment, as well as for differential diagnosis. These are complex and extensive and should

21

be performed by specially trained personnel, e. g. neuropsychologists.

The MMST is used to classify the severity of dementia in the case of Alzheimer's type of dementia. The boundaries between the different levels are only used as a guide in individual cases (here we describe the classification according to the German guideline for dementia):

- MMST 20–26 points: mild Alzheimer's disease
- MMST 10–19 points: moderate/moderate Alzheimer's disease
- MMST < 10 points: severe Alzheimer's disease

Diagnosis is supported by cerebral imaging (CT or MRI), laboratory tests and further examinations such as cerebrospinal fluid analysis, functional imaging with PET, etc., at the end of which the patient is designated to have one of the various forms of dementia.

21.3 Epidemiology of pressure ulcers in patients with dementia

The occurrence of dementia is an established risk factor for the development and chronification of pressure injuries, which is due to a variety of causes. In the setting of patients cared for in nursing homes (n = 323) with advanced dementia, decubital or pressure ulcers (stage ≥ II) were detected in 38.7% of patients in an observation period of 18 months. In an Israeli study of 172 patients with advanced dementia, 66.5% of the patients examined had a pressure ulcer when admitted to the nursing home; only 33.5% of the patients had no detectable pressure ulcer. It did not matter from which setting (hospital, home, nursing home) the patients were referred to the nursing home. The median survival time of patients with advanced dementia and pressure ulcers was significantly shorter compared to patients who did not have an ulcer: 96 days vs. 863 days; the odds ratio (OR) was 2.81 (95% CI: 1.51–5.22, p < 0.01). When additional variables (age, gender, Norton score, albumin and haemoglobin) were included in the model, the odds ratio increased to 3.86. Patients with dementia suffering from sacral pressure ulcers were also found to have a higher risk than patients who did not suffer from cognitive impairment. In another study by the same working group, 63 days median survival time was reported in patients with dementia vs. 117 days in patients without dementia.

There is little valid data available on the prevalence of pressure ulcers and their outcome in patients in the different stages of dementia in the ambulatory care setting.

In principle, dementia is an important risk factor for the occurrence of pressure ulcers in older adults which must be considered clinically. Association studies from several clinical studies also show this. In an outpatient setting, an adjusted risk ratio of 2.01 for patients with Alzheimer's type dementia was demonstrated in a study involving a total of 1,211 people with pressure ulcers (of a total of 75,168 older adults examined). Factors associated with the occurrence of pressure ulcers in nursing homes are advanced dementia (OR: 3.0; 95% CI: 1.4–6.3), use of urinary catheters (OR: 2.25; 95% CI: 1.06–4.70), reduced BMI (OR: 0.82; 95% CI: 0.86–0.99) and anaemia (OR: 0.7; 95% CI: 0.058–0.9). In a general outpatient setting, anxiety and neurosis in men (OR: 2.19; 95% CI: 1.84–2.60) and chronic wounds in women (OR: 2.89; 95% CI: 2.38–3.53) were the diseases with the highest dementia-associated probability. In men, the OR for the occurrence of pressure ulcers was 2.05.

Currently, the available data only allow a statement on patients with advanced cognitive disorders, as early stages of dementia have been insufficiently investigated.

21.4 Assessment

As with all geriatric patients, a structured assessment of the patient with dementia and pressure ulcers should be performed (➤ Table 21.2). This assessment can be done according to the guidelines of, e. g. AGAST for geriatric patients, but should be supplemented by specific estimates. Shah et al. have formulated 2014 a proposal for this. The evaluation of pressure ulcers should be carried out as described in ➤ Chap. 13 described above.

The assessment, adapted from Shah et al., should include at least four domains (physical, cognitive, psychological/psychiatric, social):

Table 21.2 Basic geriatric assessment. For a detailed description of the scales to be applied, please refer to the literature

Assessment	
Screening	Geriatric screening according to Lachs
Everyday activities	Barthel index
Ability to help yourself	Money counting test
Indication of risk of injury due to falling	Fall risk assessment
Cognition	Mini-mental state examination (MMSE)
	Clock-drawing test
Mobility	Timed up and go test (TUG)
Risk of falling	Tinetti test
Emotions	Geriatric depression scale (GDS)
Social care	Social status according to Nikolaus

1. The evaluation of the physical area should consist of the following points:
   a. Care setting of the patient (outpatient, hospital, nursing home)
   b. Status of mobility (strength, gait, balance)
   c. Presence of comorbidities (PAD, neuropathy, etc.)
   d. Development of complaints and findings
   e. Nutritional status (albumin deficiency, vitamin deficiency, etc.)
   f. Physical limitations (amputations, contractures, etc.)
2. The evaluation of cognitive domains should include the following points:
   a. Medical history, type and severity of dementia
   b. In Alzheimer's dementia, the loss of cognitive faculties; in frontotemporal dementia, the loss of judgement and behavioural problems are the main symptoms
   c. Evaluation of the executive functions (EXIT-25)
   d. Assessment of the ability to be self-sufficient or to adhere to treatment
   e. Capacity assessment
   f. Understanding the basic facts of treatment options
   g. Adequate evaluation of the current situation
   h. The patient can justify the decision/choice of treatment.

i. The patient can communicate his choice of treatment.
3. The assessment of the psychological/psychiatric domains should include:
   a. Presence and extent of depression
   b. Apathy, self-neglect, anorexia with nutritional deficiencies
   c. Delirious/psychosis
   d. Difficulties with relationships, etc.
   e. Anamnesis with personality disorders (influences compliance/adherence)
4. The evaluation of the social field should include the following points:
   a. Advanced instructions
   b. Support
   c. Power of attorney
   d. Objectives of care
   e. Level of health literacy
   f. Level of family support
   g. Conflicts in the family

It is also helpful to survey the perception of pain in the respective patients. More than 28 different scales for pain assessment are available for evaluation in dementia patients. The following scales are used in German-speaking countries. However, it must be acknowledged that there is limited evidence for their reliability, validity and clinical utility, and no single instrument can currently be recommended as a preference:

- PAINAD (Pain assessment in advanced dementia)
- ECPA (in French – Echelle comportementale de la douleur pour personnes âgées non communicantes)
- Doloplus

A systematic literature search shows how scant our current knowledge is about the effect of systemic therapies of various diseases on wound-healing. However, it does seem that the influence of individual medications on wound-healing is not entirely unexplored. With further research, drug therapy could in future play a more critical role in addition to optimised local treatment and make it possible, for example, to control the collagen content or epithelialisation specifically.

Also, it is imperative that in future studies on wound-healing, all drugs must always be carefully documented, even if they have nothing to do with essential wound-healing. As a regulation, this could significantly influence the results of the studies.

21.5 Special features of therapy for patients with dementia

Nursing measures for people with dementia usually place high demands on everyone involved in wound care. On the one hand, doctors and nursing staff are rightly expected to provide professional, targeted wound therapy that is adapted to current medical and nursing knowledge. On the other hand, there is the patient, who in the best case tolerates the wound care, accepts advice and recommendations and thus facilitates positive conditions for wound-healing. This compliance and ability to cooperate is often not present or expected in people who have dementia. The increasing loss of cognitive skills in the course of dementia development can, for example, lead to a situation in which a wound that does not hurt is simply forgotten or even denied by the person affected (anosognosia: the pathological failure to recognise an apparent physical disorder). For this reason alone, it must be expected that necessary wound treatment will be refused or associated with defensive behaviour. In people with dementia and challenging behaviour, frequent running away, verbal or physical aggression, or loud screaming during wound care, are particularly common.

While healthy people look for solutions in crises and think in terms of context, it is often observed in people with dementia, especially in the moderate stage of the disease ➤ Fig. 21.1), that the ability to think logically is compromised. Also, the ability to think and weigh up a situation sequentially, or the ability to adapt to changing situations has been limited or lost. It is often no longer possible to recognise the consequences of one's behaviour. It must therefore not be assumed that the person concerned will adhere to agreements with or recommendations made by doctors or nursing staff concerning wound treatment because he or she has forgotten them or has not understood the context. A similar situation is familiar from studies on the drug treatment of patients with dementia. For example, 73% of patients with Alzheimer's dementia need help in obtaining and taking medication.

21.5.1 Wound care

There are as yet no generally accepted standards or recommendations on wound care for people with dementia and challenging behaviour. Possible options for action are based primarily on experience in dealing with people with dementia and their individuality. Some options for work for process design are presented below.

The prompt assessment of wounds is an essential basis for further wound care. A joint wound assessment by a doctor, nurse and a wound expert is the optimal solution. At the forefront is the question of modern wound therapeutics and wound dressings which, for example, make dressing changes possible with a frequency of 2–3 or more days, thus reducing the burden on the patient with dementia. The use of highly adhesive plasters for the fixation of wound dressings should be avoided as far as possible, as these plasters contract over time and cause 'pulling' on the skin. People with dementia often cannot interpret this tugging sensation and find it very unpleasant and disturbing. It is therefore not uncommon for patients to remove bandages themselves. This often happens in the evening or at night. Patients with problems falling asleep and sleeping through the night, sometimes accompanied by restlessness, have ample time, especially at night, to fiddle with the vital bandages. A so-called placebo or distraction bandage, which is applied at an easily accessible place, e. g. on the forearm, can provide relief. In this way, attention and activity can be directed at the placebo bandage, which may have to be renewed, but this is certainly less problematic than reapplying the true wound dressing under sterile conditions. Elastic gauze bandages can be used for this purpose, e. g. wrapped around the patient's wrists and secured with wide strips of plaster or pieces of fixative fleece cut to size. The bandage can then be wrapped with a coloured cohesive bandage, as the colour distracts attention from the actual bandage.

Temporary donning of gloves during periods of restlessness can also be discussed but must be well justified and documented in each case, as it can be classified as a restrictive measure. Mittens made especially for this purpose are suitable (➤ Fig. 21.2). Their use should be limited to the night-time, as the gloves are often perceived as disturbing and would restrict the patient too much in daytime. Before utilising the gloves, an opinion should be obtained

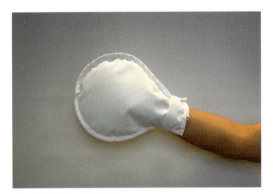

Fig. 21.2 Mitten. [P589]

from the authority responsible for the care facility. Authorities have quite different views as to whether the measure has the effect of restricting freedom and therefore requires authorisation, or whether it is to be regarded as an appropriate and moderate measure for the protection of the patient and therefore does not require judicial approval.

Furthermore, regular dressing changes should ideally be carried out by a limited number of familiar people, e. g. caregivers, to reduce the anxiety, restlessness or defensiveness of the person affected, while ensuring objective wound assessment. A dressing change with two nurses can be constructive here if the nurse in charge provides the information and addresses the patient. The second nurse takes over the handling of, or assisting with, the task. Complete preparation of the required material and a brief agreement on the planned procedure between the people involved are advisable. The time frame needed for wound care should be as generous as possible. If necessary, pain medication should be discussed in a timely manner with the attending physician before dressing changes. A standardised pain assessment (see above) can be used as an instrument for assessing pain before, during and after wound care. This pain assessment is particularly necessary if the patient affected by advanced dementia is unable to provide coherent information on their own pain perception.

21.5.2 The wound care setting

Another critical aspect for the wound care of patients with dementia is the setting in which the wound care

should be performed. A calming and empathetic atmosphere needs to be created for the dementia patient during wound care. Creativity is required here. Taking into account the great variety of requirements of people with dementia in terms of the cognitive, emotional and social effects of the disease, it is advisable to try to ascertain to which measures the patient reacts positively. This could, for example, be the care and approach of the second carer or a close relative. A validating basic attitude and the ability to validate communication are prerequisites and have an important influence on the success of wound care. However, the number of people present should be limited to what is necessary and meaningful. Fear of pain during wound care should not be ignored but should be accompanied by empathic, validating communication. Patient involvement is recommended, e. g. by instructing the patient to remove the dressing independently, if possible, or by holding the nurse's arm to influence the pace of the procedure.

Calming and continuous body contact with the patient lying in a horizontal position can be helpful in wound care.

In terms of basal stimulation, consideration may also be given to playing music, e. g. the patient's favourite music, or using soothing aromatic oils.

A hand massage accompanying or concluding the wound treatment often has a calming effect and can thus positively influence the patient's behaviour. The insistence of the patient to attend to the necessary wound care by themselves should be considered as a last resort and avoided as far as possible. Once a framework has been found in which the essential wound care is possible and feasible, it should be turned into a routine to ensure continuity for the patient. Visits and dressing change times can be correlated to avoid unnecessary dressing changes, for the benefit of the patient.

21.5.3 Drugs for the treatment of Alzheimer's dementia

The approved medicines for the treatment of Alzheimer's dementia in Europe are cholinesterase inhibitors – donepezil, galantamine and rivastigmine for the mild and moderate stages, and NMDA antagonist memantine for the moderate stage of Alzheimer's dementia. They have established their secure place in the treatment of Alzheimer's dementia. In a few studies, an influence on the healing process after hip surgery could be proven. Also, we are unable to find any reviews for memantine that shows any impact on wound-healing in pressure ulcers. Since the CNS influences skin remodelling after lesions via adrenergic and cholinergic innervations of the autonomic nervous system, positive interaction with cholinesterase inhibitors can be assumed.

In addition to the cholinesterase inhibitors, ginkgo biloba preparations are frequently used for the treatment of Alzheimer's dementia. These can lead to a slightly increased bleeding tendency, although this could not be proven in all studies.

Due to the age prevalence of dementia, patients with dementia are more likely to be given anticoagulants, and often there are inadequate combinations of drugs (polypharmaceuticals) which can impede wound-healing but also increase the likelihood of bleeding during wound care. This must be taken into account for adequate wound care.

21.6 Conclusion

Wound care requires a high degree of patient cooperation. Without this, the appropriate therapy is hardly achievable and results in high recurrence rates. In patients with dementia, collaboration and understanding are limited by the underlying disease. A multi-modal therapy approach is indicated and necessary to achieve adequate care and prevent complications. The older person with cognitive disorders represents a patient who requires special attention in everyday clinical practice.

REFERENCES
Denzer S. Chronische Wunden: Beurteilung und Behandlung. Stuttgart: Kohlhammer; 2014.
Freund H. Geriatrisches Assessment und Testverfahren. Stuttgart: Kohlhammer; 2014.
Jaul E. Assessment and management of pressure ulcers in the elderly: current strategies. Drugs Aging 2010; 27: 311–325.
Jessen F (Hrsg.). Handbuch Alzheimer-Krankheit. Berlin: De Gruyter; 2018.
Mitchell SL, Teno JM, Kiely DK, et al. The clinical course of advanced dementia. N Engl J Med 2009; 361: 1529–1538.
Morris JC, Mohs RC, Rogers H, Fillenbaum G, Heyman A. Consortium to establish a registry for Alzheimer's disease (CERAD) clinical and neuropsychological assessment of Alzheimer's disease. Psychopharmacol Bull 1988; 24 (4): 641–652.
Shah P, Aung TH, Ferguson R, Ortega G, Shah J. Ethical consideration in wound treatment of the elderly patient. J Am Coll Clin Wound Spec 2014; 6: 46–52.
Voisin T, Vellas B. Diagnosis and treatment of patients with severe Alzheimer's disease. Drugs Aging 2009; 26 (2): 135–144.

22

Joachim Dissemond, Knut Kröger

Systematics of wound treatment – the M.O.I.S.T. concept

──────── **Key notes** ────────

- Local treatment of chronic wounds today is mostly carried out as moist wound treatment, which is based on the phases of wound-healing.

- After T.I.M.E., a new concept for the local treatment of chronic wounds was developed with M.O.I.S.T.
- In the M.O.I.S.T. concept, 'O' and 'S' describe new and innovative treatment options.

22.1 Introduction

Today, moist wound treatment which is oriented to the phases of wound-healing is the gold standard of local treatment for most patients with chronic wounds. As an orientation guide, Wund-DACH, the umbrella organisation of German-speaking wound-healing societies, presented M.O.I.S.T. as a new concept for local treatment of chronic wounds (➤ Table 22.1, ➤ Fig. 22.1). With the M.O.I.S.T. concept, the ideas of the T.I.M.E. concept, which was first published in 2003 and is widely used internationally, were taken up and further developed. The factors described with 'T', 'I' and 'M' were classified as still up-to-date and essential and therefore retained. The letter 'E' was initially used to describe 'epidermis' and later 'edge' (wound margin). The wound margin, like the wider wound environment, is significant but is not an integral part of wound treatment. For this reason, this letter has been omitted. Instead, many other aspects and therapeutic options have emerged in the last decade, and new and innovative therapeutic options were found to be lacking, now described with 'O' and 'S'.

Table 22.1 M.O.I.S.T. concept for local treatment of chronic wounds

M	Moisture balance
O	Oxygen balance
I	Infection control
S	Supporting strategies
T	Tissue management

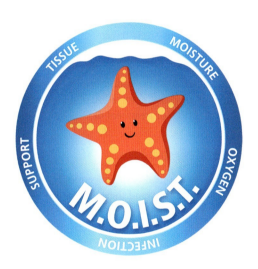

Fig. 22.1 The logo of the M.O.I.S.T. concept is called TOM. The starfish TOM stands here with its five arms as an acronym for the optimisation of wound treatment by M.O.I.S.T. (Treatment Optimisation [with] M.O.I.S.T.). [W1084]

22.2 The M.O.I.S.T. concept

M: moisture balance

Exudate management propagates a wound environment in wound treatment that is neither too moist nor too dry. In the case of very dry wounds, for example, hydrogels would be used. Very often, however, there is an excess of exudate, so that wound product such as superabsorbents are used.

O: oxygen balance

The lack of oxygen, especially in chronic wounds, leads to an undersupply of oxygen, almost independent of their genesis, which is referred to as hypoxia. Measures such as revascularisation or pressure relief have the greatest significance in treatment. If this does not lead to sufficient success, treatment options that can supply oxygen are increasingly available, such as wound dressings, haemoglobin spray as well as normal- and hyperbaric procedures.

I: infection control

Infection control describes all therapeutic measures aimed at reducing bacteria and other microorganisms. Systemic antibiotic treatment is usually only indicated for infectious diseases. On the other hand, local therapeutics with active antimicrobial substances such as polihexanide, octenidine or silver are used for infection prophylaxis, eradication of multi-resistant organisms (MRO) or treatment of local infections.

S: supporting strategies

If wounds do not heal despite seemingly adequate treatment, specific wound therapeutics can be used temporarily to intervene actively in the disturbed wound-healing process. This interaction takes place, for example, by modulating matrix metalloproteinases (MMP), pH or growth factors.

T: tissue management

All necessary wound conditioning measures are described as tissue management. Here, for example, neutral wound dressings, biosurgery or physical aids such as wound vacuum devices, electricity, plasma or ultrasound are used to improve wound-healing. Depending on the method, the application can support the processes of debridement, wound-cleansing, granulation or re-epithelialisation.

22.3 Conclusion

The M.O.I.S.T. concept is an easy-to-remember acronym that describes the various components of local treatment for chronic wounds and can thus be a help in selecting the appropriate wound treatment.

REFERENCES

Dissemond J, Assenheimer B, Gerber V, et al. M.O.I.S.T. – a concept for the topical treatment of chronic wounds. J Dtsch Dermatol Ges 2017; 15: 443–445.

Dissemond J, Augustin M, Eming S, et al. Modern wound care – practical aspects of non-interventional topical treatment of patients with chronic wounds. J Dtsch Dermatol Ges 2014; 12: 541–554.

Schultz GS, Barillo DJ, Mozingo DW, Chin GA. Wound Bed Advisory Board Members. Wound bed preparation and a brief history of TIME. Int Wound J 2004; 1: 19–32.

IV Factors which support wound-healing

23
Gunnar Riepe, Anke Bültemann

Systematic wound treatment – the WundUhr®

--- Key notes ---

- WundUhr® is an illustrated pocket guide to individual modern wound care.
- Progressive wound-healing is positioned on the outer ring, and the exudate level is placed within the clock's face.
- WundUhr® is a communication aid for patients, relatives and health care professionals with

different experience in wound care. It helps demystify the graphics and language, dialect and picturesque model landscapes via the internet.
- The indispensability of causal treatment for wound-healing is emphasised by the red, 'ticking' second hand of the WundUhr®

23.1 Introduction

The WundUhr®, German for 'wound clock', is an illustration of a clock, created to demystify modern wound treatment for patients and professionals (➤ Fig. 23.1). The continuous cycles of a clock resemble the recurrence of formation and healing if the causative factor of the wound is not eliminated. Six segments resembling the phases of wound-healing

divides the clock face. Two rings of sand and water represent the dry and wet state of the wound. Three hands are inscribed with debridement, margin protection and cause of the wound. Suggestions for the choice of therapy or dressing are placed in the corresponding phase and state of the wound. The WundUhr® can be acquired as a postcard for the clinician's pocket, as larger prints for the wall, or visited on the webpage www.wunduhr.de.

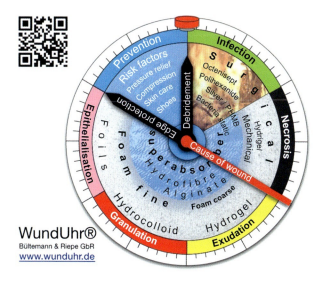

WundUhr®
Bültemann & Riepe GbR
www.wunduhr.de

Fig. 23.1 The WundUhr®. [W1093, W1094] To find on YouTube, Facebook and Instagram

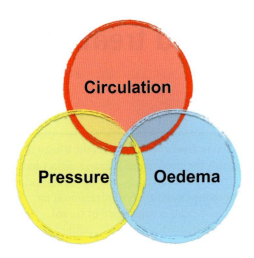

Fig. 23.2 Three major causes of chronic wounds. [W1093, W1094]

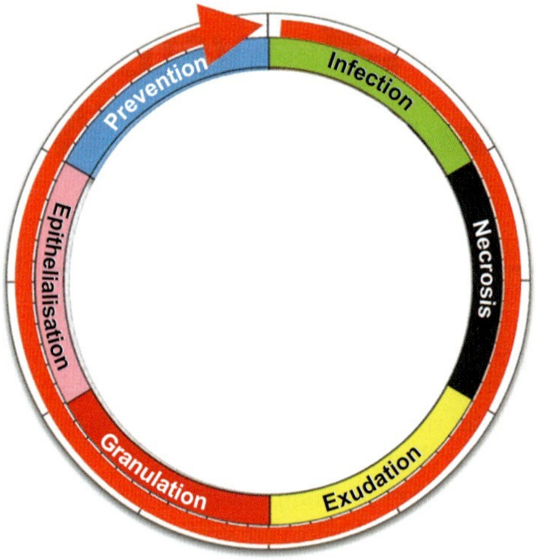

Fig. 23.3 Phases of wound-healing. [W1093, W1094]

23.2 Causal treatment

Wound closure requires the detection and treatment of the cause of the wound. The red second hand is named 'cause of wound'. It constantly reminds us to check that we treat the cause sufficiently. To simplify the process, we defined three major causes: insufficient circulation, external pressure, and internal tension due to oedema (➤ Fig. 23.2).

23.3 Debridement and edge protection

The two other hands named 'debridement' and 'margin protection' remind us that in all phases of wound-healing, we have to clean the wound bed and take care of the margin. Debridement is performed surgically or mechanically. Surgical debridement uses a scalpel, scissors, curette, hydrosurgery, electric dermatome or ultrasound. Mechanical cleansing of the wound uses drug-free rinsing, forceps, swabs, microfibre fabrics, coarse foams, hydrogel, enzymatic substances or maggots. Margin protection requires active removal of hyperkeratosis, scales and scabs as well as moisture control through skin protection, hydrofibres or superabsorbers.

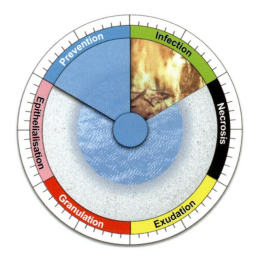

Fig. 23.4 State of the wound – dry, wet, infected. [W1093, W1094]

23.4 Phases of wound-healing

In WundUhr®, we define six phases of wound-healing (➤ Fig. 23.3, ➤ Fig. 23.4). Each segment has its corresponding name and colour in the outer ring of the clock's face.

• Infection is the phase between 12 and 2 o'clock, and its colour is green. The centre of this segment is a picture of a fire, resembling the vital danger of infection and the need to extinguish the fire quickly, within days. Written into this section is the preliminary treatment by surgical debridement followed by the antiseptics octenidine, polihexanide (PHMB) and silver. Finally, 'bacteriostatic' represents dressings which bind with bacteria and remove them from the wound.

- Necrosis falls between 2 and 4 o'clock and is coloured black. As mentioned above, surgical debridement is followed by mechanical cleaning and the use of hydrogel.
- Exudation falls between 4 and 6 o'clock and is shown in yellow, the colour of fibrin slough. In the dry state, dressings with coarse foam and hydrogel are used to loosen and bind slough and exudate, and in the wet state, dressings with alginate, hydrofibre and superabsorber are used.
- Granulation is between 6 and 8 o'clock and is red. The wound is cleaner and needs rest. Hydrocolloids and soft foams treat the dry state, with alginate, hydrofibre and superabsorber treating the wet state.
- Epithelialisation is between 8 and 10 o'clock and is pink. The wound is in its final phase of healing. Foil or soft foams are sufficient on dry wounds; superabsorbers keep wet wounds dryer.
- The sixth phase is called prevention and is coloured blue. Here again, the cause of the wound has to be taken into account, and preventive measures such as the reduction of risk factors, pressure relief, compression, skincare and appropriate shoes are written into this segment.

23.5 Individualised therapy

The content of the WundUhr® is based on many years of experience in wound treatment, and gives recommendations. Personal experience warrants individual therapy at any time. The illustrated clock allows us to identify the phase and state of the wound and helps to justify an appropriate treatment. A sudden change in the phase and state of the wound requires a change of treatment. Using the simplified graphic helps patients, health care professionals with varying levels of knowledge, and experts to discuss wound assessment and treatment. We must remember that patients with chronic wounds have experience in dealing with their wounds. Many of them have pointed out that not all health care professionals have experience in wound-healing. The clarity of the WundUhr® can help to pick this up.

The webpage www.wunduhr.de has an interactive picture of the WundUhr®. By a click of the mouse, explanations of phases, dressings and treatments (www.wunduhr.de/EN/start.html) can be seen. The interactive WundUhr® is available in German, English and French. In the German version, products of most companies on the German market are integrated, allowing one to look up the names, size and reference numbers of dressings.

The WundUhr® has been translated into 35 dialects and languages, which allows patients to feel at home or to have fun with local pronunciations. (www.wunduhr.de/mundart.html). A feeling of revulsion and rejection sometimes requires us to talk about our wounds in picturesque parables. In WundUhr® dioramas (➤ Fig. 23.5), representations

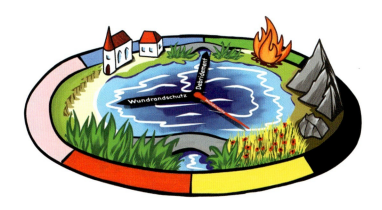

Fig. 23.5 The WundUhr® diorama. [W1093, W1094]

of wound-healing allow an abstracted and sometimes more understandable explanation of phase, state and change of treatment (www.wunduhr.de/3D/index.html).

The first WundUhr® was printed in February 2010. Since then it has been available as a postcard for bedside use or as a poster for wound treatment rooms. Currently over 39,000 printouts have been bought, predominantly in Germany, Austria and Switzerland. The web version, as well as short films on YouTube ('Wunduhr'), support the use of the WundUhr® for patients and health care professionals.

REFERENCES

Riepe G, Bueltemann A. Die WundUhr – Ein interprofessioneller Pfadfinder im Dschungel der modernen, feuchten, phasengerechten Wundbehandlung. Wundmanagement 2011; 5: 130–133.

Riepe G, Bueltemann A. Im Zeichen des Kreislaufs. Altenpflege Dossier 06, Chronische Wunden. 2016. Aus: www.altenpflege-online.net.

24

Joachim Dissemond

Systematics of debridement

── **Key notes** ──

- In the context of symptomatic therapy, debridement should, if necessary, be the first step in phase-adapted wound therapy.
- A single correct debridement process does not exist. Using the various debridement methods is as individual as the patients and the causes of the underlying wound-healing disorders.
- Choosing the appropriate debridement process depends on several factors.
- In individual cases, it may make sense to use a succession of debridement methods.

24.1 Introduction

According to the current expert consensus of the European Wound Management Association (EWMA), debridement is the removal of adhering, dead or contaminated tissue from wounds. Taken into consideration along with the treatment of the underlying causes, debridement is usually the first step in phase-adapted wound treatment. Various treatment methods are usually suitable for the practical implementation of debridement in patients with chronic wounds.

24.2 Autolytic debridement

Autolytic debridement refers to selective necrolysis by releasing the body's proteolytic enzymes, such as collagenase, elastase, myeloperoxidase, acid hydroxylase or lysozyme, and the activation of phagocytes. Also, bacteria are lysed, which releases further proteases such as hyaluronidase. These enzymes dissolve and decompose necrotic tissue and coatings so that they can be cleared away by macrophages.

For the practical implementation of autolytic wound debridement, hydrogels, gel compresses, alginates, hydrofibers, hydrocolloids or so-called wet therapeutics can be used.

Autolytic debridement is selective, painless, safe and straightforward. However, more extended periods are usually required compared to physical methods. With some products, care must also be taken to protect the wound environment, otherwise macerations may occur.

24.3 Proteolytic debridement

For proteolytic debridement, enzymes are usually used to hydrolyse peptide bonds. A gel containing streptokinase and streptodornase is currently available for wound treatment. Streptokinases catalyse the generation of plasmin from plasminogen. Plasmin degrades fibrin, fibrinogen, factor V and factor VIII into polypeptides and amino acids. Streptodornase is a deoxyribonuclease having endonucleolytic activity against double-stranded DNA. The result is fibrin degradation that promotes the removal of avital cell material.

Another wound product is an ointment with a clostridiopeptidase A. It is a collagenase. Collagenases are zinc-containing metalloenzymes from the group of matrix metalloproteinases (MMP) and the only endoproteases that can degrade human collagen. With 70–80% of the dry weight of the skin, collagen is the main component of the human dermis and thus a significant part of the detritus.

Proteolytic debridement is also painless, safe and straightforward. However, it is difficult to apply a high-fat ointment to a moist wound surface. Galenic gels are usually better suited for this purpose.

24.4 Osmotic debridement

In osmotic debridement, absorbent wound products are used. Hyperosmolar sugar derivatives such as dextranomer, in the form of pastes, cadexomer granules, or honey preparations, are used here.

For dextranomer, 1 g can absorb up to 4 ml liquid, for cadexomer it is 7 ml. The currently available cadexomer preparations usually also contain iodine for concurrent antimicrobial therapy. The antimicrobial effectiveness of honey in medical products is under discussion over the osmotic dehydrogenation, a low pH value (3.0–4.5), as well as the release of hydrogen peroxide and methylglyoxal. As honey is a natural product, its effectiveness and composition vary greatly depending on its origin.

Osmotic debridement can be performed quickly and safely. The most notable side-effect is the marked pain, which can already occur during treatment and the removal of bandages.

24.5 Mechanical debridement

For mechanical debridement, sterile cotton compresses or special disposable products can be used, for example.

Sterile cotton compresses are a traditionally used, inexpensive and safe method of removing loose coatings. One modification is the so-called wet-to-dry method. Moistened cotton compresses are applied to the wound. The pre-moistened cotton dries out, hardens and sticks to the compress, which is then removed with the adhesive material.

So-called monofilament fibre products are currently produced as pads and a Lolly. They are made of unbleached polyester with bevelled fibre tips. According to the manufacturer, the pad (10 × 10 cm) consists of a composite of 18 million fibres. Using a wound irrigation solution, the soft fibre side is moistened and used to wipe the wound and the periwound skin in circular movements with gentle pressure (➤ Fig. 24.1). Deeper wounds or wound cavities can also be treated with the Lolly.

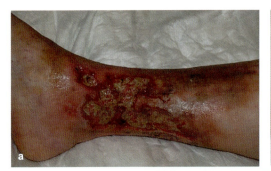
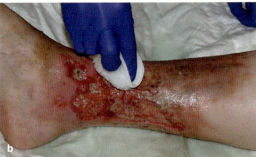
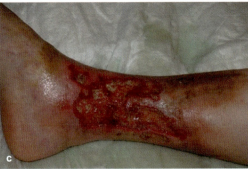

Fig. 24.1 Monofilament fibre pad. [P580]

There is also a ready-to-use, sterile and premoistened wound cleansing wipe. The wipe consists of viscose with a cleaning solution of poloxamer, allantoin and aloe vera extracts. The manufacturer recommends it not only for cleaning wounds but also for the wound margin and the care of the wound environment.

Mechanical debridement can usually be carried out safely and in a short time. Only with the wet-to-dry method are longer time intervals necessary. The use of sterile cotton compresses is the cheapest method of debridement. The most crucial limitation in mechanical debridement is the resulting pain. In this case, appropriate considerations for adequate analgesia must be made before performing the procedure (➤ Chap. 44). Compared to other mechanical debridement options, the use of monofilament fibre products often results in less pain. Mechanical debridement is usually not suitable for the removal of very firmly adhering coatings or necroses.

24.6 Surgical debridement

For surgical debridement, scissors, surgical forceps, so-called sharp spoons, scalpels or ring curettes can be used (➤ Fig. 24.2). The surgical incision does not allow exact selection of the vital tissue so that residual necroses may remain in the wounds or bleeding may occur. Following surgical debridement, alginate dressings, for example, can be applied to the wounds, for a haemostatic effect.

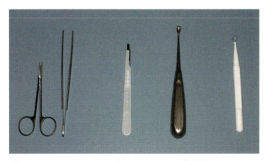

Fig. 24.2 Scissors, surgical tweezers, so-called sharp spoons, scalpels or ring curettes can be used for surgical debridement. [P580]

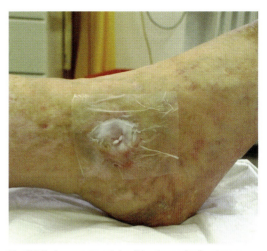

Fig. 24.3 A cream containing lidocaine and prilocaine was applied to a leg ulcer one hour before a planned surgical debridement and then covered with an occlusive foil dressing. [P580]

Surgical debridement is usually the first method chosen for treating more extensive chronic wounds with necroses or firmly adhering coatings as extensively and quickly as possible. Always ensure sufficient analgesia before surgical debridement. For smaller operations, topical therapy with local anaesthetics is often enough (➤ Fig. 24.3; ➤ Chap. 41). In severe cases, surgical debridement should be performed in an operating theatre with appropriate anaesthesia.

24.7 Biosurgical debridement

Biosurgery is the treatment of wounds with fly larvae bred under sterile conditions. The commercial rearing of fly larvae today takes place following disinfection of the eggs on a special sterile culture medium. The hatched larvae can be stored at 7–8 °C for up to five days. The larvae of the gold fly (*Lucilia sericata*), for example, are suitable for use in wound treatment. In biosurgical debridement, selective necrolysis occurs due to the extracorporeal digestion of the larvae. Ingredients of the digestive secretion are ammonia, calcium carbonate, allantoin, urea, trypsin and chymotrypsin-like proteases, collagenases and various

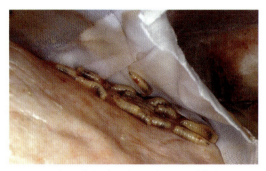

Fig. 24.4 Three days after the application of fly larvae, the bandage of the biosurgical debridement is removed. [P580]

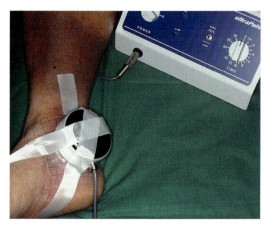

Fig. 24.5 Low-frequency ultrasound is applied to a leg ulcer by a hydrogel dressing. [P580]

antibacterial peptides such as lucifensin. Due to these properties, biosurgery is also suitable for patients in whom gram-positive bacteria, including MRSA, are to be reduced. However, it should be noted that *Lucilia sericata* larvae are sensitive to *Pseudomonas aeruginosa* and may die on contact.

The larvae can be applied to wounds either as loose larvae or in biobags. Larvae require approx. 5–10 larvae/cm^2 of the wound surface. A kind of cage has to be built in this instance with a net and stoma paste (➤ Fig. 24.4). Indications for the use of larvae are, for example, ragged and irregularly configured wounds. In the case of biobags, the larvae are already inside a polyester mesh bag, so that application and removal are much less time-consuming. However, the biobags may have to be positioned on different wound areas during treatment, as they only work where there is direct contact with the wound.

The dressing is changed after 3–4 days. The initial 2–3 mm large larvae are already 10–15 mm large at this time. The movement of the larvae stimulates exudate production, which contributes to better flushing of the wound and removal of bacteria. Here it must be checked whether the secondary dressing should be changed more frequently. With the wound dressings, it is to be noted that the larvae need sufficient liquid, are not suffocated or crushed. Further problems can result from the concomitant extremely unpleasant smell caused by proteolysis or from pain. It is debated whether the pain is caused by larvae movement or pH shift. Otherwise, biosurgery is a safe method that can also be performed on an outpatient basis.

24.8 Debridement with ultrasound or hydrotherapies

Various qualitative forms of ultrasound can be used for wound debridement. The coupling of low-frequency ultrasound is applied directly or indirectly and either continuously or pulsed via a transducer at the site of action. The application types available are, for example, a water bath (➤ Fig. 24.5) or a hydrogel dressing. With a so-called ultrasonic dissector, low-frequency power ultrasound can be used via a handpiece (➤ Fig. 24.6). The coupling takes place via the liquid flowing through the handpiece.

The mode of action of ultrasound can be subdivided into mechanical effects, in particular on tissue surfaces, mechano-acoustic/bio-acoustic effects, in particular on microorganisms, and thermal and non-thermal effects, in particular on deeper tissue layers. The essential mechanism in mediating the effect of ultrasound on wounds is the phenomenon of cavitation. Cavitation describes the formation of minute bubbles in a liquid medium by ultrasound-induced compression-tension forces that oscillate (stable cavitation) and implode (transient cavitation), resulting in microflows and pressure gradients.

Hydrotherapies are various methods in which liquids are used for debridement. The simplest treatment option is to use a shower. When using tap water, it should be noted that sterile filters should be used. The methods are known variously as high-pres-

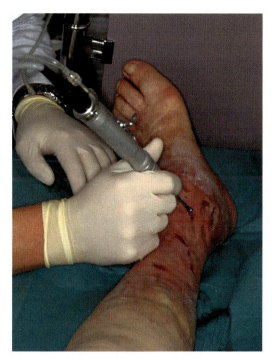

Fig. 24.6 Debridement of leg ulcers with low-frequency power ultrasound. [P580]

Table 24.1 Some of the factors to be considered in choosing a suitable debridement method for chronic wounds
The patient's pain
The patient's preferences
Cofactors and co-morbidities of patients
The skills and resources of health care professionals
Treatment setting
Economic aspects
Regulations and guidelines

sure irrigation, waterjet cutting or waterjet dissection, and apply liquids that have been accelerated to speeds of up to 1,000 km/h by high-pressure, up to 800 bar.

It is propagated that these physical wound treatments not only lead to a relatively selective removal of coatings but that microorganisms can also be effectively removed. The advantages of these devices are the good controllability and the easy handling, which can partly be taken over by patients or relatives. Disadvantages are among other things the regular disinfection required of the devices (also of the environment to some extent), the expenditure of time and the costs.

24.9 Discussion

The current European expert consensus has defined debridement as the profound removal of adherent, dead or contaminated tissue from wounds. Wound cleansing differs in focusing on the removal of contaminants, such as non-adherent metabolic waste products. Both terms should be used separately. For all wounds, it should be checked whether and which debridement is necessary at the beginning of wound treatment. In the further course of wound treatment, it may then be advisable to carry out wound cleansing regularly.

A retrospective analysis of 154,644 patients and 364,534 wounds of different entities showed that frequently debrided wounds resulted in faster wound-healing. There were patients who had gone through up to 138 debridements. This study is a good example of the different use of terms. Wound cleansing and debridement were considered in combination.

When necessary, debridement is an essential part of wound treatment. This fundamental principle has now been well proven in numerous scientific studies. However, debridements should not be carried out in the longterm and indiscriminately. Various factors should be taken into account in choosing a suitable debridement method (➤ Table 24.1).

24.10 Conclusion

Debridement is often the first step in phase-adapted wound treatment, and which therapeutic option is used depends on several different individual factors. Several methods are also suitable for the application of combined or successive therapy.

REFERENCES
Dissemond J, Goos M. Options for debridement in the therapy of chronic wounds. J Dtsch Dermatol Ges 2004; 2: 743–51.
Edwards J, Stapley S. Debridement of diabetic foot ulcers. Cochrane Database Syst Rev 2010; 1: CD003556.

Gethin G, Cowman S, Kolbach DN. Debridement for venous leg ulcers. Cochrane Database Syst Rev 2015; 9: CD008599.

Strohal R, Dissemond J, Jordan O'Brien J, et al. An updated overview and clarification of the principle role of debridement. J Wound Care 2013; 22 (Suppl.): 1–52.

Wilcox JR, Carter MJ, Covington S. Frequency of debridements and time to heal: a retrospective cohort study of 312 744 wounds. JAMA Dermatol 2013; 149: 1050–1058.

25 Systematics of infection control

Andreas Schwarzkopf

Key notes

- From an infectiological point of view, contamination (where potential pathogens adhere to the wound surface, initially without multiplication) is distinguished from colonisation (with augmentation but without signs of infection) and infection (with the symptoms of dolor, calor, rubor, tumour and functio laesa as well as possibly septic or lymphatic scattering).
- From the point of view of microorganisms and viruses, humans are the hosts that provide them with everything they need to reproduce. Host disposition describes the general condition and, to a certain extent, the behaviour of a wounded patient. The wound condition is directly dependent on this.

- Wound irrigation solutions are differentiated from antiseptics. Although the composition is partly identical, there is a different legal definition. Flushing solutions support mechanical debridement and can be preserved with antimicrobial substances. As a rule, they are sold as medical devices. Antiseptics are intended to kill bacteria in wounds and should be marketed as drugs.
- Local, easily accessible and open wound infections can be treated antiseptically after debridement or, at least, extensive mechanical cleansing. Systemic antibiotic therapy is indicated if, for example, lymphadenitis or phlegmon or erysipelas occur.

25.1 Introduction

Billions of potential pathogens populate our environment. Whatever we do, we absorb reproductive microorganisms and viruses. Our food is full of bacteria and fungi, every surface around us is more or less contaminated, just as every living entity, from the annoying housefly to the domestic cat or the family dog, up to one's own partner as well as the children, of course.

The fact that infections generally do not take up a lot of space in our lives is due to our millennia-old immune system. Macrophages, granulocytes and the complement system, as well as the secretory IgA on all mucous membranes, ensure a balance that usually prevents infections. Even our bacteria contribute to our protection through various mechanisms, such as the family flora, which fights enemy pathogens with defensins and makes disinfection in the household not only superfluous but also harmful.

Another essential mechanism is the barrier effect of our skin, which is disrupted when a wound

appears. Thrombocytes carry out an emergency closure, and bacteria of the skin surface create a colonisation resistance through rapid colonisation. Even if the skin is injured, an immediate balance is sought. As a rule, the skin heals quickly. However, factors such as diabetes, microcirculation disorders and oxygen deficiency can make the situation so unfavourable that a chronic wound develops (➤ Fig. 25.1). It is the task of the wound experts to avoid the transition from colonisation to infection and to ensure rapid treatment in the case of infection. Impulses for these treatment strategies are given in this chapter.

25.2 Infection of wounds

Each wound allows mostly bacteria and not so many fungi to settle there. Whether the **contamination** (potential pathogens adhering to the wound surface, initially without multiplication) becomes **colo-**

25

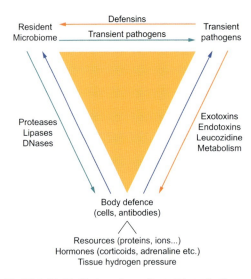

Resident Microbiome — Transient pathogens — Defensins — Transient pathogens

Proteases
Lipases
DNases

Exotoxins
Endotoxins
Leucozidine
Metabolism

Body defence
(cells, antibodies)

Resources (proteins, ions...)
Hormones (corticoids, adrenaline etc.)
Tissue hydrogen pressure

Fig. 25.1 Model of balance (according to Schwarzkopf, 2002). [P583/L231]

Table 25.1 Examples of factors influencing host disposition

(General) Condition	Wound condition
Age, protein synthesis	Delayed wound-healing due to relative protein deficiency
Mobility, muscle pump	Supply of the wound with oxygen and nutrients
Nutrition, e.g. lack of protein, calories, trace elements such as zinc, selenium	Decreased activity of cellular defence (macrophages, neutrophilic granulocytes, T-cells)
Underlying diseases, e.g. diabetes mellitus, malignancies, hypercholesterolemia	Reduction of microcirculation (partial oxygen pressure of the tissue)
Therapies, e.g. immunosuppressants, dialysis	Reduced function of the immune system
Recreational and other drugs, e.g. nicotine, alcohol, drugs	Oxygen deficiency in the tissue, nutrient deficiencies
Lack of health and medical care	Sequestrum, biofilm, necroses
Lack of pain therapy	Distress and delay in healing

nisation (with augmentation but without signs of infection) or **infection** (described in ancient times as dolor, calor, rubor, tumor and functio laesa) and possibly becomes a septic or lymphatic scattering, depends on several factors. The term 'critical colonisation', which is usually still seen as halfway between colonisation and infection, must be viewed with scepticism and must not neglect a consistent causal search. Bacteria are the beneficiaries rather than the causes.

25.3 Host disposition

From the point of view of microorganisms and viruses, humans are the hosts that provide them with everything they need. Host disposition describes the general condition and, to a certain extent, the behaviour of a wounded patient (➤ Table 25.1). The condition of the wound is directly dependent on this. Increasingly, some findings suggest that specific human genes also facilitate access for pathogens.

An essential factor for any wound treatment is also, from the point of view of preventing infection, that the condition of the wound should, as far as possible, be kept undisturbed – the risk of a possible infection

results from potential pathogens coming into contact with the wound.

In chronic wounds, in particular, a **balance** between colonising pathogens and the immune system is usually established, preventing infection but also delaying healing, or making it almost impossible, which is the case for example with pronounced **biofilm formation.** Biofilm is a protective mucous formed by bacteria into which existing material such as exudate residues and micronecroses are incorporated. It is also known as matrix or glycocalyx and, to a certain extent, protects the microorganisms living in it from the effects of antiseptics and antibiotics.

The microbial colonisation of the wound, according to the invading species, is relatively unspecific relative to the cause of the wound. In most cases, they are potential pathogens from the patient's flora or its environment, including tap water used for body cleansing, but also the flora of relatives and pets.

Balanced colonisation is therefore microbiologically characterised by a variety of bacteria and possibly fungi, which coexist relatively peacefully with the body's defence system. However, therapeutic measures and situational conditions lead to shifts. For example, *Pseudomonas aeruginosa,* which with its two green dyes pyoverdin and pyocyanin, is a potent disinfectant against annoying competitors, and poses a typical risk for large-scale burn injuries. This one-sided infestation holds a bigger infection-risk than a colourful bacteria-mix, with which the individual representatives also hold each other in check. Relatively high germ counts are not necessarily detrimental to wound-healing. The relationship between the microorganisms shifts when an infection is present; the colourful diversity gives way to one or two dominant strains, the actual infectious agents.

Wound infection is a clinical diagnosis and can therefore only be supported by microbiological and laboratory findings on inflammation markers such as the C-reactive protein.

Overheating, redness, pain, swelling of the wound margins, signs of lack of healing or stagnation characterise this condition as a rule.

Also, complications can occur, such as the spread of infection by specific pathogens in the skin or the spread via the lymphatic system or the bloodstream, which can lead to metastases elsewhere in the body and requires systemic antibiotic therapy. At this point it is possible to react therapeutically with the use of anti-infectives.

Anti-infectives are the generic term for antibiotics and antiseptics.

Antibiotics always have a spectrum, i.e. no antibiotic covers all possible pathogens, some even only act on certain groups. For example, vancomycin, linezolid and daptomycin can only be used against gram-positive bacteria. The effect of the antibiotics is based on a selective disturbance of the bacterial cell metabolism, which becomes possible after cell contact. As a rule, however, the bacteria have time to develop resistance, so that antibiotic resistances are not uncommon.

Antiseptics do not have a spectrum, i.e. they detect practically all possible bacteria. The effect is based on the depolarisation of the bacterial cell wall and rapid blocking of bacterial enzymes. In both cases, the metabolism breaks down, and the bacteria have no time to develop resistance, so that antiseptic resistances are still very rare.

The following conclusions can be drawn from the above:

- Additional exposure of the wound surface to other pathogens, e.g. through prolonged exposure to air or the use of non-sterile materials in the treatment, should be avoided.
- Local antimicrobial measures must cover the entire spectrum of potential pathogens settling on the wound to avoid disturbing the fragile balance and thus increasing the risk of infection. This means that local antibiotics cannot be administered on their own, as no antibiotic covers the entire spectrum in question. Exceptions to this rule are high, locally applied doses of gentamicin or vancomycin, for example in Palacos chains, sponges or spacers.

25.4 Laboratory diagnostics

Microbiological diagnostics can provide valuable information on treatment and occupational safety, especially for chronic wounds. Even if modern examinations show that not all pathogens present on the wound may be detected in a wound swab, an examination is always useful if multi-resistant organisms (MROs) are suspected or signs of infection are present.

Wound swabs are most effective when taken from the wound bed. A large area of the swab should be moistened. In preparation, the wound can be carefully wiped with a sterile compress, or if this is too painful for the patient, rinsed with sterile saline solution (without antiseptic additives). This method is not necessary if screening for MROs is all that is required.

Finally, it is recommended to smear or touch several different wound areas with the obtained swab (as the distribution of the bacteria to be detected on the wound surface is not always uniform), which is guaranteed when using the 'Essen Rotary technique' (➤ Fig. 25.2). Swabs and tissue samples obtained intraoperatively must be marked to trace their localisation. If numbers, e.g. 1–5, are used, it must be ensured that all colleagues who care for the patient should know the numbers, to be able to evaluate the findings reliably.

In case of dry wounds and suspected infestation with non-tuberculous mycobacteria (NTM, mycobac-

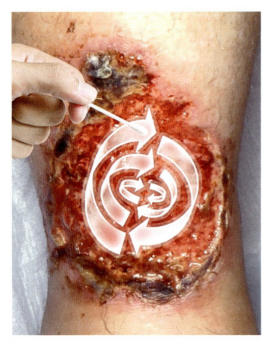

Fig. 25.2 'Essener Rotary technique'. [P583]

teria other than tubercle bacilli), suspicion of leishmania or repeatedly ambiguous smear findings, a **wound biopsy** or a **sample excision** is more useful (➤ Table 25.2). In this case, place the material in a sterile tube with a drop of distilled water (to prevent dehydration). The examination for NTM or leishmania

must be explicitly requested from the laboratory on the examination order.

In general, swabs and biopsies should be brought to the respective laboratories as quickly as possible. When it is not possible, storage at room temperature may lead to an increase in the pathogen numbers and thus to a shift in the image. If the smear is stored in the refrigerator, however, a loss of anaerobes is to be expected. This is because anaerobic pathogens are often not very tolerant to cold and die, while the facultative anaerobes survive in the refrigerator with approximately the same initial bacterial count.

Additional inflammation markers are often determined. The C-reactive protein proves to be a useful, albeit unspecific, marker that, in contrast to procalcitonin, also reacts to local processes. In abscesses, the number of neutrophil granulocytes in the differential blood count will increase only slightly. If the infection spreads in the sense of lymphadenitis or haematogenic scattering, leucocytosis will occur, and procalcitonin will also increase to a greater or lesser extent.

Since diabetes mellitus is a significant risk factor for the spread of infections, diabetes control should be regularly monitored, and the patient asked to comply/adhere.

The question of pus formation can also say something about the pathogens (➤ Table 25.3).

Table 25.2 Summary of indications and practical implementation of microbiological diagnostics in patients with wounds

Bacteriological swab without prior wound-cleansing
Detection/exclusion of multi-resistant pathogens → screening
Bacteriological swab with prior wound-cleansing
• Detection of causal pathogens in wound infection • Colonisation/infection with yeast fungi
Biopsy/Excision
• Wound infection in patients with deeper ulcerations, e.g. diabetic foot ulcer • Fistula tissue, if no fistula content can be obtained • Suspected pathogens: mycobacteria, leishmania, actinomycetes, nocardia, moulds • Wound infection without pathogen detection in the smear

Table 25.3 Sample presentation of some pathogens

Pathogen more likely to cause purulent wound infections	Pathogen more likely to cause non-purulent wound infections
Staphylococcus aureus *Streptococcus*, especially *Streptococcus pyogenes* (Group A)	*Pasteurella multocida*
Enterococci	*Alcaligenes* *Flavobacteria* *Aeromonas*
Enterobacteriaceae, such as *E. coli, Proteus*, …	*Clostridia*, such as *C. perfringens*
Pseudomonas aeruginosa, Burkholderia cepacia, Stenotrophomonas maltophilia	Yeast fungi such as *Candida albicans* Moulds such as *Alternaria* and *Aspergillus*

25.5 Wound-cleaning and disinfection

With the initial mechanical cleaning of wounds, care must be taken to ensure that cleaning is always carried out from the inside out and beyond the wound margins, followed by gentle rinsing, if necessary, with subsequent antibacterial treatment.

A distinction must be made between wound irrigation solutions and antiseptics. Although the composition is partly identical, there is a different legal definition.

Flushing solutions support mechanical debridement and can be preserved with antimicrobial substances. As a rule, they are sold as medical devices.

Antiseptics are intended to kill bacteria in wounds and are to be marketed as drugs.

The requirements for a **wound irrigation solution** are defined in the European Pharmacopoeia (Ph. Eur.). They should be kept in single-use, sterile containers. If the quantity required for rinsing is in a container, e. g. with physiological saline solution or Ringer's solution, this condition is fulfilled. If instead, infusion solutions are provided in litre bottles, and multiple doses for different rinsing cycles are taken from them over a more extended period, this will constitute a violation of pharmaceutical law as the so-called multidose containers must be preserved and provided with an expiry date from the first piercing.

This manufacturer's information must be observed; therefore, the date and time of the first opening or puncture must be marked. Before any further use, check that the expiry date has not already been reached. The draining rinsing solution is contaminated and must be collected safely.

Tap water is recommended in the literature as a wound irrigation solution. However, it should be noted that most of the relevant studies originate from the USA with correspondingly higher chlorination of the tap network. According to the Drinking Water Ordinance, 100 CFU (colony-forming unit = one reproducing bacterium) per ml are permissible directly from the pipeline. In the case of older pipeline networks and calcified fittings, higher bacterial counts must be expected, especially in residential areas, including *P. aeruginosa* as a known coloniser and wound infection pathogen. Only sterilised tap water is recommended for use in wound treatment, which is possible with the use of connected sterile filters with a pore size of 0.2 μm.

With **wound disinfection using antiseptics,** reference is made to the 2018 update of the Consensus on Wound Antisepsis. There is also a Consensus recommendation on polihexanide. In principle, the colourless antiseptics octenidine and polihexanide are now recommended for wound disinfection and cleansing, with different galenic preparations such as rinsing solutions and gels available. Silver can be used in dressing materials (> Table 25.4). The application of all antimicrobial substances should be critically examined after 14 days at the latest. The manufacturer's instructions must be observed concerning prolonged use.

Table 25.4 Properties of important antiseptics

Active substance	Application time	Contraindications	Remarks
Alcohol (70%)	15–30 seconds	Alcohol disease	Burns, protein coagulation
Octenidine	1–5 minutes	Wound cavities, fistulas	Use also in remanent skin disinfection
Polihexanide	About 20 minutes	Cartilage contact	Extensive use in cosmetics, therefore allergies are possible, MRSA sanitation
Chlorhexidine	About 20 minutes	Considered obsolete!	Delayed effect in the gram-negative range
Povidone-iodine (PVP)	2–5 minutes	Hypothyroidism	Discolouration from brown to yellow when the effect is over
Silver	Depending on shape, minutes to about half an hour	Pseudomonas infections	Tolerance/resistance in *P. aeruginosa* and *E. coli* considered relatively cytotoxic
Sodium hypochlorite	1–5 minutes	Not sufficiently evaluated	Effect results from the elimination of chlorine ions, complete decay

PVP iodine is assessed more cautiously due to its brown colouration and comparatively higher in vitro cell toxicity, but remains an approved drug. The relatively new cadexomer iodine has different release kinetics and is available as dressing material.

Maggot therapy (biosurgery) with larvae of the gold fly *Lucilia sericata* represents a combination of moderate bacterial reduction and proper necrosis removal but is only available in hospitals.

Enzymatic or **autolytic** cleansing procedures usually have little effect on the colonisation of wounds.

25.6 Therapy of wound infections

Local, easily accessible and open wound infections can be treated antiseptically after debridement or, at the least, extensive mechanical cleansing. Systemic antibiotic therapy is indicated if, for example, lymphadenitis or phlegmon or erysipelas occur. In the case of postoperative infections in the surgical area, antibiotic treatment is also required for deep infections.

Initially, antibiotics against gram-positive bacteria are recommended in this situation. These pathogens account for about 70% of the pathogens in question. Combinations of group 1 cephalosporins with rifampicin or fosfomycin i. v. are also suitable – especially when implants are involved. Vancomycin or linezolid are also frequently used. Linezolid is also available orally but should be used cautiously due to the risk of resistance formation, especially in the case of vancomycin-resistant enterococci.

In erysipelas, mostly caused by *Streptococcus pyogenes*, penicillin remains the first choice. Since other accompanying pathogens often maintain the necrotising fasciitis, a broad coverage, e. g. with meropenem, is recommended in this emergency situation, in addition to the immediate operation. According to the new guidelines, the combination of beta-lactam antibiotics with the aminoglycoside gentamicin is recommended again, whereby 240 mg can be given once as a short infusion for three days in the absence of the possibility of determining serum levels.

A calculated antibiotic dose must be evaluated after 72 hours at the latest. If the results are available by then, the procedure will be adjusted or de-escalated. If the findings are not yet available and the condition worsens, a renewed debridement, an escalation and additionally the local use of antiseptics is recommended (note contraindications such as cartilage contact).

In chronic wounds, systemic use of antibiotics is less successful due to the combination of biofilm and microcirculation disorder and should, therefore, be strictly indicated. After debridement, the application of antiseptics makes sense. The ICW e. V. recommends a critical evaluation of antiseptic administration after 14 days at the latest. If there is no effect, the cause must be looked for again. The aim of such an examination can be microcirculation disorders but also sequesters, necroses, abscesses and fistulas. As a rule, only a renewed surgical intervention can lead to a lasting improvement.

Also, metabolic diseases such as diabetes mellitus should be treated as well as possible. Affected patients should smoke as little as possible and eat a balanced diet.

25.7 Conclusion

The treatment of wound infection takes place in three important steps:
1. Diagnostics, typical symptoms, microbiology
2. Therapy, locally with debridement and antiseptics, only in the case of systemic spread antibiotics
3. Prevention of recurrence, establishment or improvement of microcirculation.

However, this also requires the cooperation of the patients concerned, who must be motivated accordingly.

REFERENCES

Dissemond J, Gerber V, Kramer A, et al. Praxisorientierte Empfehlung zur Behandlung kritisch kolonisierter und lokal infizierter Wunden mit Polihexanid. Wundmanagement 2009; 2: 62–68.

Jassoy C, Schwarzkopf A (Hrsg.). Hygiene, Infektiologie, Mikrobiologie. 3. A. Stuttgart, New York: Thieme; 2018.

Kramer A, Dissemond J, Kim S, et al. Consensus on wound antisepsis: an update. Skin Pharmacol Physiol 2018; 31: 28–58.

Schwarzkopf A, Dissemond J. Indications and practical implementation of microbiologic diagnostics in patients with chronic wounds. J Dtsch Dermatol Ges 2015; 13: 203–209.

Schwarzkopf A. Wunde auswischen – aber wie? Wundmanagement 2017; 11: 304–305.

Wysocki AB. Evaluating and managing open skin wounds: colonization versus infection. AACN Clin Issues 2002; 3: 382–397.

25

26

Kerstin Protz, Joachim Dissemond

Systematics of wound therapeutics

26.1 Wound dressings

Kerstin Protz

Key notes

- Although an optimal wound dressing can support wound-healing, it is only possible to initiate the healing process adequately by engaging with causal therapy, treatment and elimination of the causes and successful patient education.
- Adequate wound-cleansing is the prerequisite for optimal wound assessment and the basis for successful healing. Only a clean wound can heal. Therefore, at the beginning of any wound care, the focus is on adequate debridement.
- Products that can cancel each other out in their physical effect should not be used in combi-

nation. For example, alginates, hydrofibre, fine-pored polyurethane foam dressings or nonwoven dressings with superabsorbers absorb the moisture of hydrogels. Justified exceptions should be weighed up in individual cases.
- One product is often sufficient for wound care. For economic reasons, the rule of thumb is to use a maximum of two products, as well as fixative materials if necessary, such as elastic gauze bandages, tubular bandages or film dressings.

26.1.1 Introduction

Various decision criteria need to be taken into consideration for the selection of an individually adapted wound dressing. The standard today is phase-specific moist wound care. The following measures should be taken into account when selecting an individual wound dressing: wound stage and phase, possible signs of infection or an already existing infection, exudate quantity and condition, condition of wound margin and periwound skin, continence situation of the patient as well as existing odours. Further aspects are cost-effectiveness, manageability and the patient's acceptance of the dressing. The change interval depends on the healing state of the wound and the correct ratio between exudation of the wound and absorbency of the wound dressing.

26.1.2 Treatment options in different wound stages

In the following, various local treatment options are presented, each of which is based on wound stages and conditions.

NOTE
The information compiled here provides a brief, practice-oriented overview and does not absolve the reader from reading the respective manufacturer's informations carefully!

Necroses and fibrin coatings

Adequate wound-cleansing is the prerequisite for optimal wound assessment and a basis for successful healing. The methods of wound-cleansing and debridement are already described in ➤ Chap. 24. Therefore, only local wound-cleansing with certain wound products which remain on the wounds is discussed here.

When treating wounds with dressings, a distinction must be made between dry and moist surfaces. First of all, the possibilities of using the product for wounds with slightly dry surfaces are described.

C A V E

Dry necroses, e. g. in the case of peripheral artery disease (PAD), should only be removed after successful revascularisation or to relieve acute infections. Under no circumstances should they be softened by wound products before such an treatment. Until then, only dry dressing changes should be performed.

In autolytic wound cleansing, the body's own self-cleaning processes are supported and accelerated by the supply of moisture. As a result, necroses and coatings lose their firmness and detach from the wound bed. This autolysis process is gentle but slow and can be supported by products such as hydrogels or hydro-responsive wound dressings (HRWD).

Hydrogel as tube gel or as hydrogel dressing

Hydrogels are available as tube gels (➤ Table 26.1), or hydrogel dressings (➤ Table 26.2). They consist of up to 95% of water; further components are gelling agents and alginates in part. Hydrogels are insoluble in water and have an action duration up to three days as tube gels, and up to seven days as dressings. Preserved tube gels, e. g. with polihexanide or octenidine, are increasingly available. Their economic advantage is the prolonged usability after opening (see package insert).

Table 26.1 Hydrogel as tube gel (➤ Fig. 26.1)	
Goals and characteristics	• Autolytic effect: supported by the release of moisture, it breaks down necroses and fibrin coatings, among other things. • Promotes granulation • Can partially store exudate • Stable (only unpreserved gels); can thus be applied well to difficult body parts such as the heel region without flowing away • Keeps the wound surface moist, hydrates dry wounds • Initially cooling effect • Atraumatic dressing change
Indications	• Dry wounds • Necroses and coatings • 2Nd-degree burns • Exposed tendons, bones, cartilage, muscles
Contraindications	• Known hypersensitivity to the product or its ingredients (**cave:** preservatives, e. g. propylene glycol) • Necroses and coatings for untreated PAD • Severe weeping and bleeding wounds • 3rd and 4th-degree burns • Not approved for the treatment of infected wounds • Some products are contraindicated for surgical implants • Some products with antiseptic ingredients may not be used in the area of cartilage and joints
Application notes	• Length of use: 1–3 days depending on the thickness of the coatings • Apply to a thickness of approx. 0.3–0.5 cm. • Secondary dressing required; for slightly dry coatings with a sterile transparent film (increased autolytic effect), for slightly moist coatings with a fine-pored polyurethane foam dressing to absorb excess wound exudate; to save on costs with daily dressing changes, cover with a wound contact layer and sterile (suction) gauzes • Gel residues can be removed with a sterile wound irrigation solution
Complications	• Incompatibility/allergy • Overdose, lack of skin protection or too long a change interval can all lead to maceration • Wound pain and burning, especially in patients with inflammatory or arterial wounds

Table 26.2 Hydrogel dressings (➤ Fig. 26.2)

Goals and characteristics	• Good wound control through transparency • Pain-relieving due to initial cooling effect • Light cushioning function • Granulation-promoting • Rehydration of dry wounds • Autolytic effect • Can partially store exudate
Indications	• Slight to moderately exuding wounds • Superficial, clean abrasions • Clean wounds at risk of drying out • Wounds in the granulation and epithelialisation phase • Split skin removal points • 2nd-degree burns • Cleansing of chronic, stagnant wounds
Contraindications	• Known hypersensitivity or allergy to the product or its ingredients • Clinically infected wounds, deep fungal infections • Strongly exuding or bleeding wounds • 3rd- and 4th-degree burns
Application notes	• Length of use: 1–7 days depending on exudation • Can also be used for wounds on paper-thin skin, due to cortisone damage or age, but only without an adhesive framing or adhesive dressing • The initial cooling effect may be painful for patients with arterial wounds • Wound dressing can be removed without leaving residues
Complications	• Lncompatibility/allergy • Maceration of the periwound skin • Hypergranulation

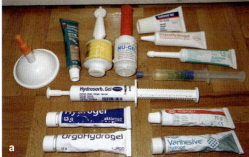

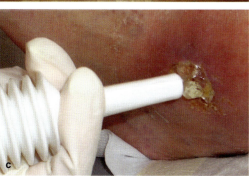

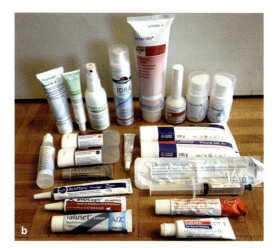

Fig. 26.1 a Exemplary product overview of unpreserved hydrogels as tube gels; **b** exemplary product overview of preserved hydrogels as tube gels; **c** application of a hydrogel. [M291]

26

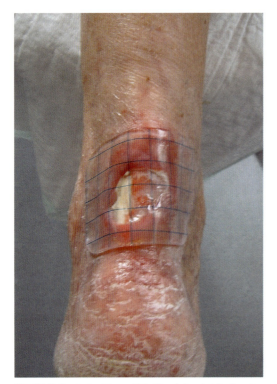

Fig. 26.2 Exposed tendon with hydrogel dressing for keeping moist. [M291]

These products, however, are mostly liquid compared to unpreserved tube gels. The latter are to be used only once, recognisable by the pictogram with the crossed-out 2.

Hydro-responsive wound dressings (HRWD)

The hydro-responsive wound dressing (HRDW) is a multi-layer, cushion-shaped wound dressing and consists of an absorbent cushion with superabsorbent polyacrylate embedded in cellulose and cellulose fibres (➤ Table 26.3). This wound dressing is already activated with Ringer's solution, ready for use. The wound contact side consists of a polypropylene knitted fabric to which silicone strips are applied. This is to prevent sticking to the wound bed. The side facing away from the wound contains a waterproof

Table 26.3 Hydro-responsive wound dressings (➤ Fig. 26.3)

Goals and characteristics	• Delivers Ringer's solution to the wound for up to three days, keeping the wound constantly moist • Absorbs wound exudate in turn; in addition, toxins, cell debris, proteases and bacteria-contaminated wound exudate are absorbed and removed from the wound during the change of the dressing • Promotion of granulation
Indications	Deep, fissured wounds and wound cavities (applies to the 'Cavity' product support for wound-cleansing)
Contraindications	Known hypersensitivity/allergy to the product or its ingredients
Application notes	• Length of stay: 1–3 days depending on wound condition • Never cut or damage the wrapping • Establish contact of the dressing to the wound bed • If necessary, cover with a second dressing and cover or fix with elastic gauze bandage/tubular bandage or adhesive fleece • If the wound dressing adheres to the wound bed, rinse with Ringer's solution before removing • Do not introduce topical medication or disinfectants into the wound or combine them with the product
Complications	• With initial application of the product, the wound may be enlarged by the degradation of avital tissue • The supply of moisture can lead to maceration (→ skin protection) • Reddening of the wound margins due to reactivated blood circulation

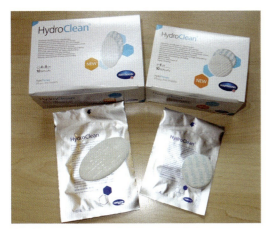

Fig. 26.3 Overview of hydro-responsive wound dressings. [M291]

polypropylene film together with a hydrophobic polypropylene nonwoven fabric on top.

If moist wound coatings are present, wound dressings are used which support the cleansing of the wound but do not add more moisture to it. These include special cleaning cloths, sponges and pads, soft-adherent dressings with poly-absorbent fibres, alginates, hydrofiber/gelling fibre dressings and a polymer membrane dressing.

Soft-adherent dressing with poly-absorbent fibres

Soft-adherent dressing with poly-absorbent fibres and polyacrylate are available with and without silver as a sterile fleece dressing with a micro-adhesive lipid colloid matrix (TLC), or as a tamponade (but without silver) with a sterile application aid (➤ Fig. 26.4; ➤ Table 26.4).

Alginate

Alginates can be used well for the cleaning of moist coatings – both superficially and in cavity wounds – if they have sufficient moisture (exudative cleaning phase). Alginates can only be tamponated loosely and must not overlap the wound margin → risk of maceration. These products are described in detail below (➤ Table 26.13).

Hydrofibre/gelling fibre dressings

Hydrofibre/gelling fibre dressings can also be used well for the cleaning of damp coatings – both on the surface and in cavity wounds – with sufficient moisture (exudative cleaning phase). These products are also described in detail below (➤ Table 26.14).

Polymeric membrane dressing

Polymeric membrane dressings are medium-pored foams which are available with or without an adhesive facing, with or without added silver and for different quantities of exudate (from little to a lot) optionally with superabsorbents (➤ Table 26.5). They contain glycerine and the surfactant F68, a non-ionic, non-toxic, mild wound cleanser. This enters the wound bed with gradual release of moisture and supports autolytic wound cleansing.

Infected wounds

The most common complication in wound-healing is local infection, which in individual cases can lead to systemic infection or even sepsis (➤ Fig. 26.6).

Fig. 26.4 Cleansing with a soft-adherent dressing with poly-absorbent fibres before (**a**) and after (**b**) one day of dressing change. [M291]

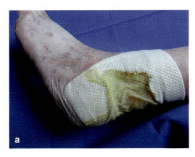
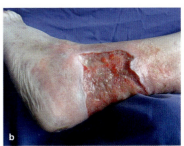

Table 26.4 Soft-adherent dressing with poly-absorbent fibres

Goals and characteristics	• When in contact with wound exudate, the polyacrylate fibres form a gel which binds and absorbs fibrin coatings and thus promotes the cleansing of fibrinous wounds (autolytic wound-cleansing) • The silver-containing variant is also said to have an antibacterial effect
Indications	From the cleansing phase for fibrinous, exuding wounds and potentially fibrinous wounds, such as acute wounds
Contraindications	• Known hypersensitivity to the product or its ingredients • Do not use together with hydrogen peroxide or antiseptics from the family of organic mercury compounds or hexamidine • A fistula whose diameter is smaller than the sterile application aid of the tamponade • Do not use a tamponade on a dry wound • Do not use the tamponade as an endonasal tamponade during paranasal sinus surgery
Application notes	• length of use: 1–2 days in the cleansing phase, afterwards (depending on exudation and wound condition) maximum of seven days • Clean the wound with sterile wound irrigation solution before use • If necessary, clean the wound mechanically in advance • The gently adhesive facing of the dressing is applied directly to the wound • The tamponade is inserted loosely into the wound with the applicator stick (cut to size and shorten if necessary) • Adapt secondary dressing according to exudation quantity • Product is not absorbable; always remove residues thoroughly
Complications	When initially applying the product, the wound may become enlarged with the removal of the fibrinous tissue

Table 26.5 Polymeric membrane bond (➤ Fig. 26.5)

Goals and characteristics	• Wound cleansing and moistening • Filling wound cavities • Oedema-reducing effect
Indications	• Usable in all phases of wound-healing Deep, fissured wounds and wound cavities • 2nd-degree burns • Depending on foam properties, appropriate for heavily, moderately or slightly exuding wounds • Split skin and extraction area • Can be applied to exposed bone, tendon and cartilage tissue
Contraindications	• Known hypersensitivity to the product or its ingredients • Bite wounds, fungal infections • 3rd and 4th-degree burns
Application note	• Length of stay: 1–7 days depending on wound condition • In the beginning, the cleansing effect can cause a lot of moisture, so that the wound dressing may have to be changed more often • Maceration due to late changing of saturated wound dressings (→ apply skin protection) • Depending on used product secondary dressing required
Complications	• Incompatibility/allergy • Maceration of the periwound skin, hypergranulation • Tissue damage due to tamponing too tight

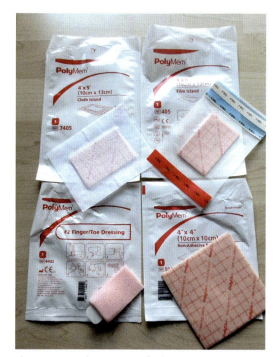

Fig. 26.5 Exemplary overview of polymeric membrane dressings. [M291]

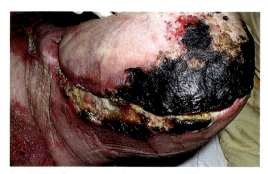

Fig. 26.6 Infected amputation stump. [M291]

> **N O T E**
> Infected wounds are cleaned with modern antiseptics, e.g. colourless octenidine or polihexanide solution, at the beginning of every treatment.

The following wound dressings are available for the treatment of infectious, critically colonised and infected wounds: silver-containing wound dressings, activated charcoal or activated carbon dressings with silver, hydrophobic wound dressings, or wound dressings with polihexanide (PHMB). Silver-containing

alginates, tamponades of hydrophobic wound dressings, tamponades of HydroBalance wound dressings made of moist cellulose with PHMB, gauze dressings with PHMB, or silver-containing cavity foams are suitable for filling infected or infection-prone deep, fissured wounds and pockets.

Wound dressings containing silver

These wound dressings use the bactericidal effect of silver, which has been known since ancient times. Many silver-containing wound dressings release elemental silver to the wound or, on contact with wound exudate, release silver ions which then have a bactericidal effect. These attach themselves to the cell wall of the bacteria and penetrate the microorganisms, disrupting their cell function and impairing cell division by hindering DNA replication. Some silver wound dressings contain only bound silver, which has a catalytic effect when the germs penetrate.

Silver in wound dressings
• Elemental silver: e.g. silver metal, nanocrystalline silver,
• Inorganic compounds: e.g. silver oxide, silver phosphate, silver chloride, silver sulphate, silver calcium sodium phosphate, silver zirconium compound, silver sulfadiazine (SSD),
• Organic complexes: e.g. silver-zincallantoinate, silver alginate, silver carboxymethylcellulose.

The silver component can be integrated into dressings in various ways:
• Nanocrystalline or elemental silver as a coating on one or both sides of the dressing,
• Silver alginate within the dressing as part of the structure,
• Elemental silver, ionic silver or silver compounds as a coating within the dressing or in the spaces between the materials,
• Combinations of these.

Silver-containing wound dressings (➤ Table 26.6) differ according to manufacturer and product with regard to the silver content, the quantity released, structure and composition as well as indication and contraindication. For example, there are alginates, hydrofibre/gelling fibre dressings, wound contact layers, alginate gels, fine-pored polyurethane foam dressings, cavity polyurethane foam dressings for

Table 26.6 Silver wound dressings (➤ Fig. 26.7)

Goals and characteristics	• Broad spectrum of action against gram-positive and gram-negative bacteria, including MRSA, VRE and fungi • Depending on the product, release of elemental silver or silver ions to the wound; the silver content of the products differs in some cases by several hundred per cent • Sometimes it is necessary to moisten the silver-containing wound dressing (see package insert) to bring the elementary silver into its ionic form
Indications	Infectious, critically colonised and infected wounds
Contraindications	• Known hypersensitivity/allergy to the product or its ingredients • Products containing sulfonamides (= silver sulfadiazine: SAg or SSD) must not be used in women who are pregnant or breastfeeding or in newborns/premature babies; sulfonamides can cause nuclear jaundice
Application notes	• Length of use depending on product, exudation and wound: 1–7 days • Partly temporary black colouration of the wound and periwound skin due to the released silver ions. Since infected wounds exudate heavily, materials with a high absorption capacity should always be used for covering, e.g. superabsorbent dressings. Besides, no film-coated wound dressings should be used as these keep the wound additionally warm and moist and may promote the progression of infection; however, it is possible to use film to fix the wound dressings to the margins. • Some products are not compatible with Octenisept, and others are not compatible with Ringer-/NaCl-0.9% solution. • Partly not compatible with MRI-imaging techniques • No contact to electrodes or conductive gels with electronic measurements • In part, not to be used along with oil-based products, such as paraffin wax • Some silver-containing wound dressings require a secondary dressing
Complications	• Incompatibility/allergy • Can stick to the wound with weak exudation • Black-grey pigment residues on healing scars (dirt tattoos) • In very large areas of application, casuistic reports on argyria (very rare)

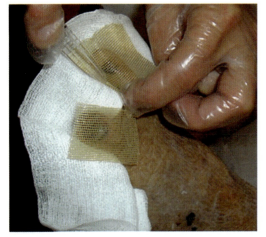

Fig. 26.7 Application of a wound contact layer with silver. [M291]

tamponing, and polyethylene tissue embedded with nanocrystalline silver.

The use of wound dressings containing silver requires a clear indication and is not a permanent solution, not least for economic reasons.

NOTE

Silver-containing wound dressings are not used for wound healing, but primarily for local wound antisepsis or local treatment of infections. Therefore, they should not be used continuously. As a rule, a local infection should be successfully treated within 14 days. Afterwards, the wound dressing should be changed to hydroactive wound dressings free of active ingredients.

Activated charcoal/activated carbon dressing with silver

This wound dressing consists of a 100% activated charcoal/carbon knit impregnated with elemental silver and covered with a polyamide fleece (➤ Table 26.7). The antiseptic effect of silver in combination with the odour-binding function of

Table 26.7 Activated charcoal/activated carbon dressing with silver (➤ Fig. 26.8)

Goals and characteristics	• Binds odours and toxins • Broad spectrum of action against gram-positive and gram-negative bacteria, including MRSA, VRE and fungi • Wound-cleansing
Indications	• Wounds with increased risk of infection, e.g. due to immunodeficiency, ulcerating tumour wounds, anal fistulas, abscesses and other therapy-resistant chronic wounds • Wounds at risk of infection, critically colonised, infected or foul-smelling wounds
Contraindications	• Known hypersensitivity to the product or its ingredients • Exposed bones, tendons, muscles
Application notes	• Length of use: a change of dressing at least once a day for infected wounds, otherwise every 1–3 days • Soft, snug and easy to tampon • May not be cut or torn, otherwise charcoal particles may enter the wound. • Depending on the product, secondary dressing may be required; for heavily exuding wounds, it is recommended to use superabsorbent dressings as secondary dressing.
Complications	• Incompatibility/allergy • The dressing can stick to the wound bed = traumatisation of granulating tissue when removing the dressing; moisten therefore with Ringer's or physiological NaCl solution before removal

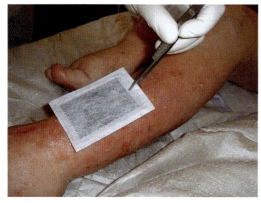

Fig. 26.8 Application of an activated charcoal dressing with silver. [M291]

charcoal is specially tailored to the requirements of active wound therapy for infected wounds. Elemental silver is bound to an activated carbon compound to take advantage of the antiseptic effect of silver in the fight against wound pathogens. This means that no free silver is released into the wound.

The activated charcoal dressing with silver has a very large surface, with which a high absorption capacity is achieved. Toxins, which are permanently released by living bacteria (exotoxins) or which remain in the wound as residues when gram-negative bacteria are destroyed (endotoxins), are deactivated in the activated charcoal by absorption. The silver ions then kill the germs bound in the charcoal fleece by damaging the cell membrane and cell wall of the bacteria. Cell metabolism is no longer possible, which prevents cell division and proliferation.

Hydrophobic wound dressings

These wound dressings are all coated with the insoluble vapour-deposited active ingredient dialkylcarbamoyl chloride (DACC), which is hydrophobic and binds bacteria and fungi. Hydrophobic wound dressings have a green colour and are available as swabs, gauzes, gel dressings, tamponades, polyurethane foam or superabsorbent dressings, absorbent dressing pads and as hydroactive wound dressings with a highly porous hydropolymer matrix (➤ Table 26.8). Swabs and gauzes consist of impregnated acetate fabric; the absorbent dressing pads additionally contain an absorbent cellulose layer (white). The tamponade consists of an impregnated cotton fabric.

Wound dressings with polihexanide (PHMB)

The following wound dressings utilise the antiseptic effect of polihexanide, which is effective against gram-positive and gram-negative bacteria, including MRSA, VRE and fungi.

Table 26.8 Hydrophobic wound dressings (➤ Fig. 26.9)

Goals and characteristics	• Bind the hydrophobic wound bacteria and fungi to the active ingredient DACC in a moist environment • The bound microorganisms are removed from the wound with each dressing change • No development of resistance, no cytotoxicity
Indications	Infectious, colonised and infected wounds of different genesis
Contraindications	• Known hypersensitivity or allergy to the product or its ingredients • Not to be used alongside oxidising solutions such as hypochlorite or hydrogen peroxide* • Dry wounds*
Application notes	• Length of use: a change of dressing at least once a day for infected wounds, otherwise every 1–4 days depending on the product and condition of the wound • Not to be used in combination with oils, fats, ointments or fatty gauzes, as the hydrophobic interaction cannot take place in this way • For wounds at risk of drying out, use of the gel compress or combined use with a hydrogel as a tube gel to prevent the wound from drying out or pain during dressing changes caused by an adhesive wound dressing • To be able to remove the tamponade from deep cavities/fistulas easily, it should protrude about 3–4 cm from the end of the opening • Depending on the product a secondary dressing is required
Complications	• Incompatibility/allergy • If the wound dressing has unexpectedly dried out due to insufficient wound exudation, the wound dressing can be atraumatically removed using Ringer's or physiological NaCl solution

* applies to polyurethane foam with superabsorber

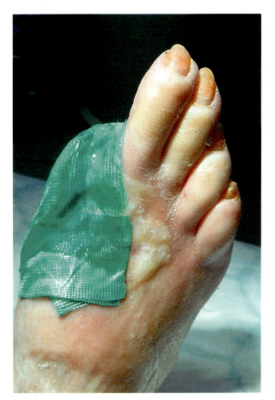

Fig. 26.9 Treatment with the hydrophobic wound dressing as a gel dressing. [M291]

HydroBalance wound dressing made of moist cellulose plus PHMB

This wound dressing consists of a fine net of moist cellulosic fibres woven in several layers from biosynthetically obtained cellulose and water (➤ Table 26.19). The dressing is also available as a tamponade. With the antimicrobial additive PHMB (**polih**exa**m**ethylene **b**iguanide = polihexanide) this product can be used for critically colonised and infected wounds. Depending on the condition of the wound, the retention period is up to seven days. A secondary dressing is required.

Other wound dressings with PHMB

This product sector is currently growing, particularly in Europe. For example, fine-pored polyurethane foam dressings containing polihexanide are also available.

CAVE

In the case of a clinically infected wound, only a conventional secondary dressing such as a superabsorbent dressing or a gauze should be used for the first few days. The dressing should be changed once or several times a day depending on the exudation. An antimicrobial wound dressing that is in direct contact with the wound and contains, e.g. silver or PHMB, may remain longer. In the

26

case of silver-containing wound dressings and hydrophobic wound dressings with a film coating (in particular foam dressings), the moist and warm environment may cause the infection to spread (except anaerobes). Also, infected wounds are often highly exudative, necessitating frequent dressing changes (= uneconomical). The use of these products is recommended after the infection is gone.

Granulating wounds

Granulating wounds are usually clean, granulated, deep red wounds with good blood circulation, a moist, shiny appearance and decreasing exudation. To avoid trauma, granulating wounds with their sensitive, vascular-rich, fresh tissue should be treated very carefully. An optimal wound environment is ensured by keeping the wound moist and ensuring that the wound dressing is in contact with the wound bed. Preference should be given to dressings which ensure atraumatic dressing changes and allow long changing intervals. The following wound dressings are available for the treatment of granulating wounds: fine-pored polyurethane foam/hydropolymer dressings/polymer membrane dressings, hydrocolloid dressings, hydrocolloid-like wound dressings and hydrogel dressings.

Fine-pored polyurethane foam, hydropolymer and polymeric membrane dressings

These wound dressings consist of fine-pored polyurethane foam and absorb exudate without changing shape or size (➤ Table 26.9). There are special shapes to better serve areas such as the knee, axilla, heel and sacral region. Some products contain additional superabsorbents to absorb larger amounts of exudate. There are also dressings with a lower absorption capacity (e. g. 'lite' products) for low exuding wounds. Fine-pored polyurethane foam, hydropolymer and polymeric membrane dressings are available with and without an adhesive facing or edge. The latter are used for sensitive, scaly, irritated and macerated periwound skin. Products with special coatings, such as silicone, soft gel, hydrogel or micro-adhesive lipid colloid mass, are also available for stressed skin. The polymeric membrane dressing also contains glycerine and the surfactant F68, which gives it a highly cleansing effect. It is also said to reduce pain and oedema.

C A V E
Viscous exudate is only insufficiently absorbed by many of these products.

Hydrocolloid dressings

Hydrocolloid dressings are semi-occlusive products consisting of a water-repellent polymer matrix in which hydrophilic particles of pectin, cellulose derivatives and gelatine are embedded (➤ Table 26.10). Depending on their thickness, they are designed to absorb different amounts of exudate (thin/lite/transparent products for low exudate). Hydrocolloids are also available in a variety of special forms, e. g. for using in the sacral or heel region. Some product types have a flat facing or an adhesive facing made of adhesive fleece or transparent film to ensure proper adhesion.

Hydrocolloid-like wound dressings

This group includes products that have different structures but support a similar mode of action. Most have a hydropolymer matrix in which superabsorbent polyacrylate particles are incorporated. The top layer consists of a breathable, semi-permeable polyurethane film. There are also products with carboxymethyl cellulose and hydrogel technology. Hydrocolloid-like wound dressings are used on superficial, weakly to moderately exuding wounds (➤ Fig. 26.12).

In contrast to hydrocolloid dressings, they do not release absorbed exudate even under pressure. These products are all relatively thin, snug and leave no gel residue. Some of these products can be cut to size if required. Depending on exudation and wound condition, the length of use is up to one week; or significantly more than seven days for one product.

N O T E
These products are a further development of hydrocolloid dressings. They have the same indications, but they have significantly fewer complications and are less time-consuming to use.

Hydrogel dressings

Hydrogel dressings consist 15–95% of water (➤ Table 26.2). They serve as semi-occlusive wound

Table 26.9 Fine-pored polyurethane foam, hydropolymer (HP) and polymeric membrane dressings (PM; ➤ Fig. 26.10)

Goals and characteristics	• HP swells on contact with wound exudate and thus dresses the wound without forming a gel or liquefying; no residues remains in the wound • Takes up germs and cell debris as well as excess wound exudate in the fine-pored foam structure • Promotes granulation through its fine-pored structure • Has a high absorptive capacity (about 20–30 times its own weight) without drying out the wound • The air-permeable membrane enables gas exchange; its thermo-insulating function ensures a warm and moist wound climate • Has good cushioning properties • Available as wound dressing and cavity/packing/WIC foams for tamponing of wound cavities/pockets
Indications	• 2nd-degree burns • For tamponing clean, granulating, deep, exuding wounds and pockets • Thin or specially coated, e.g. with silicone, soft or hydrogel, lipid colloid technique, HP for the epithelialisation phase • Special features of PM: can be used in all wound-healing phases
Contraindications	• Known hypersensitivity or allergy to the product or its ingredients • Some products should not be used on clinically infected wounds, with the exception of tamponades, which should only be covered with traditional dressings such as gauzes • Dry wounds • Bite wounds, fungal infections • As a primary layer on exposed bone/tendon/muscle tissue (does not apply to PM) • 3rd + 4th-degree burns
Application notes	• Length of use: depending on exudation and wound condition up to seven days • Some products must not be cut as this will destroy their suction structure. • When using cavity foams, the wound may only be filled up to a maximum of two-thirds, as these can swell up a lot and cause the tissue to drift apart or be squeezed. • Can also be used with compression therapy • Some products cannot absorb viscous wound exudate optimally due to blocked pores. • Although the products absorb a lot of moisture, they release it again under pressure in varying quantities → risk of maceration • Some products must not be used together with oxidising rinsing solutions (e.g. hydrogen peroxide, hypochlorite solution); this may break down the absorbent polyurethane foam • Do not release any moisture themselves, therefore sufficient exudation is necessary to keep the wound moist • Depending on the product, a secondary dressing is required
Complications	• Incompatibility/allergy • Maceration of the periwound skin • Hypergranulation • Tissue damage due to tamponing too tight

dressings for moist wound treatment and are only suitable for superficial, granulating wounds with weak to moderate exudation. Due to their transparency, these wound dressings allow good wound control. They keep wounds moist and can therefore also be used in structures at risk of drying out, e.g. tendon tissue. Hydrogel dressings without an adhesive coating are suitable for the thin skin in older people or skin which has been damaged by cortisone. Due to their cooling effect, they also give pain relief. They can be used for up to seven days, depending on wound exudation.

Additional fixation

The edge or sides of fine-pored polyurethane foam/hydropolymer/polymer membrane dressings, hydrocolloid dressings, etc. can be additionally fixed at the edge with a non-sterile, semi-permeable transparent film at difficult body

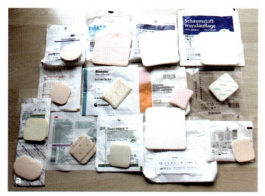

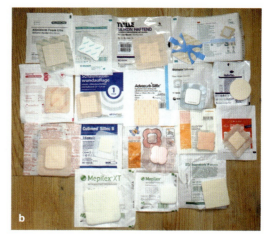

26

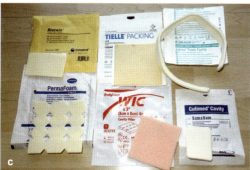

Fig. 26.10 a Exemplary overview of fine-pored polyurethane foam dressings; **b** exemplary overview of coated fine-pored polyurethane foam dressings with silicone or soft gel; **c** exemplary overview of cavity foam dressings. [M291]

sites such as the sacral region. This prevents a premature slipping or rolling up of the applied dressing. A complete sticking over with transparent film dressings bears the risk of loss of semi-occlusivity and thus possibly the formation of a moist chamber. These film dressings are moisture-repellent so that they can be wiped off when soiled.

A special adhesive technique achieves a stronger adhesive effect: the wound is first covered with strips of a semi-permeable transparent film dressing before applying the dressing. The adhesive surfaces of the wound dressing adhere to the film and not to the skin. Finally, the all-round fixation of the wound dressing with transparent film additionally ensures a secure hold.

Table 26.10 Hydrocolloid dressing (➤ Fig. 26.11)

Goals and characteristics	• Promotes granulation • Keeps the wound moist • Is water-repellent • Lyses superficial coatings • Absorbs wound exudate only to a limited extent, thereby forming a gel, recognisable by the blister which forms within the wound dressing • Protects against external contamination
Indications	• Superficial, light to moderate exuding wounds • Granulating and epithelialising wounds • Primary healing wounds
Contraindications	• Known hypersensitivity/allergy to the product or its ingredients (**cave:** colophony) • Exposed tendons, bones, muscles • Clinically infected wounds, deep fungal infection, osteomyelitis • 3rd and 4th-degree burns • Tumour wounds, ischaemic ulcers

Table 26.10 Hydrocolloid dressing (➤ Fig. 26.11) *(cont'd)*

Application notes	• Length of use: 1–7 days • The periwound skin should be dry and free from grease; shave hair • To achieve good adhesion, it is recommended that this wound dressing is moulded/shaped at body temperature • Change of dressing if a blister has formed which has migrated to the edge of the dressing • Due to the formation of blisters, the product must be applied over a large area, overlapping the wound margin by at least 2–3 cm • Forms a yellow, unpleasant-smelling gel that can be mistaken for pus. After removal of the dressing, wound cleansing is necessary • Suitable for showering • Strong adhesion on dry skin = remove carefully, especially on sensitive skin
Complications	• Incompatibility/allergy • Irritation, maceration of the periwound skin • Hypergranulation • If the hydrocolloid dressing is applied too tightly, exudate leaks out at the edge after only a few hours

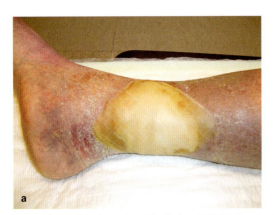
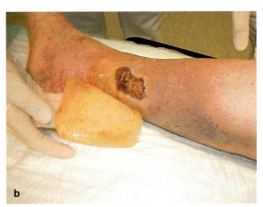

Fig. 26.11 a Blister formation with a hydrocolloid dressing; **b** gel residues and maceration when a hydrocolloid wound dressing is removed. [M291]

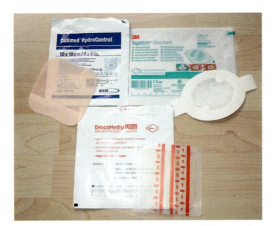

Fig. 26.12 Exemplary overview of hydrocolloid-like wound dressings. [M291]

C A V E

These product groups have the function of keeping wounds sufficiently moist and warm during the granulation phase. In individual cases, however, this milieu can also promote the formation of hypergranulation. In such a case, the treatment is adjusted appropriately, e.g. with gauzes and wound contact layers (➤ Table 26.12) to reduce the amount of moisture.

Epithelialising wounds

If a wound has a new epithelial layer forming from the margin, it produces only little wound exudate. The epithelial tissue looks pink, light pink to whitish (➤ Fig. 26.13). It is particularly important to keep

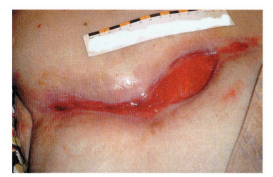

Fig. 26.13 Granulation with epithelialisation progressing from the margin. [M291]

the surface moist to ensure the migration of the epithelial cells. The wound dressing must not have any suction effect during this wound phase and must not stick to the wound. The focus is now on a long rest of the wound and a gentle, atraumatic dressing change.

Various wound dressings can be used here: transparent or thin hydrocolloid dressings, hydrocolloid-like wound dressings, hydrogel dressings, thin fine-pored polyurethane foam/hydropolymer dressings or foam dressings with special coatings, semi-permeable transparent film dressings, wound contact layers.

Transparent/thin hydrocolloid dressing

These wound dressings are a thinner, transparent variant of the hydrocolloid dressing (➤ Table 26.10), some of which allow good wound observation. Due to their elastic consistency, they can be easily moulded/shaped and have only a very low absorption capacity. Depending on the exudation, they remain in the wound for up to seven days (➤ Table 26.20).

Hydrocolloid-like wound dressings

See above and ➤ Fig. 26.12

Hydrogel dressings

➤ Table 26.2

Thin, fine-pored polyurethane foam/hydropolymer dressings ('Lite' variants)

For application on weakly exuding wounds, these wound dressings are also available in a thinner, partly specially coated, version (➤ Table 26.9).

Semipermeable transparent film dressings

The semipermeable (= permeable to water vapour and oxygen) transparent film dressing consists of a polyurethane film of varying elasticity and is often coated with a hypoallergenic polyacrylate adhesive (➤ Table 26.11). It is generally well tolerated by the skin. These products are also available with a skin-friendly silicone coating or without polyacrylate adhesive, and as a latex-free variant.

Fatty gauzes and wound contact layers

Fatty gauzes (paraffin gauze dressings) are coarse-meshed nets which, depending on the product, consist of natural or synthetic fibres with applied hydrophobic ointment and are intended to prevent sticking to the wound bed (➤ Table 26.12). Daily dressing changes are necessary when using them. Wound contact layers are a modern alternative to fatty gauzes (➤ Table 26.12). They are more finely meshed and either not at all coated or provided with skin-friendly, e. g. silicone or hydrocolloid-like coatings, which prevent sticking to the wound bed. They can be left longer on wounds compared to the classic fatty gauzes. In general, these products do not meet the criteria for moist, warm wound care. They are suitable for superficial, weakly exuding wounds and acute minor injuries. In addition, there are wounds that require dry treatment, e.g. ulcerated neoplasms or fresh burn wounds (in order not to produce after-burning).

C A V E

Viscous, sticky exudate cannot or only poorly flow through fine-meshed grids. Also, greasy ointments may clog the pores of the skin, hinder the exchange of gases and lead to maceration of the periwound skin.

Table 26.11 Semipermeable transparent film dressings (➤ Fig. 26.14)

Goals and characteristics	• Protects against secondary infection (germ barrier) • Proper wound monitoring possible due to transparency of the dressing • Supports the patient's independence and mobility, e.g. showering is possible with this dressing • Does not absorb exudate • Self-adhesive • Can be used as a secondary dressing (sterile) or for fixation of wound dressings (non-sterile) • A distinction must be made between sterile packed film dressings and non-sterile rolls of film.
Indications	• Dry, primarily healing wounds • Epithelialising wounds • Split skin removal points • Use as a secondary dressing over, e.g. hydrogels, alginates • As surgical drape material • Well suited for the occlusive application of topical local anaesthetics, e.g. EMLA cream • For fixing cannulas, i.v. catheters
Contraindications	• Known hypersensitivity or allergy to the product or its ingredients • No use in undermined, deep wounds without wound filling • Clinically infected wounds • Bleeding or heavily exuding wounds • 3rd and 4th-degree burns
Application notes	• Length of use: 1–7 days depending on wound condition; the film dressing dissolves by itself if left on the wound for too long • Atraumatic peeling of the film by piecewise overstretching parallel to the skin; to avoid shear forces, the skin underneath the film is supported by pressing down with the hands; it does not adhere to moist skin (incontinent/ heavily sweating patients) • If used to fix other wound dressings, fix only the edge of these dressings; complete over-ticking a dressing leads to loss of semi-permeability/occlusivity and thus possibly to the formation of a moist chamber.
Complications	• Incompatibility/allergy • Strong adhesion to dry skin → risk of injury, especially in the case age/ cortisone skin ('tape-stripping') and repetitive application • Formation of a moist chamber with film dressings glued on top of each other

Crepey skin/thin skin in older people

Special care is required for cortisone-damaged, crepey or thin aged skin, which is very susceptible to traumatic damage. Optimal care is difficult because many wound dressings adhere to the wound, and dressing changes can lead to further tearing of other skin areas. Hydrocolloid dressings, hydrocolloid-like wound dressings as well as many fine-pored polyurethane foam or hydropolymer dressings are not suitable for this purpose; better is the use of **hydrogel dressings** without adhesive or an adhesive surface. In some cases, however, wound contact layers or appropriately coated, fine-pored polyurethane foam dressings with a silicone coating, for example, are also suitable for this type of treatment.

Deep or undermined wounds

For the adequate treatment of undermined wounds (➤ Fig. 26.16), contact of the products with the wound bed is essential. Therefore, existing wound cavities, pockets or fistulas must first be filled or tamponed before they are covered with a suitable secondary dressing. Proper tamponing prevents the wound from closing over an unobserved cavity and from developing an undetected infection. Alginates, hydrofibre/gelling fibre dressings or fine-pored polyurethane foam/HP/PM, as so-called cavity or packing products, are suitable for lining undermined wounds.

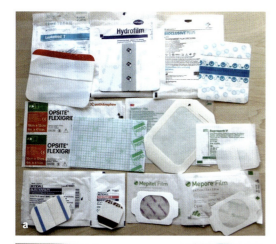

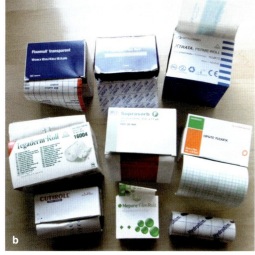

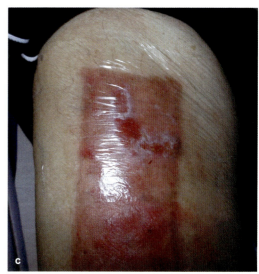

Fig. 26.14 a Exemplary overview of sterile transparent film dressings; **b** exemplary overiew of non-sterile transparent film dressings; **c** sterile transparent film dressings at split skin removal point. [M291]

Table 26.12 Fatty gauze and wound contact layers (➤ Fig. 26.15)

Goals and characteristics	Products should prevent the dressing from sticking to the wound bed. Some of these products swell through wound exudate on.
Indications	• Superficial abrasions and lacerations, ulcerating neoplasms, burn wounds • Fatty gauze for covering hydrogels • Coverage of skin grafts
Contraindications	Known hypersensitivity or allergy to the product or its ingredients (**cave:** propylene glycol)
Application notes	• **Length of use with fatty gauze:** daily dressing change required • **Length of use with wound contact layers:** 1–7 days; some products may remain on the wound for up to 14 days • Strips of fatty gauze must not be not be laid twice or on top of each other → formation of a moist chamber • Secondary dressing with absorbent products, e.g. superabsorbent dressings or gauzes, essential
Complications	• Incompatibility/allergy • Some products stick to the wound bed with low exudate levels

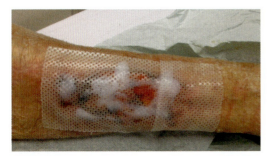

Fig. 26.15 Applied silicone-coated wound contact layer. [M291]

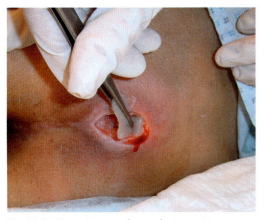

Fig. 26.16 Tamponing an undermined category III pressure ulcer with an alginate. [M291]

Alginates

Alginates (➤ Table 26.13) are made from cultivated marine brown algae. They contain alginic acid, calcium and possibly trace elements such as zinc and manganese or gelling agents. They are available as dressings and tamponades. Alginates are well suited for filling undermined, deep and fissured wounds. They are soft and easy to drape and adapt to the wound surface due to their gel form. As fresh granulation

tissue can be crushed by the swelling process, alginates should only be tamponed loosely.

It should be noted that alginates store fluid not only vertically, but in all directions and thus swell. Therefore, it is important to ensure that the application is accurately fitting to the wound; otherwise, there is a risk of maceration at the wound margin and periwound skin. Alginates are exogenous substances and must therefore be completely removed from the wound during dressing changes. They should only be used in clearly visible areas.

C A V E
A combination of alginates with hydrogels is not recommended, as the alginate absorbs the gel and is then saturated.

Hydrofibre/gelling fibre dressings

This wound dressing consists of sodium carboxy-methyl cellulose, cellulose-ethyl sulfonate fibres or polyvinyl alcohol fibres and is available as a dressing and tamponade (➤ Table 26.14). The wound exudate is only absorbed in the vertical direction. Thus, in contrast to alginates, hydrofibre/gelling fibre dressings swell only in height but not in width. This dressing is applied with 2–3 cm overlapping the wound margin. This keeps the wound and the periwound skin dry, as the moisture does not spread beyond the edge of the wound. This reduces the risk of maceration.

Cavity/packing polyurethane foam dressing/WIC-Polymeric membrane dressing for deep or undermined wounds

A characteristic feature of these fine-pored foams is their high absorption capacity. They are particularly

Table 26.13 Alginate (➤ Fig. 26.17)	
Goals and characteristics	• In contact with wound exudate, an exchange of calcium ions from the alginate and sodium ions from the wound exudate takes place. The alginate swells and the fibres transform into a hydrophilic gel that fills the wound and keeps it moist; depending on the alginate, the gel can look yellowish, brownish or greenish. • High absorption capacity → absorbs approximately 20 times its own weight of liquid; exudate absorption includes germs, cell debris and waste products into the gel structure • Haemostatic effect • Wound-conditioning and cleansing • Granulation promotion

Table 26.13 Alginate (➤ Fig. 26.17) *(cont'd)*

Indications	• Medium to severely exuding wounds • Moist, coated wounds in the cleansing phase • Undermined, fissured, deep or extensive wounds as well as fistulae and abscess cavities • Split skin removal points • 2nd-degree burns • Infected wounds in case of undermining to fill the wound pocket (wound cover, e.g. gauzes + fixation with adhesive fleece) • Wounds in trauma and tumour surgery
Contraindications	• Known hypersensitivity or allergy to the product or its ingredients • Dry wounds, necroses, encrusted coatings • Severe bleeding, surgical implants • 3rd and 4th-degree burns
Application notes	• Length of use: depending on exudation and wound, product and manufacturer, 3–7 days • Daily dressing changes in case of infected wounds • Despite high absorption capacity under pressure, almost entirely releases the absorbed liquid again, which can lead to problems especially under compression therapy → maceration of wound margin/environment • For slightly dry wounds, alginates can be moistened with Ringer or physiologic NaCl solution before use; however, it should be noted that this reduces the absorption capacity accordingly! • If alginate components remain dry, the wound produces too little wound exudate → changeover to a suitable treatment option, e.g. hydrogels • Carefully remove any fibre residues stuck to the wound margin with NaCl 0.9% or Ringer's solution • Secondary dressing required
Complications	• Incompatibility/allergy • Odour development due to trapped waste materials • Maceration of the periwound skin

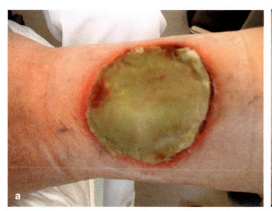 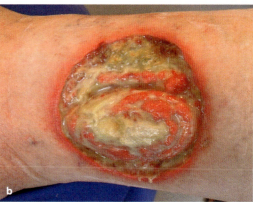

Fig. 26.17 a Saturated alginate; **b** progress of wound cleansing through alginate use. [M291]

suitable for tamponing larger wound cavities and pockets with a higher amount of wound exudate (➤ Table 26.9). Many of these products swell considerably and thereby increase their volume. They should therefore be cut under sterile conditions and only fill a maximum of two-thirds of the wound cavity. Too firm tamponing carries the risk that the swelling dressing will squash the surrounding tissue. A secondary dressing, e.g. a semi-permeable transparent film dressing, possibly in combination with a sterile gauze, is additionally required. Depending on the wound and exudation, it can remain in place for up to seven days.

Table 26.14 Hydrofibre/gelling fibre dressings (➤ Fig. 26.18)

Goals and characteristics	• Is soft and easy to tampon • Converts into a transparent, dimensionally stable gel by absorbing wound exudate; wound exudate and cell debris are trapped (also under compression therapy) • Supports autolytic wound-cleansing • Has a high absorbency and absorption capacity; can absorb 25–30 times its own weight in wound exudate
Indications	• Strong to moderately exuding wounds • Acute and chronic wounds • 2nd-degree burns • Postoperative wounds, split skin removal points • Undermined, tunnelled wounds
Contraindications	• Known hypersensitivity or allergy to the product or its ingredients • Dry wounds, dry necroses • Heavily bleeding wounds
Application notes	• Length of use: 3–7 days, depending on wound condition • Gel residues from the wound dressing must be removed from the wound or rinsed out • Secondary dressing required
Complications	• Incompatibility/allergy • Risk of the wound bed drying out in rather dry wounds with moderate exudation

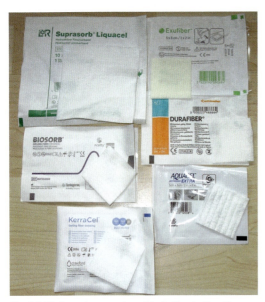

Fig. 26.18 Exemplary overview of hydrofibre/gelling fibre dressings. [M291]

Adjusting the wound dressing

For the filling of undermined wounds, sterile cutting of the wound dressing in a spiral form is a good way to line pockets and cavities.

Foul-smelling wounds

Unpleasant wound odour mean a serious restriction of the patient's quality of life, because they reduce their social contacts and the odour can also represent a considerable psychological burden up to body image disorders (disgust with oneself). Especially with infected wounds and ulcerated neoplasms, such malodours are common side effects. Adequate control, containment and elimination of wound odours are essential for the patient's increased well-being. The treatment for the causative factors of the odour, e. g. curing the infection, is always at the forefront.

Activated charcoal dressings or activated carbon dressings with/without silver

These terms cover a large group of very differently structured products (➤ Table 26.15). As a primary common feature, they all have an odour-binding activated charcoal/carbon layer. These wound dressings usually have a multi-layer structure. Depending on the product, they have an ethylene methyl acrylate film, an absorbent pad, an acrylic fibre wound contact layer, hydrofibre, cellulose or an outer layer of nonwoven fabric. The products consist of 100% pure, activated

Table 26.15 Activated charcoal dressing/activated carbon dressing (➤ Fig. 26.19)

Goals and characteristics	• Odour absorption • Large suction capacity • Protein molecules and bacteria are absorbed, but not directly killed off
Indications	• Unpleasantly smelling wounds • Acute and chronic wounds, including ulcerative neoplasms
Contraindications	Known hypersensitivity/allergy to the product or its ingredients
Application notes	• Length of use: 1–3 days depending on odour development and amount of exudate; the product made of pure carbon fibre can remain for up to one week • Do not cut the product (exception: a product made of pure carbon fibre), otherwise carbon particles can get into the wound; this will cause the wound to turn black (= no more observation possible) • Depending on the product, cover with a secondary dressing
Complications	Intolerance/allergy

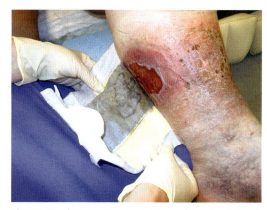

Fig. 26.19 Changing an activated charcoal dressing. [M291]

charcoal fibres. Activated charcoal dressings are also available, which are additionally impregnated with silver (➤ Table 26.7).

C A V E

In the case of direct wound contact, there is a risk that the activated charcoal dressing will stick to the wound bed. To avoid unnecessary pain and traumatisation of the tissue, a combined wound contact layer or, depending on exudation, hydrogel can be used in direct wound contact. In principle, these wound dressings should be moistened before removing if dry.

In ulcerating neoplasms, film-coated wound dressings must be avoided, otherwise there is a danger of promoting the growth of tumour cells. Conventional secondary dressings, e.g. gauzes, are preferable here. The use of superabsorbent dressings is particularly recommended for severe wound exudation (➤ Table 26.16) to reduce unnecessary and above all painful and frequent dressing changes.

Severely exuding wounds

In addition to the physical complaints, a severely exudating wound will seriously impair the patient's quality of life. High amounts of exudate especially limit the choice of clothing, reduce social contacts and increase psychological stress. In the case of extremely exuding wounds, many wound dressings are quickly exhausted and require dressing changes several times a day. The cause of wound exudate must always be treated, which means, for example, in the case of oedema, the application of appropriate and professional compression therapy. Also, wound care and dressing-changing intervals must be adjusted according to the amount of exudate.

At this stage, superabsorbent dressings, hydrocapillary dressings or fine-pored polyurethane foam dressings with superabsorbers or the additive 'plus' should preferably be used.

Superabsorbent dressings

Superabsorbent dressings (➤ Table 26.16) are composed differently depending on the product. Some contain a cellulose core or cellulose flakes in which superabsorbents (sodium polyacrylate) or liquid-storing polymers are embedded. In addition, a layer of activated carbon is sometimes embedded to bind toxins and odours. The wrapping or sheath consists of nonwoven fabric. Some products have a specially coated 'wound contact layer', e.g. of perforated polyethylene, to prevent sticking to the wound bed. In some products, the side facing away from the wound

Table 26.16 Superabsorbent dressings	
Goals and characteristics	• High and fast absorption power while maintaining a moist wound climate • High absorption power leads to an increase in volume and weight of the wound dressing • Ensured wound rest and reduced risk of contamination: longer change intervals due to high absorption power • Wound margin protection: exudates of the wound no longer damage the periwound skin • Wound-cleansing: excess wound exudate, coatings, bacteria, cell debris are actively absorbed into the wound dressing • Odour reduction
Indications	Heavily to moderately exuding wounds and fistulas
Contraindications	• Known hypersensitivity or allergy to the product or its ingredients • No use/contact on mucous membranes, in the eye area • Not for use in tunnel-forming wound pockets, as the product can expand considerably when wound exudate is absorbed. • Dry or slightly exuding wounds: risk of dehydration and pain from the wound drying out
Application notes	• Length of use: depending on exudation, 1–4 days • Due to the high absorption power, the wound dressing may weigh several 100 g; this may result in a pressure load on the wound/periwound skin → check absorption of the wound dressing at appropriate intervals • May not be cut or opened • Should not be folded (→ performance reduction, because expansion is inhibited) • The high level of absorption/suction of the wound dressing may cause pain • If there is a risk of sticking to the wound bed, use a wound contact layer or use a product already equipped with such a contact layer
Complications	• Incompatibility/allergy • Risk of drying out in moderately exuding wounds

also has a laminated fleece to protect clothing from moisture penetration. Some of these products also have an adhesive side. This seals wound margins and prevents macerations.

Although all superabsorbent dressings are available in sizes of 10 × 10 cm, only the inner core of one product actually has these dimensions (> Fig. 26.20). When prescribing these products, therefore, it must be ensured that the size of the inner absorbent core matches the size of the wound.

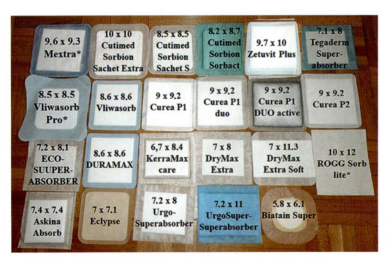

Fig. 26.20 Overview of super-absorbent dressings and the size of their superabsorbent pad. [M291]

Hydrocapillary dressing

The hydrocapillary dressing consists of a wound pad in which cellulose fibres with polyacrylate superabsorbent particles are embedded (➤ Table 26.17). The wound contact layer is a polyethylene net. The outer layer consists of a polyurethane film. The wound dressing is available with and without a hydrocolloid adhesive edge.

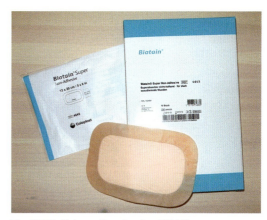

Fig. 26.21 Hydrocapillary dressing. [M291]

Fine-pored polyurethane foam dressings with superabsorbents

Another option for treating heavily exuding wounds is the use of fine-pored polyurethane foam dressings with an extra absorptive function. These usually contain superabsorbents and can be identified by the suffix 'plus' (➤ Table 26.9).

Other special wound dressings

In addition to the wound dressings mentioned above, of which all can be assigned to the different wound stages, there are further dressings with some special indications. These include the fine-pored polyurethane foam dressing with ibuprofen, a cellulose film or a HydroBalance wound dressing made of moist cellulose with/without the preservative PHMB.

Fine-pored polyurethane foam dressing with ibuprofen

This fine-pored polyurethane foam dressing (➤ Table 26.18) contains 0.5 mg ibuprofen per cm^2, which is released continuously for up to seven days on contact with the wound exudate. It is available in two variants: non-adhesive and soft adhesive with a spiderweb-

Table 26.17 Hydrocapillary dressing (➤ Fig. 26.21)	
Goals and characteristics	• Highly absorbent wound dressing with superabsorbents • Containment of germs and cell debris in the hydrocapillary wound pad • Promotion of granulation
Indications	• Moderately to severely exuding wounds • Greasy, fibrin-covered wounds • 2nd-degree burns
Contraindications	• Known hypersensitivity or allergy to the product or its ingredients • Dry wounds • 3rd and 4th-degree burns
Application notes	• Length of use: 1–7 days depending on wound condition and exudation; if the wound pad is completely swollen, a change should always be made • Can also be used with compression therapy • Can be used as a primary and secondary dressing on top of other wound products, such as alginates • Wound dressing should be removed before radiation therapy
Complications	• Incompatibility/allergy • Drying out of weakly exuding wounds

26

Table 26.18 Fine-pored polyurethane foam dressing with ibuprofen (➤ Fig. 26.22)	
Goals and characteristics	• Pain relief over the entire period of use and during dressing changes • Effective exudate management → rapid absorption and binding of wound exudate
Indications	Treatment of exuding, painful wounds
Contraindications	• Known hypersensitivity or allergy to the product or its components. **Cave:** ibuprofen and cross sensitivity need to be taken into consideration) • Do not use during pregnancy and in children under 12 years of age • Wounds that affect deeper layers than the skin, e.g. bone, muscle or tendon tissue
Application notes	• Length of use: 1–7 days • Do not use alongside oxidising solutions such as hypochlorite, PVP iodine or hydrogen peroxide • Do not use alongside other products containing active ingredients • The wound dressing can be applied up to a total area of 1,200 cm² =, e.g. three dressings of 20 × 20 cm each; dressing changes not more frequently than two per day = corresponds to 2,400 cm² of a total dressing area for a maximum application • The wound dressings should be stored horizontally • Removal of the wound dressing before radiation therapy • In the case of weakly exuding wounds, moistening the wound dressing with NaCl 0.9% or Ringer's solution is recommended. The release of ibuprofen depends on the amount of exudate • Can also be used with compression therapy
Complications	Incompatibility/allergy

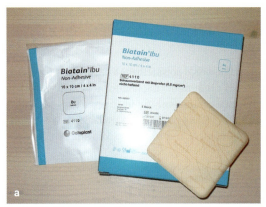 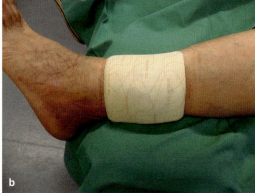

Fig. 26.22 a Fine-pored polyurethane foam dressing with ibuprofen; **b** applied fine-pored polyurethane foam dressing with ibuprofen. [M291]

like adhesive layer applied to the polyurethane foam (but without an adhesive edge). Use is indicated for patients who suffer from pain despite regular use of analgesics.

CAVE
Wound dressings containing ibuprofen may only be used as a supplement and are not a substitute for any systemic pain therapy that may be necessary, in accordance with the step-by-step plan of the WHO.

Cellulose film

This product is a biological cellulose film, bacterially produced cellulose film to promote epithelialisation, especially at split skin removal sites and 2nd-degree burns (➤ Fig. 26.23). It is only applied once and supports immediate pain reduction. The cellulose films are wound dressings that act as a germ barrier and have a high water vapour permeability. They are transparent and are additionally covered with a secondary dressing, e.g. a gauze, during the first few days. Fixation by using light compression, e.g. with

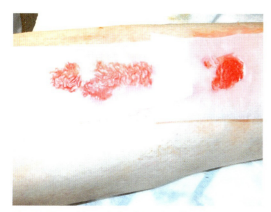

Fig. 26.23 Freshly applied cellulose film. [M291]

an elastic gauze bandage, is necessary. If the cellulose film dressing is dry, no additional dressing or fixation is required. Friction and movement usually cause the dressing to come off after 14–16 days, and the wound has healed (➤ Fig. 26.23).

HydroBalance wound dressing made of moist cellulose

This wound dressing consists of a fine net of multi-layered interwoven moist cellulose fibres from biosynthetically-obtained cellulose and water

(➤ Table 26.19). The dressings are also available as tamponades. A version of this product also contains PHMB (➤ Table 26.20), so that it can also be used for critically colonised and infected wounds. The duration of use is up to seven days. A secondary dressing is required.

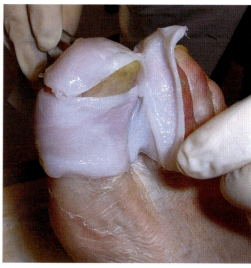

Fig. 26.24 Application of a HydroBalance wound dressing made of moist cellulose. [M291]

Table 26.19 HydroBalance wound dressings made of moist cellulose with/without PHMB (➤ Fig. 26.24)

Goals and characteristics	• Depending on the condition of the wound, releases moisture into the wound or absorbs excess wound exudate. • Maintenance/creation of a moist wound environment • Ensuring an atraumatic dressing change • Subjectively cooling effect is partly perceived as pain-relieving
Indications	• Weak to moderately exuding wounds • Superficial and deep wounds • With the addition of PHMB, additionally applicable for critically colonised and infected wounds
Contraindications	• Known hypersensitivity or allergy to the product or its ingredients • 3rd and 4th-degree burns • Exposed bone or cartilage (applies to PHMB products!) • For infected wounds, the wound dressing (incl. PHMB) should not be used as the sole therapeutic measure
Application notes	• Length of use: depending on wound exudation, product and degree of colonisation up to three or seven days • For infected wounds, use HydroBalance wound dressings made of moist cellulose + PHMB • Use of systemic antibiotic therapy (for clinical infection): no occlusive secondary dressing may be used here! Additional strict medical control
Complications	Intolerance/allergy

26.1.3 Tabular overview of the use of wound dressings

➤ Tab. 26.20 provides a simple and quick overview of the wound dressings described in this chapter. It explains their practical use, as appropriate to the respective wound stages and conditions.

26.1.4 General selection criteria for wound dressings

The use of modern wound dressings is only justified if they are not changed daily. In addition to the manufacturer's instructions, dressing changes are always based on the extent of healing of the wound and the exudation. Modern wound dressings are designed to remain on the wound for two to seven days. Therefore, as a rule, a dressing change should not be performed more than 3 ×/week. Exceptions are the treatment of infected wounds, heavily exuding wounds at the beginning of compression therapy in the decongestion phase, or for the treatment of ulcerating neoplasms. In these cases, the dressing is usually changed daily.

Since the wound goes through various phases in the healing process, it is not advisable to prescribe wound dressings over a period of several weeks. When transitioning from the clinical to the outpatient area, a maximum of ten wound dressings should therefore be prescribed as a rule of thumb.

Tab. 26.20 Appearance of the wound and possible treatment options*

Appearance of the wound	Options for wound dressings
Necrosis 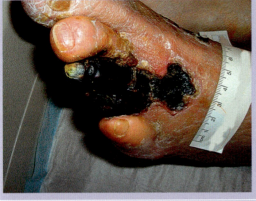	**Cave:** necroses, e.g. in PAD, must only be removed after successful revascularisation. Under no circumstances should they be softened before such an operation. Until then, only dry dressing changes should be carried out!
Dry coating 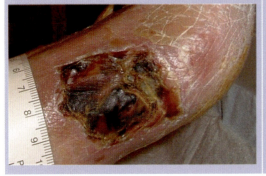	• Hydrogel as tube gel/hydrogel dressing • Hydro-responsive wound dressings

Tab. 26.20 Appearance of the wound and possible treatment options* *(cont'd)*

Appearance of the wound	Options for wound dressings
Moist coating 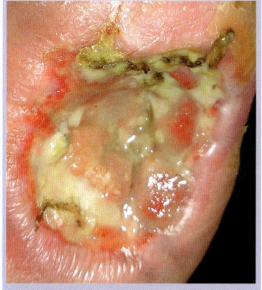	• Alginate • Hydrofibre/Gelling fibre dressings • Soft-adherent dressing with poly-absorbent fibres • Polymeric membrane dressing
Infected wound 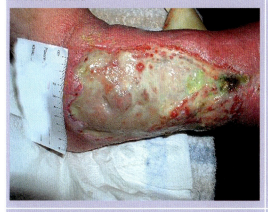	• Silver wound dressings • Activated charcoal dressing or activated carbon dressings with silver • Hydrophobic wound dressings • Wound dressings with PHMB
Strongly exuding wound 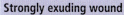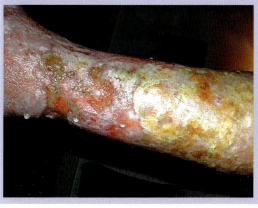	• Superabsorbent dressings • Hydrocapillary dressing • Fine-pored polyurethane foam dressings with 'plus' function

Tab. 26.20 Appearance of the wound and possible treatment options* *(cont'd)*

Appearance of the wound	Options for wound dressings
Wound odour 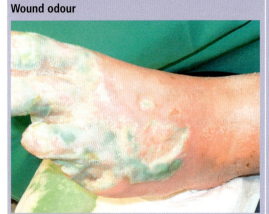	Activated charcoal dressing or activated carbon dressing with/without silver
Undermined wound 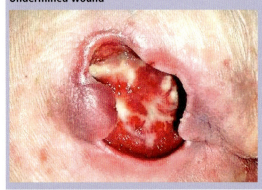	• Alginate • Cavity/packing polyurethane foam/WIC polymeric membrane dressing • Hydrofibre/gelling fibre dressings
Granulating wound 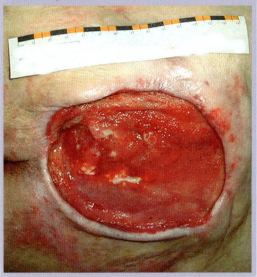	• Fine-pored polyurethane foam/hydropolymer/polymer membrane dressing • Hydrocolloid dressing • Hydrocolloid-like wound dressings • Hydrogel dressing

Tab. 26.20 Appearance of the wound and possible treatment options* *(cont'd)*

Appearance of the wound	Options for wound dressings
Epithelialising wound 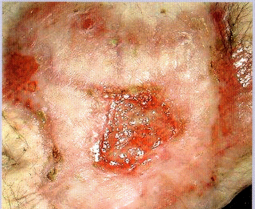	• Thinner/transparent hydrocolloid dressing • Thinner or specially coated (e.g. with silicone or hydrogel) fine-pored polyurethane foam/hydropolymer dressing • Hydrocolloid-like wound dressings • Hydrogel dressing • Semipermeable transparent film dressing • Fatty gauze/wound contact layer (e.g. silicone-coated)
Split skin donor site 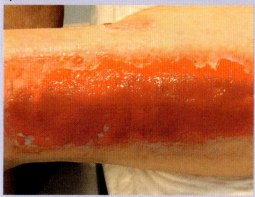	• Cellulose film • Alginate • Semipermeable transparent film dressing • Silicone-coated fine-pored polyurethane foam/hydropolymer dressing

* Photos: [M291]

The following treatment applications, among others, are uneconomical:
• A combination of products which absorb others and thus cancel out their physical effect, i.e. no joint use of hydrogel as a tube gel with alginate, hydrofibre/gelling fibre dressings or superabsorbent dressings.
• If a hydrogel is needed several times, no preservative-free hydrogels (single-use products – recognisable by the circled and crossed out 2) should be used, only preservation products.
• As single-use products for small wounds, alginate tamponades are unnecessarily costly, since a large residual quantity must be discarded. An economical alternative is the use of small alginate dressings, e.g. 5 × 5 cm in size.

REFERENCES
Deutsche Gesellschaft für Wundheilung und Wundbe-handlung (DGfW). S3-Leitlinie Lokaltherapie chronischer Wunden bei Patienten mit den Risiken periphere arterielle Verschlusskrankheit, Diabetes mellitus, chronische venöse Insuffizienz. 2012. AWMF-Leitlinien-Register Nr. 091/001. Aus: www.awmf.org/uploads/tx_szleit-linien/091-001m_S3_Lokaltherapie_chronischer_Wunden_2012-ungueltig.pdf (last accessed 12 October 2020).
Dissemond J, Bültemann A, Gerber V, Jäger B, Kröger K, Münter C. Diagnosis and treatment of chronic wounds: current standards of Germany's Initiative for Chronic Wounds e.V. J Wound Care 2017; 26: 727–732.
Dissemond J, Augustin M, Eming S, et al. Modern wound care – practical aspects of non-interventional topical treatment of patients with chronic wounds. J Dtsch Dermatol Ges 2014; 12: 541–554.
Protz K. Moderne Wundversorgung. 9 A. München: Elsevier; 2019.
Vasel-Biergans A. Wundauflagen für die Kitteltasche. 4. A. Stuttgart: Wissenschaftliche Verlagsgesellschaft; 2017.
Wundzentrum Hamburg e.V.: www.wundzentrum-hamburg.de/standards.

26.2 Active wound therapeutics
Joachim Dissemond

─────────────── **Key notes** ───────────────

- Active wound therapeutics are a very heterogeneous group of products whose propagated primary goal is to have an active influence on the wound environment.
- Matrix metalloproteinases, pH-value, oxygen/reactive oxygen species, cytokines, macrophage activity or growth factors are to be influenced therapeutically.
- Active wound therapeutics are used in particular for otherwise therapy-refractory wounds.

26.2.1 Introduction

There are many other products for wound care which cannot be allocated to one of the groups described in ➤ Chap. 26.1. Of particular interest here are the so-called active wound therapeutics, which are also referred to as wound-starters. This is a very heterogeneous group whose propagated primary goal is to influence the wound environment actively. Through interaction with the wound, wound-healing which promotes modulation of the wound environment should take place. We here look at some of the points of attack propagated as examples. The topic of oxygen is described in detail in ➤ Chap. 31.

26.2.2 Targets for wound products

Matrix metalloproteinases

Matrix metalloproteinases (MMP) are a group of zinc-dependent endopeptidases that catalyse the cleavage of peptide bonds. Currently, 23 different MMPs are known in humans. They can be subdivided into further subfamilies such as collagenases, gelatinases and stromelysins. The expression of MMPs is regulated by a complex interplay of inducers and suppressors. Tissue inhibitors of metalloproteinases (TIMPs) are of great importance here. The central role of MMPs in the physiological healing of wounds was primarily described in the context of the degradation of extracellular matrix proteins. MMPs also have numerous other functions in the regulation of physiological and pathological processes. They are essential for angiogenesis, tumour growth and as signalling molecules.

Binding of MMPs in the wound environment is to be achieved by products containing, for example, collagen and cellulose, polyhydrogenated ionogens (PHI-5) or sucrose octasulfate. These wound products are available with various carrier materials and additives such as silver and are usually left on the wound for 1–3 days. Good evidence with several RCTs exists for the sugar sucrose-**octasulfate,** which is also referred to as nano-oligo-saccharide factor (NOSF) in wound treatment products. In a double-blind RCT with 240 patients with neuroischaemic DFU, it was shown that complete wound closure was achieved significantly more frequently within 20 weeks in the intervention group with 48% compared to 30% of the patients in the control group.

Extracellular matrix proteins

The extracellular matrix (ECM) is the substance between the cells in the intercellular space. It consists of a primary substance and fibres which are synthesised and secreted by cells. The ECM is essential for cell adhesion, cell migration, cell proliferation, signal transduction as well as for the construction, reconstruction and degradation of tissue. Further functions are shaping, water content, elasticity, tensile strength and stability of tissue. The degradation and remodelling of ECM are controlled centrally by MMPs.

Hyaluronic acid as glycosaminoglycan is a physiological component of the ECM of connective tissue and can bind substantial amounts of water. Various cell surface receptors interact with hyaluronic acid and trigger several cell reactions that are believed to have a positive effect on various aspects of wound-healing. In a meta-analysis, in 2016, a total of nine RCTs with 865 patients with chronic wounds were analysed. No sound evidence was found that the use of hyaluronic acid can accelerate wound-healing. However, there was evidence of pain reduction, especially in patients with a venous or mixed leg ulcer.

Amelogenin is an ECM used in wound treatment. It is a protein that is involved in amelogenesis (development of dental enamel), among other things. Therefore, most of the published studies come from dentistry. In an RCT with 123 patients with venous leg ulcers, the use of a viscous amelogenin solution compared to a drug-free alginate solution resulted in significantly better wound-healing, especially in larger and older wounds.

Growth factors

Growth factors are proteins that are either transferred as signals from cells or act as membranes. There are different families of growth factors that are divided into fibroblast growth factors (FGF), transforming growth factors (TGF), hedgehog, wingless, delta and serrate, and ephrins. Growth factors regulate various intracellular processes and play a central role in the development of tissue. Signal transmission is usually via binding to specific receptors of the cell membrane. Thus, only cells that carry the specific receptor for the respective growth factor can react to the signal. The receptor-binding leads to a conformational change that leads to the activation or deactivation of genes via further signal transmissions. Angiogenesis is a well-investigated field for the mode of action of growth factors.

The platelet-derived growth factor (PDGF) in a gel and the epidermal growth factor (EGF) in a wound dressing are currently offered as growth factors for wound treatment. A meta-analysis of four RCTs with 922 patients with DFU showed that the additional use of a gel with PDGFbb (Becaplermin) improved healing times by about 30% and healing rates by 12% in wounds with an area of $\leq 5 \text{ cm}^2$.

β-Glucan

The β-glucans are high-molecular polysaccharides that occur in nature, for example, in the cell walls of cereals, bacteria and fungi. They bind to the receptors dectin-1, complement receptor three and toll-like receptors. The toll-like receptors play an important role in innate defence and are expressed in particular by dendritic cells and macrophages. They are used, among other things, for the recognition of PAMPs (pathogen-associated molecular patterns), which occur exclusively in pathogens. For wound-healing, it is propagated that products with β-glucan should activate macrophages, especially in cases of chronic, stagnant wound-healing.

In an RCT with a total of 60 patients with type 1 or 2 diabetes and ulcers in the lower extremities, the patients received either a gel with β-glucan or a reference product of methylcellulose 3 x/week over 12 weeks, in addition to the conventional treatment regimen. A trend of 36 vs. 63 days was observed for shorter average cure rates in the group treated with the β-glucan.

pH value

The centrally important aspects and interactions of the pH value within the framework of wound-healing are described in detail in ➤ Chap. 8.1. Each wound product has a pH value and can, therefore, potentially influence the pH value in wounds. In a study of 15 exemplarily-selected wound products, it was shown that the pH value of wound products could lie in an extensive range between 2.13 (Promogran®) and 11.7 (Acticoat®). For the fewest wound products, the pH value is specified by the manufacturer. One of the few wound-healing products that promote the active lowering of the pH value is a paste containing modified starch, poloxamer and macrogol. In a clinical study, the reduction of the pH value in patients with leg ulcers could be shown by the one-time application of this paste from an average of 7.7 to 6.7. However, there is no evidence that this active lowering of the pH value accelerates wound-healing.

Chitosan

Chitosan is a naturally occurring biopolymer of poly-aminosaccharides that can be produced from chitin – obtained from the shells of shrimps, for example. In wound treatment, it is mainly the bleeding and pain-relieving as well as antimicrobial properties that are supposed to promote wound-healing. Chitosan also activates and stimulates various cells and collagen type IV synthesis. The majority of the numerous published research results on chitosan originate from basic research. Here there are indications that chitosan is fundamentally suitable for promoting wound-healing. In an RCT in China, 90 patients with therapy-refractory chronic wounds of different genesis were treated with chitosan or vaseline gauze. After four weeks, a significantly better wound area reduction (66% vs. 40%) and pain reduction were observed in the group treated with chitosan.

26.2.3 Perspective

Current treatment concepts assume that the underlying mechanisms of wound-healing disorders are the same in almost all patients with chronic wounds. For example, patients with pressure ulcers, venous leg ulcers or DFU receive the same wound products. Although many differences between the different entities can be identified today, this plays virtually no role in the implementation of wound-healing concepts about local therapy. The same applies to cofactors and comorbidities, such as drugs, obesity, diabetes, old age or reduced mobility, which are hardly considered.

However, new knowledge about molecular processes has considerably broadened our understanding of health and disease. This trend, which is still relatively new in medicine, is referred to by catchwords such as 'individualised', 'targeted' or 'personalised'. The idea behind this is that patients, as well as their illnesses, can be individually very different. These individual differences are to be determined by specific test procedures to determine a corresponding tailor-made therapy strategy. The necessary diagnostic options for wound treatment are lacking in everyday clinical practice. In this respect, it would be desirable in the future to integrate test systems into wound dressings which continuously take measurements. In addition to the factors mentioned above of the wound environment, it could also be helpful to obtain information on the saturation of the wound dressing, temperature or pressure, for example.

In the second step, the optimal wound environment could be adjusted explicitly by releasing substances. Such wound products are also referred to as smart wound dressings (➤ Fig. 26.25). If it is possible to read out information contactless via a smartphone, this information could be transmitted telematically to a wound centre. From there, the nursing service could be informed with appropriate urgency, for example, or the patient could be admitted as an inpatient. However, these developments, which are supported by the newly enacted E-Health Act, still require considerable progress with new findings in wound-healing research.

The central goal of personalised medicine is an individually adapted, improved prevention, diagnosis and therapy. In summary, the smart wound dressings already in research offer an exciting perspective for better future wound treatment. However, individualised medicine also raises fundamental ethical, legal and economic questions that have not yet been fully clarified.

26.2.4 Conclusion

Many factors, such as pH value, oxygen, MMPs or growth factors, play a central role in wound-healing. At present, however, it is not possible to reliably measure these aspects in everyday clinical practice. Besides, there is a lack of meaningful studies that prove when values have to be actively changed and what the 'optimal' values should be. In this respect, these certainly exciting wound-healing products are mostly used for otherwise therapy-refractory wounds according to the 'trial and error' principle. If the scientific database improves, however, it is conceivable that such products could be used at an early stage based on individual diagnostics.

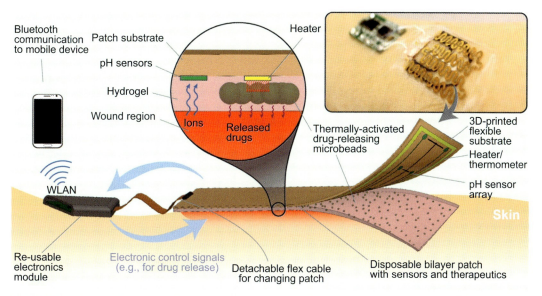

Fig. 26.25 Smart-wound dressings should continuously measure various factors and modify them if necessary. This information should then be read contactless and sent telematically. [F1024-001]

REFERENCES

Derakhshandeh H, Kashaf SS, Aghabaglou F, Ghanavati IO, Tamayol A. Smart bandages: The future of wound care. Trends Biotechnol 2018; 36: 1259–1274.

Edmonds M, Lázaro-Martínez JL, Alfayate-García JM, et al. Sucrose octasulfate dressing versus control dressing in patients with neuroischaemic diabetic foot ulcers (Explorer): an international, multicentre, double-blind, randomised, controlled trial. Lancet Diabetes Endocrinol 2018; 6: 186–196.

Kiaee G, Mostafalu P, Samandari M, Sonkusale S. A pH-mediated electronic wound dressing for controlled drug delivery. Adv Healthc Mater 2018; 7: e1800396.

Mostafalu P, Tamayol A, Rahimi R, et al. Smart bandage for monitoring and treatment of chronic wounds. Small 2018; 6: e1703509.

Powers JG, Higham C, Broussard K, Phillips TJ. Wound-healing and treating wounds: Chronic wound care and management. J Am Acad Dermatol 2016; 74: 607–625.

27 Systematics of surgical treatment

Ingo Stoffels

Ingo Stoffels

Key notes

- Today, an extensive range of surgical methods is available for ulcer surgery.
- Venous surgery and endovenous techniques are suitable for the elimination of primary or secondary varicosis as a causal therapy for venous leg ulcers.
- Shave therapy is the method of choice with a presentation of dermatolipo(fascio)sclerosis.

- In individual cases, surgical techniques involving the fascia cruris (fasciotomy, fasciectomy) can also be used.
- Both local surgical treatment and extended surgery, dealing with the causes of wounds, play a crucial role in the interdisciplinary overall therapy concept of wound treatment.

27.1 Introduction

For poorly healing, persistent wounds, the term 'therapy-resistant' plays an important role. If wounds do not show any healing tendencies after three months despite seemingly adequate diagnostics and therapy, or an ulcer has not healed after 12 months, the indication for surgical treatment should be examined.

27.2 Operational procedure

Depending on the severity of sclerosis, different surgical procedures with three treatment approaches are available for the operative therapy of pronounced ulcers that persist for years or decades despite sufficient conservative therapy:

1. Elimination of insufficient epi- and transfascial venous sections
2. Local ulcer surgery
3. Procedure involving the fascia cruris

27.2.1 Venous surgery

The overall concept of modern surgical treatment of chronic wounds also includes surgery of the causative

pathologies. In the context of a venous leg ulcer, this includes direct treatment of chronic venous insufficiency (CVI).

In venous leg ulcers, the elimination of insufficient epi- or transfascial venous sections normally leads to permanent healing of the ulcer without further specific measures. If the leg ulcer is more extensive and spontaneous healing is not to be expected, local surgical measures can be combined. A common example of a single-stage combination intervention is a Shave therapy with a subsequent mesh split skin graft transplantation. In the case of a postthrombotic leg ulcer, the elimination of insufficient epifascial and transfascial reflux lines can also be performed without significant risk after prior diagnosis of venous haemodynamics. Here, too, combinations with local surgery on the ulcer, in particular Shave therapy, are possible.

Endovenous therapy

Endovenous procedures such as laser therapy, radio wave therapy and foam sclerotherapy are increasingly becoming good alternatives to traditional vein surgery. The choice of the procedure must be made in the context of a patient-related individual case decision. Currently, the best-established methods are thermal ablation methods, such as laser and radio wave therapy, and chemical occlusion methods, such as foam sclerosing.

Scientific long-term results concerning ulcer-healing and recurrence rates are still pending for the endovenous procedures due to the shorter follow-up times. However, comparable results are expected. The less invasive endovenous procedures can be used to reduce surgical and postoperative risks, especially for special diagnostic constellations such as the combination of a venous leg ulcer with morbid obesity. Ageing and multimorbid patients are also a target group for endovenous therapy.

Perforator vein treatment

The therapy of insufficient perforator veins plays a unique role in the haemodynamic concept of ulcer development. Due to the short connection distance between the deep and superficial venous system, a relevant volume shift into the epifascial venous system can occur in the case of an existing insufficiency. The consequences are oedema formation and trophic disturbances leading up to the development of the ulcer. Open surgical procedures with paratibial longitudinal incision of the lower leg and selective binding of all perforator veins are no longer in use due to the large trauma, subsequent wound-healing disorders and lymphatic complications.

Today, insufficient perforator veins with minor trophic disturbances are usually directly epifascially dissected or ligated. If there is advanced dermato-lipofasciosclerosis in the ulcer region that prevents direct access, subfascial techniques are available. In addition to uncontrolled subfascial dissection by finger, spatula or scissors, Hauer in 1985 introduced the endoscopic subfascial dissection of perforator veins (ESDP). Using the ESDP technique, it is possible to choose an approach other than the actual ulcer and the peri-ulcer skin changes and to cut through perforator veins under endoscopic visual control or to ligate them using a clip. However, this procedure must be critically evaluated based on clinical studies and experience. Postoperative, partly persistent accompanying complications (sensitivity disorders, the tendency to oedema, pain, subfascial infection) and high recurrence rates (40–75% after ESDP) led to a significantly reduced use of the method. A possible indication is several extensive perforator insufficiencies of the medial lower leg with an associated regional manifestation of CVI and necessity for endoscopic paratibial fasciotomy.

27.2.2 Ulcer surgery

Shave therapy

The principle of the so-called shave therapy involves the layerwise tangential resection of epifascial necrotic and sclerotic tissue with immediate coverage of the defect by split skin grafts if necessary. It therefore belongs to the surgical methods for local ulcers. Due to the promising long-term results and low traumatisation in comparison to other local surgical procedures, it is often the method of choice in the surgical treatment of those therapy-resistant venous leg ulcers (➤ Fig. 27.1). The fascia cruris is usually not opened. No other procedure can currently achieve better long-term results. Quaba et al. reported as early as 1987 on the successful layered shaving treatment for therapy-resistant venous leg ulcers. The technique was further scientifically established by Schmeller et al. (1996).

Various dermatome models are available for split skin removal and shave therapy. Battery-operated or shaft-operated systems allow precise removal of necrosis and sclerosis and enable comfortable and fast surgery. The layered, controlled removal of all necroses and sclerotic parts of the ulcer creates a fresh wound that should be as flat as possible and provides the ideal graft site for the prepared split skin. The skin is preferably removed in the area of the lateral thigh. The thickness of the split skin should be 0.3–0.4 mm. Thicker grafts have a more reduced healing rate, and thinner split skin grafts are less stable under pressure. The same applies to the expansion ratio of any mesh graft used – an expansion of 1:1.5 is more stable under pressure than a graft with an expansion ratio of 1:3. Finally, the split skin is applied stress-free to the wound and fixed with individual sutures, clasps, adhesives, or vacuum therapy. There is no valid data on the total layer depth to be removed. Significant preparation of a wound bed with small capillary bleeding is important.

Bradytrophic structures such as tendons may have to be excised. The required layer depth is ultimately also dependent on the actual ulcer depth and is subject to the training curve of the surgeon. Lymph drainage

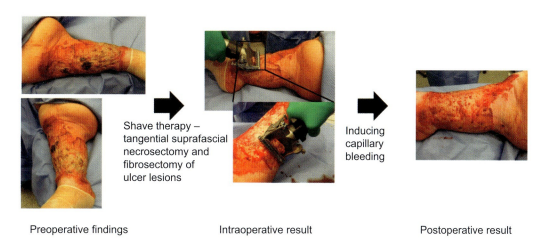

Shave therapy –
tangential suprafascial
necrosectomy and
fibrosectomy of
ulcer lesions

Inducing
capillary
bleeding

Preoperative findings · · · · · · · · · · · · · · · Intraoperative result · · · · · · · · · · · · · · · Postoperative result

Fig. 27.1 Shave therapy of a venous leg ulcer. [F1024-001]

should be used in postoperative aftercare. Consistent and sufficient compression treatment in the long term is obligatory with underlying CVI.

With healing rates of over 90%, excellent results are achieved in ulcers due to primary varicosis. However, with postthrombotic syndrome or vein insufficiency of another genesis, the probability of ulcer recurrence is increased due to the persisting underlying disease. By shaving the necrotic or sclerotic ulcer and preparing a well-vascularised wound bed, even therapy-resistant ulcers with a history of several decades can be healed. The average time of ulcer duration up to surgical treatment in these patients is about 16 years. Comparable procedures, such as basic wound-conditioning by promoting granulation tissue and subsequent split skin transplantation, lead to worse results and lower healing rates of about 30–50%. Granulation tissue as a graft site is not optimal compared to a well-vascularised ulcer base after shaving. In the evaluation of the long-term results of up to 84 months follow-up, healing rates of up to 80% could be determined.

27.2.3 Fascial surgery

In the presence of consecutive trophic disorders of the skin, subcutaneous fatty tissue and muscle fascia, fascial surgery for leg ulcer is becoming increasingly important in addition to local surgical measures.

Paratibial fasciotomy and fasciectomy are surgical procedures that involve the fascia cruris in the treatment of chronic leg ulcers. By opening the subfascial space and the associated pressure relief in the lower leg compartments, fascial surgery represents the causal therapy approach in the concept of chronic compartment syndrome.

Paratibial fasciotomy according to Hach

Wolfgang Hach first described paratibial fasciotomy (PTF) – by splitting the fascia cruris and opening the subfascial compartments, the pressure is relieved, leading to faster healing. A paratibial incision opens the skin, subcutis and fascia cruris. The fascia cruris is then split with scissors or a fasciotomy up to the inner ankle. A proximal fascia cleavage generally follows. A fasciotomy can also be performed endoscopically and can be combined with perforator restructuring.

Retrospective analyses or prospective studies have not yet been published. A permanent reduction of elevated subfascial pressure values after fasciotomy could not be proven. Since paratibial fasciotomy has often been combined with other procedures such as endoscopic subfascial perforator vein dissection or stripping, its exclusive mechanism of action is still unknown.

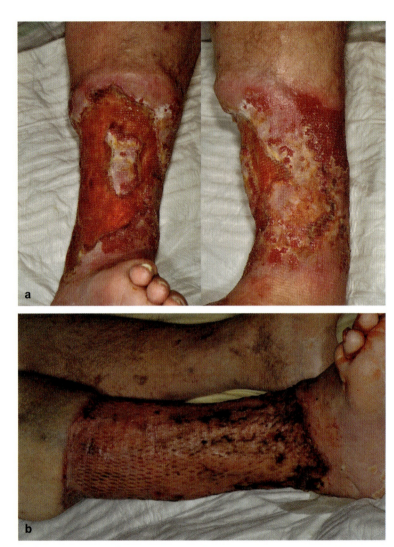

Fig. 27.2 A 57-year-old female patient with venous leg ulcer and pronounced dermatolipofasciosclerosis who has been refractory to therapy for 17 years. **a** Result after crural fasciectomy and split skin transplantation in mesh technique; **b** result four weeks after surgery. [P584]

Fasciectomy

The therapeutic principle of crural fascial resection includes the resection of the entire necrotic and sclerotic tissue on the lower leg, involving the fascia and necrotic tendons. At the same time, all perforator veins in the affected area of the lower leg are removed. Resection of the fascia removes the separation of the compartments and relieves the lower leg muscles of pathological pressures. If there is a circular ulcer, this is referred to as a crural fasciectomy. Crural fascial resection is indicated in patients with stage IV

chronic venous stasis syndrome according to Hach, with circular dermatolipofasciosclerosis, circular or extensive ulcerations and chronic fascial compression syndrome (> Fig. 27.2). The musculature represents a sufficiently good basis for extensive split skin transplants. The ulcer should be incised proximal and distal to the lower leg in the healthy, mostly fibrosis-free area. The fascia can then be incised lengthwise in the full length of the ulcer and sclerosis. The skin fascia flap can then be circularly removed from the lower leg muscles, tendons, tibia and fibula. Necrotic tendons, possibly also the Achilles tendon, should be resected.

The extensive soft tissue defects can then be well covered with split skin implants in mesh technique. It should be noted that surgical techniques such as fasciectomy require sufficient experience on the part of the surgeon. Vascular and nerve injuries are possible complications.

Fascial resection can cure otherwise refractory leg ulcers in up to 80% of cases. It should be noted that surface sensitivity is often reduced after such procedures, but depth sensitivity generally remains unaffected. Fascial resection is more traumatising, and the operation times are longer due to increased preparation effort, in comparison to shave therapy. The indication range for fasciectomy has changed in recent years due to the good results following shave therapy. Primary crural fascial resections in exclusively epifascially localised ulcerations are no longer indicated today. If primary transfascial necroses with exposed tendon parts are present, these can be successfully treated by resection of the lower leg fascia, including the necrotic tissue and tendon parts. Recurrences after multiple shave therapies are today also an indication for fasciotomy.

Split skin transplantation

Areas similar in structure and pigmentation to the recipient region are favoured as donor areas for the removal of split skin. Since hypopigmentation of the donor region may occur after removal of split skin, sites covered by clothing are preferred. It is also possible to remove the split skin from the capillitium since the removal of thin split skin does not destroy the hair follicles, and the donor area is covered by regrowing hair. The epidermis is removed together with the uppermost layer of the dermis, usually 0.2–0.4 mm thick, with the use of a motor-driven dermatome. Thicker grafts have a poorer healing rate, and thinner split skin grafts are less stable under pressure. The same applies to the expansion ratio of the mesh graft if used. An expansion of 1:1.5 is more stable under pressure than a graft with an expansion ratio of 1:3. Finally, the split skin is applied stress-free to the wound and fixed by individual sutures, clasps, adhesives, or vacuum therapy. It is essential that in conventional split skin

transplants, perforations are made with the scalpel to guarantee drainage of the wound fluid. The split skin must be transplanted onto tissue with sufficient blood supply. For this reason, a superficial debridement in the area of the ulcer to be treated can be carried out directly before transplantation, so that temporary bleeding is induced and the split skin can be treated by diffusion.

Reverdin skin grafting

Especially with leg ulcers, tiny wounds, or elderly and multimorbid patients, the possibility exists of skin transplantation as Reverdin pinch grafting. Small island grafts of up to 1 cm in size are transplanted as split skin flaps. These skin flaps are obtained by tangential excision. They do not have to be fixed at the recipient site by sutures or staples. It is usually sufficient to apply a dressing with a non-adhesive wound dressing and sufficient contact pressure. One advantage of this method is, among other things, that the graft places fewer demands on the recipient site and is less susceptible to shear forces during the healing process. Also, the Reverdin skin grafting technique can shorten the intervention time and, if necessary, the operation can also be performed on an outpatient basis.

Reverse corium grafting

Bradytrophic structures such as exposed tendons may have to be excised. If this is not possible or if bony structures are exposed, reverse corium plastic surgery may be helpful (➤ Fig. 27.3). Deepithelialised corium components are applied reversely to the functional structure which prepares the wound bed for subsequent split skin transplantation. The corium graft is removed in a layer with a thickness of 0.3–0.4 mm in the same way as the split skin is removed using a dermatome. After reverse corium transplantation using the sheet or mesh fixation technique, sufficient healing with subsequent granulation can be expected. Split skin transplantation can also be performed in the course of the procedure.

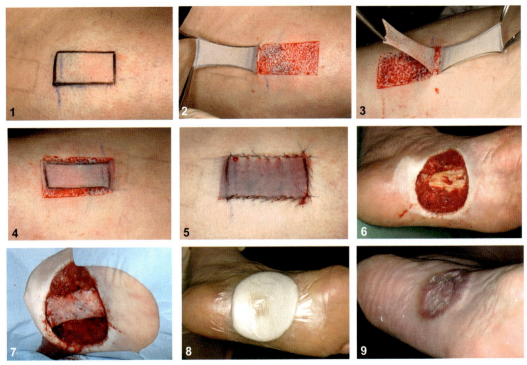

Fig. 27.3 The reverse corium graft was removed from the thigh and transplanted onto the wound with the tendon of the sole exposed. Fixation was performed with negative pressure wound therapy (NPWT). [P584]

27.3 Conclusion

Operative procedures have gained in importance in the treatment of chronic wounds in recent years. The reasons for this are, on the one hand, the more intensive scientific processing of the available methods and, on the other hand, the increasing use of surgical options. Surgical ulcer surgery should only be performed after the possible conservative measures have been exhausted. For poorly healing or persistent ulcers, the concept of therapy resistance plays a decisive role. Only if there is no healing tendency within three months after all conservative possibilities have been exhausted or if an ulcer has not healed after 12 months should the indication for surgical measures be considered. The indications for the various surgical procedures must be set individually. The often advanced age of the patients and the associated additional risks must be taken into account in the decision-making process.

In surgical treatment, shave therapy and fasciectomy are established, especially with chronic per-sistent venous leg ulcers. They are also promising if, due to the extensive ulcerations, neither varicose vein surgery alone nor fasciotomy with or without endoscopic subfascial dissection of the perforator veins are promising, especially in the case of extensive and long-standing ulcers. The results after shave therapy can only be explained by the elimination of pathophysiological trophic disorders in the dermis and subcutis (dermatoliposclerosis) next to and under the ulcers. In crural fascial resection, a positive postoperative effect on the improvement of compartment pressure values can also be assumed. Due to its low invasiveness and rapid postoperative healing with good functional and esthetic results, shave therapy is the surgical therapy of choice for therapy-resistant ulcus cruris. Fascial resection can only be recommended as a more invasive procedure for deep ulcers or necrotic fascia and tendons. Even in cases of therapy failure after shave therapy, a secondary fasciectomy can still lead to therapeutic success.

The indication for ulcer surgery should be permissive, taking into account the often long-standing ulcer anamnesis of patients with considerable impairment of quality of life due to pain and also the costs of local wound treatment. However, postoperative follow-up treatment and guidance of the patient must be an integral part of the concept.

REFERENCES

Ehresmann U, Gallenkemper G. Leitlinie der Deutsche Gesellschaft für Phlebologie. Diagnostik und Therapie des Ulcus cruris venosum. Phlebologie 2008; 37: 308–329.

Hach W, Schwahn-Schreiber C, Kirschner P, Nestle HW. Die crurale Fasziektomie zur Behandlung des inkurablen Gamaschenulkus (Chronisches Faszienkompressionssyndrom). Gefässchirurgie 1997; 2: 101–107.

Schmeller W, Roszinski S. Shave-Therapie zur operativen Behandlung persistierender venöser Ulzera mit großflächiger Dermatoliposklerose. Hautarzt 1996; 47 (9): 676–681.

Schwahn-Schreiber C, Schmeller W, Gaber Y. Langzeitergebnisse (7 Jahre) nach Shave-Therapie bzw. krualer Fasziektomie bei persistierenden venösen Ulcera. Phlebologie 2006; 35: 89–91.

Stoffels I, Dissemond J, Klode J. Moderne Ulcus-Chirurgie – Chirurgische Behandlungsoptionen. Phlebologie 2013; 42: 199–204.

28 Systematics of physical wound treatment

Joachim Dissemond, Katharina Herberger, Sigrid Karrer, Christian Willy

28.1 Physical wound treatment options

Joachim Dissemond

Key notes

- There is an increasingly growing variety of treatment options available for chronic wounds.
- For many wound treatments, there are many different products from different companies, often differing technically in their application, etc., so that a 1:1 comparison is usually not possible.

- Applying different treatment methods which are integrated into an overall concept can potentially support the healing of chronic wounds.
- There is insufficient scientific evidence for most wound therapies.

For the treatment of chronic wounds, various types of therapies have been used in recent decades to support multiple aspects of wound-healing. In the following chapters, the methods are described in more detail, such as adverse pressure treatment (➤ Chap. 28.2), cold atmospheric plasma (➤ Chap. 28.3) and electricity (➤ Chap. 28.4), with an overview of other treatment options for chronic wounds given here as an introduction.

28.1.1 Ultrasound therapy

Ultrasound consists of mechanical waves of which the physiological effects are the result of interactions with transmission media. The reciprocal piezoelectric effect is used to generate low-frequency ultrasound. Ultrasounds of low-frequency areas can use low frequencies with higher intensity and are then partially reflected when hitting a medium without mediating significant thermal effects. The effects of ultrasound in chronic wounds can be divided into mechanical, mechano-acoustic/bio-acoustic and thermal or non-thermal effects. The phenomenon of cavitation is essential in conveying the ultrasound effect in wound treatment. Cavitation describes the formation of microscopic bubbles in liquid media by compression-tension forces that oscillate (stable cavitation) or implode (transient cavitation).

Low-frequency ultrasound or power ultrasound is usually used for the treatment of chronic wounds. During ultrasound therapy, patients with chronic wounds showed an increase in oxygen partial pressure (pO_2) and a reduction in pCO_2 of the cutaneous capillary blood flow. It was under discussion that this improvement of microcirculation is a result of mechanical irritation of the vascular endothelium and an increased release of nitric oxide (NO).

A 2017 updated Cochrane meta-analysis using therapeutic ultrasound in patients with venous leg ulcers analysed 11 randomised controlled trials (RCT). In the studies comparing ultrasound therapies with standard therapies, no significant differences were found in the number of wounds healed.

28.1.2 Extracorporeal shock wave therapy

In extracorporeal shock wave therapy (ESWT), sound pressure waves are used therapeutically. These shock waves are acoustic impulses of which the sound event lasts a few microseconds. Three different generator principles are currently in use – the electromagnetic, the piezoelectric and the electrohydraulic principle. For several decades shockwaves have been used in medicine, for example, for the treatment of urolithiasis (extracorporeal shockwave lithotripsy, ESWL). Here, the devices are adjusted so that energy is compressed in the centre of the concrements, where the shockwaves focus. These are then destroyed very precisely and with the highest possible protection of the surrounding tissue. In contrast to this, in wound treatment, the shockwaves are usually not focused but applied to wounds over a wide area. Improvements in wound-healing are to be achieved by promoting neoangiogenesis, tissue regeneration and the suppression of proinflammatory processes. It has been shown that ESWT increases the expression of RAS, TGF-ß1, VEGF, eNOS and PCNA and increases local blood perfusion. However, the therapy can cause considerable pain in some cases.

In the Cochrane meta-analysis published in 2018, five RCTs with a total of 255 patients with diabetic foot ulcers treated with ESWT were analysed. Here it was shown that treatment with ESWT, in comparison to standard therapies as well as hyperbaric oxygenation, resulted in significantly more wounds being healed. However, the authors consider the evidence to be insufficient. In the Cochrane meta-analysis on venous leg ulcers and ESWT, also published in 2018, no studies could be found.

28.1.3 Electromagnetic therapy

The electromagnetic therapies differ from the treatment options with electrostimulation methods (➤ Chap. 28.4), in as far that here we work with an electrically generated magnetic field and not directly with the effects of electricity.

In the two Cochrane meta-analyses updated in 2015, two RCTs were analysed for pressure ulcers with 60 patients, and three RCTs for venous leg ulcers with 94 patients. Even if there are indications of an improvement in wound-healing in individual studies, the authors see no meaningful option for evaluation in summary due to the heterogeneity and the inadequate quality of the studies. The evidence is therefore considered insufficient.

28.1.4 Phototherapy

Phototherapies are very different procedures in which light is used therapeutically.

In **photodynamic therapy (PDT),** a photosensitiser is applied first, followed by irradiation. A δ aminolevulinic acid (ALA) derivative is usually used as a photosensitiser. ALA is not a direct photosensitiser but is metabolised in the target cells into photosensitisers in the form of various porphyrins. After an exposure time of 3–6 hours, the irradiation can be carried out, which has a depth effect of a few millimetres. Reactive oxygen species (ROS) and, in particular, singlet oxygen ($^1O_2$), are produced, which directly or indirectly mediate cytotoxic effects. PDT is usually painful for patients.

Even though PDT has promoted wound-healing in smaller studies in recent years, the off-label treatment of clinically infected wounds and in particular MRSA detection seems to be a useful indication.

Water-filtered infrared A (wIRA) uses radiation with wavelengths around 760–1,400 nm to generate positive effects in the skin tissue, leading to an increase in the capillary blood flow and pO_2, due to thermal and non-thermal effects. The described bactericidal and pain-relieving effects could also be of importance in wound treatment. The contact-free treatment, which can be patient-operated, is usually carried out with table-top devices. So far, only a few clinical studies with a small number of cases exist for use in patients with chronic wounds.

In wound therapy, **gas lasers** such as helium/neon or gallium/arsenide lasers are predominantly used. Erbium:YAG or CO_2 lasers are used primarily for the ablation of necrosis or dermatoliposclerosis. Individual publications can also be found on diode lasers for wound treatment.

In **low intensity or low-level laser therapy (LILT or LLLT),** formerly synonymously referred to as soft lasers, very different devices with different wavelengths, intensities and execution intervals and times are used. One common feature is that monochromatic and coherent light is used. The propagated goal of the treatment is to promote wound-healing and to reduce inflammation and pain. However, pain can also be caused by treatments.

In a meta-analysis published by Li et al. in 2018, seven RCTs with 194 patients with DFU were analysed, which showed a statistically better wound surface reduction and healing through the additional use of LLLT. In a systematic literature analysis published by Machado et al. in 2017, four studies on LLLT in patients with pressure ulcers could be found. Significantly better results were obtained concerning the promotion of wound-healing exclusively with devices with a wavelength of 658 nm. In two of the few published RCTs with patients with venous leg ulcers (n = 24 and n = 45), no better wound-healing could be objectified.

There are also other devices for wound treatment in which polarised, polychromatic or non-coherent or ultraviolet (UV) light is used. For most methods, there are some case report series or smaller clinical studies, so that the evidence is insufficient.

Other methods such as high tone therapy (HiTop) or bio-resonance therapy (BRT) are instead offered in the context of alternative, not conventional medical treatments.

28.1.5 Conclusion

For the treatment of chronic wounds, there are increasingly various treatment options that can potentially support partial aspects of wound-healing. For many of these therapies, different products from different companies exist, which often differ technically in the way they are carried out, etc., so that a 1:1 comparison is usually not possible. It is therefore not surprising that most of the therapy options presented here have insufficient evidence. However, this is a widespread problem in wound treatment and does not mean that these methods are ineffective. Unfortunately, based on the currently available evidence, it is not possible today to objectively decide which patient will benefit from such treatment, when, for how long, etc. The results of such a decision are not available today.

REFERENCES
Aziz Z, Cullum N. Electromagnetic therapy for treating venous leg ulcers. Cochrane Database Syst Rev 2015; 7: CD002933.
Cooper B, Bachoo P. Extracorporeal shock wave therapy for the healing and management of venous leg ulcers. Cochrane Database Syst Rev 2018; 6: CD011842.
Cullum N, Liu Z. Therapeutic ultrasound for venous leg ulcers. Cochrane Database Syst Rev 2017; 5: CD001180.
Dissemond J. [Physical treatment modalities for leg ulcers]. Hautarzt. 2010; 61: 387–396.
Wang HT, Yuan JQ, Zhang B, et al. Phototherapy for treating foot ulcers in people with diabetes. Cochrane Database Syst Rev 2017; 6: CD011979.

28.2 Negative pressure wound therapy
Christian Willy

──────────────── **Key notes** ────────────────

- Vacuum therapy is also synonymously referred to as vacuum treatment, vacuum-sealing therapy or negative pressure wound therapy (NPWT) and has been performed since the early 1990s.
- NPWT is an integral part of modern wound therapy in numerous medical specialities, such as surgery, dermatology and urology.
- Advantages of this form of therapy include hygienic wound closure, continuous suctioning of wound secretion, the possibility of gaining time until plastic defect coverage without increasing the risk of infection, and the so-called reduction of the size of the wound.
- Of importance is the individually selectable negative pressure on the patient, with a possible spectrum from 50 to 200 mmHg suction.
- An extension of the therapy is possible by supplementing the NPWT with the additional, freely repeatable irrigation of the wound (instillation), e. g. with saline solution or antiseptic liquid (vacuum instillation therapy).

────────────────────────────────────

28.2.1 Introduction

Vacuum therapy, synonymously also referred to as vacuum treatment, vacuum-sealing therapy or negative pressure wound therapy (NPWT), is a method for treating acute and chronic wounds that was developed in the US and Germany at the end of the 1980s. Since the early 1990s, this method has been used clinically on an increasing scale. In Germany, vacuum therapy has been regarded as an established

28

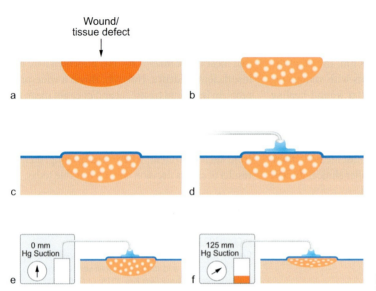

Fig. 28.1 Functional principle of NPWT. [P585/L231]

wound treatment method in everyday clinical practice since around 1995.

28.2.2 Functional principle

The principle of this form of treatment is that the narrowly defined suction effect of drainage, distributed over the entire wound cavity or wound surface via an open-pored sponge, adapted to the wound contour (➤ Fig. 28.1a, b). To prevent ambient air from being sucked in, the wound and the sponge inside it are hermetically sealed by an airtight, water vapour-permeable, transparent and bacteria-proof polyurethane adhesive film (➤ Fig. 28.1c). A 'suction cup' is then glued over a small hole in the film (➤ Fig. 28.1d), which is connected to a vacuum source through a hose (➤ Fig. 28.1e, f).

28.2.3 Effects on wound-healing

The most important clinically relevant advantages of NPWT are the following effects on wound-healing and the affected tissue, which are regarded as the result of the suction acting evenly on the entire wound surface:

- Reduction of the wound surface due to the negative pressure working on the sponge, which pulls the wound edges together (wound retraction).

- Stimulation of the formation of granulation tissue in an ideally moist wound environment even via bradytrophic tissue, such as tendons and bones.
- Continuation of effective wound-cleansing (suctioning of smaller tissue debris) after sufficient surgical primary debridement of the wound.
- Safe, continuous removal of wound secretion within a closed system with a neutral odour and hygienic dressing technology; constant soaking of the dressing, patient clothing and bed linen can be avoided (reduction in the amount of care required).
- Pressure-induced reduction of interstitial oedema with the consecutive improvement of microcirculation.
- Pathogen tightness of the wound dressing due to wound-sealing, so that no external bacteria can penetrate the wound and none of the patient's wound pathogens are spread – particularly relevant in the case of contamination with problem pathogens, e. g. MRSA-infected wounds.
- Reduction in the number of dressing changes required (need to change dressings only every 2–3 days, under controlled and sterile conditions up to seven days), which can significantly reduce the amount of care required, especially for severely exuding wounds.

28.2.4 Handling and duration

Before starting NPWT, surgical debridement of the wound with resection of avital or infected tissue must be performed. Only then can vacuum therapy be started. For this reason, the first treatment often takes place in the operating theatre. Depending on the wound, pathogen colonisation and selected sponge material, the applied dressing can remain for between two and seven days. In the infection situation, for example, a second look should be performed 24 to 48 hours after the primary intervention at the latest. In the case of 'clean' wound conditions and to prepare the wound bed, changes are usually to be made at intervals of three to five (maximum seven) days. The vacuum sponge change is carried out under inpatient conditions on the ward, in the operating theatre or under outpatient conditions, depending on wound pain, technical effort and sterility requirements. The total treatment duration depends on the success of wound-healing. It can last a few days as interim therapy to condition the wound or as definitive therapy until the wound is closed. The following aspects should be considered to avoid misuse:

- If NPWT is indicated, start as early as possible.
- A sponge change should not only be a sponge change. It should often be assessed as to whether the wound can be reduced in size, also whether another method of wound closure could be chosen, e. g. a secondary suture, split skin covering or flap surgery, and when and how the next procedure should be performed. As a rule, these decisions are not decisions that the inexperienced young surgeon can make – in contrast to the sponge change (no-error operation), which is usually easy to perform from a technical point of view. The seemingly simple procedure, often at the end of the surgical program, therefore always presents a challenge.
- Termination of the therapy as soon as possible.

28.2.5 Modifications of NPWT

The NPWT allows some parameters to be adapted to the respective wound situation in a differentiated manner. These parameters can be changed:
1. Wound filler material – polyurethane/polyvinyl alcohol sponge/gauze

2. Suction strength – values between 50 and 200 mmHg are selectable
3. Fluid application – instillation therapy

Choice of wound filler material

The sponges have different properties in pore size and stability:
- Polyurethane (PU, pore size 400–600 µm, soft, black) forms a stronger mechanical bond with the wound tissue after approx. 3–4 days due to the ingrowth of granulation tissue. Therefore, the sponge should be changed after 2–3 days.
- Polyvinyl alcohol (PVA, pore size 200–1,000 µm, white), the somewhat firmer and less deformable sponge, can remain in the wound for several days without a tendency for tissue ingrowth.

It should be emphasised that the hydrophilicity of the sponges is very different. If liquids are to be applied using vacuum instillation therapy, hydrophilic sponges in particular should be used. For rather superficial or very irregularly shaped and less secreting fissured wounds, a gauze instead of a sponge is also suitable as a wound filler.

Selecting the suction strength

According to an experimental animal trial (n = 4) by Morykwas et al., the suction of 125 mmHg should be the most favourable suction strength for tissue formation and wound-cleansing. However, the possibility of variation in the choice of suction for some modern vacuum therapy units is an advantage. It must be taken into account that every vacuum therapy is accompanied by **increased** pressure on the tissue, at least in the tissue layers directly adjacent to the sponge. For chronic wounds, patient pain, deep soft tissue injuries with localisation of the vessels close to the wound or more extensive dressings with a more circular application of the dressing to an extremity, it will be advisable to set the suction value between 75 and 100 mmHg. The same applies to wounds of children, nutritively poorly supplied tissue (subcutaneous tissue) or generally unfavourable perfusion situations (diabetes mellitus, pressure ulcer) or after an operation (status after cleavage of compartment syn-

28

drome). Care must be taken to use a suction source that compensates for the loss of suction in the event of small air leaks.

NPWT instillation therapy

Following the method of Fleischmann et al., a so-called NPWT instillation therapy (NPWTi, since the component instillation is added) can be carried out if residual contamination of the wound still exists. This modification is usually performed with an antiseptic substance [polyhexanide, polyvinylpyrrolidone iodine, super oxidised water (sodium hypochlorite and hypochlorous acid, NaOCl + HOCl)]. Individual authors even propagate vacuum instillation therapy with the use of the physiological saline solution for every wound, including non-infected, especially chronic wounds.

Testing of a recommendation for the basic equipment with three antiseptic solutions in everyday clinical life

NaOCl/HOCl
Benefit   Low toxicity, biocompatible with cartilage and CNS tissues; rapidly effective, NPWTi-usable.
Disadvantage   No remanence. Not relevant for single intraoperative irrigation, but requires an increased frequency of instillation phases for NPWTi. Since frequent instillation cycles tend to provoke leaks, it makes sense to have an additional, remanent substance available, where lower rinsing cycle frequencies are possible.

PVP iodine in alcoholic solution
Benefit   Most deeply effective substance and most effective against viral infections; indispensable therefore in our opinion for wounds with suspected virus entry [bite and stab injuries (cannulae, knife stab)].
Disadvantage   Off-label use (clarification required); no remanent effect.

Polyhexanide solution with PHMB concentration of 0.02%
Benefit   Low toxicity, promotes wound-healing, due to lower concentration (0.02% and not 0.04%), a longer-lasting application of NPWTi is also possible, with a remanent effect.
Disadvantage   Not biocompatible with cartilage and CNS tissue.

With this technique, a pre-defined and programmed quantity of the respective fluid is actively instilled into the wound via a roller pump, using a further tube system with a pre-existing sealing system, in a vacuum therapy phase without suction. The hydrophilic sponge is soaked with the fluid, and the wound is brought into full contact with it. The transparent sealing foil prevents the instillation solution from flowing off outside the wound during the instillation process. After 20 minutes, which is the usual reaction time required for an antiseptic effect, the therapy unit takes up the original suction again – the liquid is sucked off. Then the regular suction between 75 and 125 mmHg is applied again. The therapy cycle is automatically computer-assisted and carried out several times per diem. There are no clear guidelines for the number of cycles. It is pragmatic to select about 4–6 cycles, so that container changes do not have to take place every 12 hours.

Each instillation cycle corresponds to a routine dressing change. With the automated instillation system, the number of 'dressing changes' is practically unlimited, so that intensive and effective wound treatment can be carried out without interruption. The number of time-consuming, sometimes painful dressing changes is considerably reduced for the patient and the therapist thus considers instillation therapy to be a patient-friendly and cost-effective form of treating chronic wounds.

Experience with the application of instillation therapy has been gained in the following indications:

- Septic wounds after initial surgical debridement (instillation of antiseptics or saline solution). Recent studies have shown that even with sodium chloride NPWT instillation, the number of biofilms used could be considerably reduced compared to conventional negative pressure therapy.
- Infections in the area of implant sites (instillation of antiseptics).
- Uncomplicated chronic wounds (instillation of saline solution).
- Painful wounds (postoperative or infection-induced painful conditions occasionally require instillation of local anesthetics).

28.2.6 Indications and contraindications of NPWT

NPWT is indicated for extensive soft tissue defects – initial and postoperative, acute and chronic infected wounds after surgical debridement, and for fixation of skin grafts. It has also become the method of choice for sternal wound infections and a viable alternative for the temporary closure of the open abdomen. NPWT also proved its worth in the treatment of patients with pressure ulcers, venous leg ulcers and especially diabetic foot ulcers.

Pressure ulcer III and IV   After wound debridement, to prepare the wound for surgical closure. In an overall view of the more severe stage of pressure ulcer, surgical therapy must be regarded as the method of choice. The decision always includes surgical debridement, as well as the decision as to whether the optimal plastic intervention procedure can be connected directly, or whether wound-conditioning using NPWT or a second-look procedure should be performed before flap surgery. As a rule, a maximum period of two weeks seems to be sufficient for the NPWT-conditioning phase, if necessary. NPWT is preferred to other methods for wound-conditioning and is therefore of particular importance. In everyday clinical life, however, approximately 10–15% of pressure ulcers are an indication for a primarily conservative method. Compared to alternative traditional methods, NPWT is said to have a higher chance of recovery. NPWT is indicated above all when general or local operability no longer exists in very elderly patients (suction value 100 mmHg).

Venous leg ulcer   After wound debridement (e. g. shaving, fasciectomy) to prepare the wound bed for the subsequent split skin transplantation, which is then fixed again using vacuum therapy. Here, the same therapy procedure is used for two completely different purposes (wound-conditioning, skin fixation).

Diabetic foot ulcer   After wound debridement for wound bed preparation, it is particularly important not to apply too much suction (= pressure on the tissue). Suction values of 50–100 mmHg are sufficient.

Various authors have also regarded other indications, such as burns, enterocutaneous fistulas or lymphocutaneous fistulas as indicative. Acute bleeding and the risk of bleeding are specific **contraindications.** The possibility of applying vacuum therapy to exposed vessels and neoplastic tissue is controversial. In individual situations where vacuum therapy was successfully implemented, it was still acknowledged that this form of therapy can also be indicated in these controversially regarded cases. For example, in the palliative situation of malignant ulcerating wounds, the hygienic, secretion-conducting supply method using negative pressure therapy is helpful without endangering the patient.

28.2.7 Application example

The individual stages of vacuum therapy are presented using a sample presentation of a patient case. The case shows the hygienic and comfortable treatment of an infected and unstable sternal wound in a 73-year-old patient (➤ Fig. 28.2).

28.2.8 Conclusion

NPWT has been a firmly established form of treatment for acute and chronic wounds in numerous medical specialities in everyday clinical life since around 1990. The extension of the therapy with the use of an automatically controllable, freely repeatable flushing of the wound (NPWT instillation therapy), e. g. with saline solution or antiseptic liquids, opens up further areas of application for this therapy.

REFERENCES

Apelqvist J, Willy C, Fagerdahl AM, et al. EWMA Document: Negative pressure wound therapy. J Wound Care 2017; 26 (Suppl. 3): 1–154.

Argenta LC, Morykwas MJ. Vacuum-assisted closure: a new method for wound control and treatment: clinical experience. Ann Plast Surg 1997; 38 (6): 563–576.

Fleischmann W, Russ M, Westhauser A, Stampehl M. [Vacuum sealing as carrier system for controlled local drug administration in wound infection]. Unfallchirurg 1998; 101 (8): 649–654.

Isago T, Nozaki M, Kikuchi Y, Honda T, Nakazawa H. Effects of different negative pressures on reduction of wounds in negative pressure dressings. J Dermatol 2003; 30 (8): 596–601.

Willy C. The theory and practice of vacuum therapy – scientific basis, indications for use, case reports, practical advice. Ulm: Lindqvist Book Publishing; 2006.

28

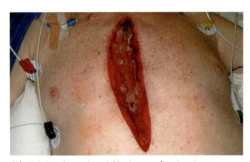

Infected sternal wound, unstable sternum after sternotomy, fibrinous membranes and necrosis, particularly in the cranial part of the wound.

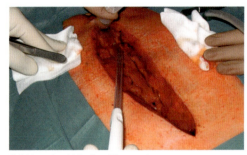

Debridement and irrigation of the wound.

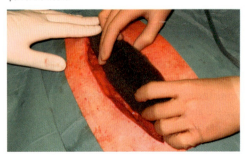

The foam is fitted to the shape of the wound (black polyurethane [PU] foam).

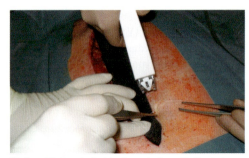

Fixation of the foam to the lateral wound edges with skin staples (alternatively, this can be done with skin suture or without any fixation).

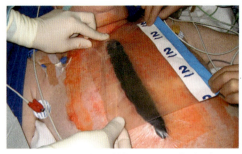

Sealing of the wound with an airtight transparent adhesive drape.

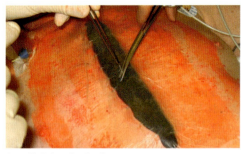

A small hole is cut into the drape.

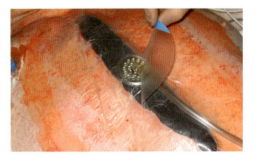

The *trac-pad connector* is applied onto this hole.

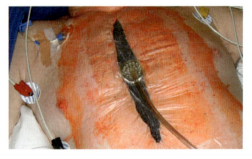

Wound after connection of the vacuum source at 125 mmHg. Compared to the initial finding (on the left), there is a distinct narrowing of the wound due to the 'shrinking' of the foam caused by suction.

Fig. 28.2 Hygienic and comfortable treatment of an infected and unstable sternal wound in a 73-year-old patient. [P585]

28.3 Cold atmospheric plasma
Sigrid Karrer

Key notes

- Plasma is an ionised gas of which the main active components are reactive species, ions and electrons, electromagnetic fields, UV radiation, visible light and heat radiation.
- Cold atmospheric plasma (CAP) is capable of effectively and rapidly combating various microorganisms and multi-resistant pathogens

and promoting wound-healing by influencing cellular functions.
- To date, no side effects have been observed in clinical studies from treatment with CAP; unlike antibiotics or antiseptics, there is also no evidence of allergies or resistance formation.
- There are already several CE-certified plasma medical devices on the market that can be used for wound treatment.

28.3.1 Introduction

A promising therapy option for the treatment of wounds has been available for several years: cold atmospheric plasma (CAP). Physically, plasma is defined as the fourth state of matter besides solid, liquid and gaseous. Plasma is an ionised gas consisting of various components, such as reactive oxygen species (ROS) and nitrogen species (NOS), ions, electrons, electric fields, visible light and UV radiation. Depending on the gas temperature, a distinction is made between 'hot' (thermal) plasma and 'cold' (non-thermal or low-temperature) plasma.

'Hot' plasmas have long been used in medical technology, e. g. for disinfecting heat-stable devices or for blood coagulation and tissue ablation. Only the development of low-temperature plasmas under atmospheric pressure made a gentle and pain-free application on humans possible. It opened up a new field of application and research – plasma medicine. Different technologies are used to generate cold plasma. With direct plasma sources [Dielectric Barrier Discharge (DBD) device], the plasma is generated between a dielectric barrier layer on the electrode and the skin, which serves as a counter electrode, with the current flowing through the body. With indirect plasma sources (plasma needle, plasma torch, plasma jet), the plasma is generated in a cavity between two electrodes and then transported contact-free to the skin with a stream of gas. Direct plasma sources, therefore, require a carrier gas such as helium or argon. So-called hybrid plasmas combine features of direct and indirect plasmas, with no current flowing through the body. The essential active components of plasma

are present in different plasma sources to varying degrees. Therefore, the results of studies conducted with different plasma devices cannot be directly compared.

Low-temperature plasmas are now used in a wide range of medical applications – be it for antiseptics or the treatment of bacterial, viral or mycotic infections, for the destruction of biofilms, for wound treatment and tissue regeneration, as well as for tumour therapy. Treatment with CAP is painless, purely physical, and does not provide a target for allergic reactions, for example. The pathogenic effect of CAP against a broad spectrum of microorganisms has been confirmed in numerous studies without there being any evidence of bacterial resistance. The plasma thus has great potential as an alternative to conventional antimicrobial therapies, such as antibiotics and antiseptics.

Some plasma devices are already approved and CE-certified as medical devices for wound treatment (e. g. Adtec SteriPlas® from ADTEC Healthcare, kINPen® MED from neoplas tools GmbH, PlasmaDerm® from CINOGY GmbH; ➤ Fig. 28.3). The development of new devices is progressing rapidly so that further innovative products will come onto the market shortly.

28.3.2 Mechanisms of action

Numerous studies show that gram-negative and gram-positive bacteria can be killed very efficiently with CAP, as can biofilms, fungi, viruses and spores. The bacteria are killed by CAP within a few seconds, regardless of their resistance status (MRSA), as are extremely radiation-resistant pathogens such as *Deinococcus radiodurans* and other human pathogenic microorganisms,

28

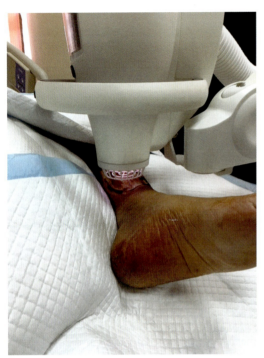

Fig. 28.3 Treatment of a chronic wound with Adtec Steri-Plas®, an indirect low-temperature plasma source. At six electrodes, plasma with argon as a carrier gas is generated and then transported to the target area via gas flow. The treatment is completely painless and takes about two minutes per area. [V859]

such as listeria, salmonella or enterohaemorrhagic *Escherichia coli* (EHEC). The antimicrobial properties of CAP are mainly due to physical mechanisms caused by the reactive species, free radicals and UV photons present in the plasma, but also to biological mechanisms such as DNA and cell membrane damage. Also, the interaction of CAP with liquids and surfaces on which the pathogens are located plays a complex role. The antimicrobial effectiveness can also be influenced by the plasma source used, the composition of the plasma, the duration of treatment and the frequency of treatment. The selectivity of CAP on prokaryotic cells against eukaryotic cells is based, among other things, on different cell metabolism and a higher cell organisation of the eukaryotic cells, which are better able to protect themselves against reactive oxygen species and external stress.

CAP not only influences wound-healing through its antibacterial properties but also influences wound-healing relevant cells. Previous in vitro and in vivo studies show that CAP intervenes very early in the wound-healing process and promotes immune cell activation (macrophages, leukocytes and neutrophil granulocytes). Furthermore, CAP reduces bacterial inflammation by activating antimicrobial peptides, the β-defensins, in keratinocytes. In addition, CAP promotes the expression of wound-healing cytokines (e. g. IL-6, IL-8) and growth factors (e. g. TGF-β1, TGF-β2) in keratinocytes and fibroblasts and induces the production of collagen due to the activation of fibroblasts. Thus CAP promotes the matrix synthesis of the connective tissue structure to be restored. Also, stimulating effects of CAP on angiogenesis by induction of angiogenesis-promoting growth factors (such as VEGF, EGF, FGF) and cytokines (such as IL-1, IL-2, IL-6, IL-8, TNFα, TGF-β) could be observed. Also on microcirculation and oxygen saturation in tissues, beneficial effects are described by CAP. In summary, it can be said that different cellular mechanisms in different cell types of the skin are activated in all phases of wound-healing, which can have a positive effect on wound-healing.

28.3.3 Clinical use

CAP applications are contact-free and painless, treatment times are short, and no allergic or toxic reactions, development of resistance or other relevant side effects have been detected so far. There are several controlled clinical trials in patients with chronic and acute wounds that have demonstrated the wound-healing and pathogen-reducing properties of CAP.

In two randomised controlled phase II studies in patients with infected ulcers of different etiologies, it was shown that once-daily supplementation with MicroPlaSter alpha® or MicroPlaSter beta® (ADTEC Healthcare) for two or five minutes, respectively, resulted in significantly higher pathogen reduction compared to plasma-free control. In an open, retrospective, randomised, controlled study, the effect of MicroPlaSter alpha® on wound-healing was investigated. In 70 patients with infected ulcers of different etiologies, no significantly greater reduction in wound size was observed compared to the control wounds. There was a significant reduction in wound size found only in a subgroup of 27 patients with venous ulcers.

Forty patients with split skin sites were treated with the MicroPlaSter beta® to investigate the plasma effect on wound-healing in similar, non-infected wounds. In this placebo-controlled study, the wound-halves treated with CAP showed faster epithelialisation and fewer fibrin deposits and blood crusts from the second day of treatment.

The DBD plasma generator PlasmaDerm® VU-2010 (CINOGY GmbH) was used in a randomised, controlled study as an add-on therapy three times a week for eight weeks in 14 patients with venous ulcers. Plasma treatment led to a significant reduction in bacterial load immediately after plasma treatment, but not over the entire treatment period. Plasma-treated wounds showed a larger but statistically not significant decrease in wound size compared to control wounds. The Plasma-Derm® FLEX9060 (CYNOGY GmbH) was also used once a week in six patients with wound-healing disorders following oral and maxillofacial surgery. All patients healed completely within an average of 15.5 weeks.

In a pilot study, the effect of a plasma jet (kINPen® MED, neoplas tools GmbH) on pathogen reduction in venous ulcers was investigated in comparison to antiseptic treatment with octenidine dihydrochloride. The treatment was carried out three times a week for two weeks, but the therapy with plasma jet was inferior to octenidine in terms of pathogen reduction.

The effectiveness of a CAP jet (Maxium® beamer, Gebrüder Martin GmbH) on the multi-resistant organism (MRO) was investigated in 11 patients with 18 chronic wounds. In all wounds, the MRO could be significantly reduced or entirely removed by additional plasma treatment.

Despite the partly promising first clinical studies and the advantages of plasma therapy over antiseptics and antibiotics, treatment with CAP has not yet found its way into the clinical routine. It is usually only offered in specialised centres and not reimbursed by health insurance companies due to the lack of billing options. Further controlled studies will be necessary to demonstrate the superiority of CAP over standard antibacterial therapies.

28.3.4 Conclusion

Thanks to interdisciplinary research in medicine, physics, chemistry, biology, microbiology and technology, plasma medicine has developed into an innovative and dynamic field of research in recent years. The treatment of chronic wounds is particularly promising since CAP not only contributes to the reduction of pathogens and biofilm but also promotes wound-healing and blood circulation. Even though the understanding of the molecular effects of CAP has grown considerably in recent years, there is still a need for further basic and clinical research with the various plasma devices to expand the potential of plasma medicine further and exclude long-term risks.

REFERENCES

Gan L, Zhang S, Poorun D, et al. Medical applications of nonthermal atmospheric pressure plasma in dermatology. J Dtsch Dermatol Ges 2018; 16: 7–14.

Heinlin J, Isbary G, Stolz W, et al. Plasma applications in medicine with a particular focus on dermatology. J Eur Acad Dermatol Venereol 2011; 25: 1–11.

Isbary G, Heinlin J, Shimizu T, et al. Successful and safe use of 2 min cold atmospheric argon plasma in chronic wounds: results of a randomized controlled trial. Br J Dermatol 2012; 167: 404–410.

Karrer S, Arndt S. [Plasma medicine in dermatology: mechanisms of action and clinical applications]. Hautarzt 2015; 66: 819–828.

Metelmann HR, von Woedtke T, Weltmann KD (Hrsg.) Plasmamedizin. Kaltplasma in der medizinischen Anwendung. Berlin, Heidelberg: Springer; 2016.

28.4 Electrostimulation
Katharina Herberger

───────────────────── **Key notes** ─────────────────────

- Electrostimulation (EST) is a local wound treatment method.
- EST promotes various wound-healing processes, including cell proliferation and migration, differentiation of the extracellular matrix and tissue perfusion and oxygenation.

- The efficacy of EST in leg ulcer, diabetic foot ulcer, pressure ulcer and chronic wounds of mixed aetiology can be evaluated as evidence-based, based on numerous clinical studies and three meta-analyses.

28.4.1 Definition

In electrotherapy, synonymously also called electro-stimulation (EST) or stimulation current therapy, electrical currents are transmitted to the skin as alternating or direct current impulses which flow through the body or body parts and thus produce physiological effects. Originally, EST methods were used for muscle and nerve stimulation. Indirect positive effects were shown in the treatment of chronic wounds. In the meantime, EST has developed into an important therapy option for poorly healing wounds.

28.4.2 Operating principle

The EST is based on the observation that the charge ratio of intact and injured skin differ. The skin has a transepithelial potential (TEP) which is maintained by chloride ions on the skin surface and sodium ions flowing into the dermal extracellular space. Thus, there is a negative charge on the skin surface, and the epidermis forms the barrier to the positive potential of the underlying dermis. If a wound occurs, the electrical barrier is lost, resulting in a so-called 'short-circuit current'. The changes in the electrical currents at the wound follow specific changes to stop again after the healing has completed. In a chronic wound, these electrical potentials which promote healing are disturbed when an electric field is applied, transferring the wound from a chronic to an acute situation.

Physiological effects

Various basic scientific studies have proven the therapeutic effects of electrostimulation on wound-healing. The observed effects include the galvanotaxis of macrophages and granulocytes as well as the promotion of proliferation, protein synthesis and directed migration of fibroblasts. Furthermore, positive effects on collagen formation and the extra-cellular matrix with a subsequent higher tensile strength of the scar tissue could be demonstrated. Also, improvement of perfusion, reduction of oedema and pain, and increased tissue oxygen saturation, as well as an antibacterial effect, were described.

Clinical efficacy

Based on numerous clinical studies and three meta-analyses, the clinical efficacy of EST can be regarded as scientifically well proven. Besides, the evidence was summarised in a national consensus paper, and a practical treatment algorithm was recommended. The literature summary by the consensus group showed that the effectiveness of the treatment of patients with ulcus cruris, pressure ulcers and diabetic foot wounds is best proven, with 25 and 18 studies respectively.

Gardner et al. carried out the first meta-analysis in 1999. For a total of 15 studies, the wound reduction in wounds of each genesis was analysed, and an average wound reduction of 22.2% was found in the 803 treatments compared to 9.1% in the controls per week. From this, Gardner et al. concluded a wound size reduction 2.4 times faster or acceleration of 144% compared to the control. In the second meta-analysis of Koel, 2013, the analysis of 15 (n = 379) randomised controlled trials on EST in different indications showed an almost doubled additional wound size reduction within four weeks from 15.6% to 37.8% ($p < 0.05$). A third meta-analysis by Kwan et al. dealt with EST in diabetic foot wounds. The investigation of three pooled studies showed a significantly higher number of healings under EST (treatment effect 2.8 [95% CI = 1.5–5.5; $p = 0.0029$]).

28.4.3 Indications

The EST is used for the treatment of various wound-healing disorders. The treatment of chronic wounds, in particular, venous leg ulcers, arterial and mixed leg ulcers, diabetic foot ulcers, pressure ulcers category II–IV according to EPUAP and chronic wounds of mixed aetiology is regarded as a reliable indication based on sufficient scientific evidence. Also, successful treatments are described for secondary wound-healing, e. g. after amputations as well as for use in wound bed preparation and follow-up, after plastic surgery, postoperative wound-healing disorders, suture dehiscence, burns and infected wounds. Further studies are necessary to classify the application in these types of wounds, as the available evidence is usually based on individual case reports.

EST is not a cause-removing treatment, but a local wound treatment procedure. For this reason, causal therapy should always be sought beforehand or as concomitant therapy.

28.4.4 Treatment prerequisites, procedure, and therapy systems

There are various low-frequency EST systems available for wounds that differ in application parameters. These include DC, interference and AC systems. Most of the experience has been with monophasic, low-frequency DC therapy, in which the impulses are applied directly to the wound and not to the healthy skin, as is the case with biphasic EST. It is a painless therapy procedure that can be patient-operated according to instructions and is recommended to be repeated over a defined period, usually as a daily treatment. As a rule, a dressing is applied directly to the wound, which consists of a hydrogel matrix and serves as an electrode. A second electrode is attached to the healthy skin at a defined distance from the first electrode to close the DC circuit. Depending on the polarity, the electrode close to the wound above the wound represents the electrical cathode (negative pole) or the anode (positive pole).

Biphasic low-frequency currents, on the other hand, are applied to healthy skin via electrodes. This procedure was borrowed from electrostimulation for muscle or nerve stimulation, for the treatment of chronic wounds. Monophasic DC pulse therapy was developed for direct wound treatment. Necroses and strong deposits should be removed before treatment to avoid disturbances of the electrical flow. Another prerequisite is not too much exudation at the wound. After granulation has been completed, the therapy is usually terminated and replaced by phase-adapted local therapy or surgical wound-covering procedures.

Contraindications exist in particular for other electrical therapy devices such as pacemakers or nerve stimulation devices. ➤ Fig. 28.4 shows a typical course of treatment of an EST in mixed leg ulcers for almost

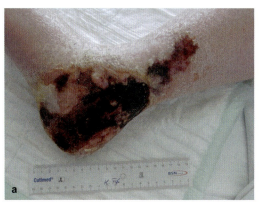
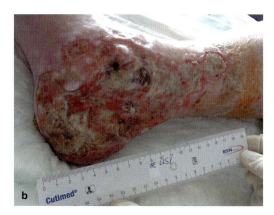
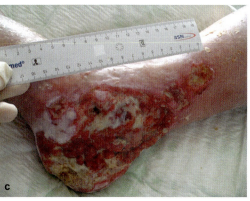

Fig. 28.4 Typical course of treatment of an EST in mixed leg ulcers for almost six weeks. [P585]

six weeks, during which a complete granulation under the EST occurred.

28.4.5 Conclusion

The EST of poorly healing wounds has become an essential therapeutic option in recent years. Several national and international guidelines recommend the use of EST for chronic wounds.

REFERENCES

Herberger K, Debus ES, Larena-Avellaneda A, Blome C, Augustin M. Effectiveness, tolerability, and safety of electrical stimulation of wounds with an electrical stimulation device: Results of a retrospective register study. Wounds 2012; 24: 76–84.

Herberger K, Heyer K, Goepel L, et al. Consensus document on electrical stimulation in treatment of chronic wounds in preparation for a national S1 guideline. Wound Medicine 2015; 9: 10–33.

Jaffe L, Vanable J. Electrical fields and wound-healing. Clin Dermatol 1984; 2: 34–44.

Kloth LC. Electrical Stimulation for wound-healing: A review of evidence from in vitro studies, animal experiments, and clinical trials. Int J Low Extrem Wounds 2005; 4: 23–44.

Pullar CE. The biological basis for electrical stimulation as a therapy to heal chronic wounds. J Wound Technol 2009; 6: 20–24.

29 Systematics of compression therapy

Stefanie Reich-Schupke

Key notes

- Compression therapy is an essential component of therapy for almost all types of leg wounds, except for critical ischaemia.
- A distinction must be made between a decongestion phase and a maintenance phase.
- Compression therapy can be performed with bandages, adaptive systems or compression stockings. Also, intermittent pneumatic compression can be used.
- The selection of the material and the implementation of the therapy should be based on the patient's symptoms, concomitant diseases and preferences.

29.1 Definition and important basic terms

Compression therapy (CT) is indispensable in the treatment of venous and lymphatic diseases. It exerts a defined pressure on the extremity or another treated part of the body due to the external contact pressure, which produces numerous effects (➤ Chap. 33.1.2).

In ➤ Table 29.1, the vital basic terms are summarised to understand the effect of CT, to provide indications and to select the right materials.

29.2 Mode of operation

➤ Table 29.2 summarises the mode of action of the CT proven in studies, which goes far beyond a purely mechanical effect.

When applying CT, a distinction is made between two phases of CT: the initial decongestion phase and the subsequent maintenance phase. Compression bandages or adaptive systems should be used as long as there is considerable oedema and also that a change in circumference can be assumed under CT. For bandages, underpadding should be used to avoid tissue damage. In the case of severe swelling in the forefoot area, the wrapping of individual toes has proven to be effective in analogy to lymphatic

dressings for other indications. If the extremity has attained a stable shape, it is advisable to change to a stocking treatment for reasons of practicality in everyday life; the adaptive systems used, if necessary, can continue to be used here.

29.3 Indications and contra-indications

CT has proven to be effective and safe for numerous oedema and vascular diseases (➤ Table 29.3). There are *de facto* few absolute contraindications. In the field of relative contraindications, the use of compression with selected materials and special caution is usually possible without problems (➤ Table 29.3). In the area of relative contraindications, special measures for skin protection and measures to avoid pressure peaks should be applied. In this case, the padding underneath the bandages is particularly important.

29.4 Materials

Modern CT can be performed with bandages, adaptive systems, medical compression stockings and air cuffs (so-called intermittent pneumatic compression). The

Table 29.1 Overview of important basic terms for compression therapy

Term	Definition	Reference
Resting pressure	The pressure that the material exerts on the extremity at rest – without muscular work.	After the resting pressure in the ankle area, for example, the classes of medical compression stockings are defined.
Working pressure	Pressure built up between material and working muscle	The medically relevant parameter for an effective CT is the working pressure. It can be influenced both by changing the resting pressure and by changing the material strength.
Material strength	Compression materials consist of elastic components that are more or less elastic. The lower the elasticity and the stronger the knitted fabric, the higher the material strength.	Compression stockings with identical resting pressure can have completely different properties due to a change in material strength.
Knitting style	Compression stockings can be manufactured as round and flat knit material. The number of stitches in the circular knitting material does not differ from beginning to end, but the stitch size does. With flat knitting material, a different number of stitches can be knitted in each row.	Circular knitting materials are only partly variable in shape; flat knitting materials can be produced individually and adapted to any body shape.
Decongestion phase/maintenance phase	The decongestion phase defines the CT up to the maximum and stable reduction of a possibly existing oedema, which is followed by the maintenance phase to ensure the condition of the system.	In the decongestion phase, dressing systems or adaptive systems have proven themselves. In the maintenance phase, compression stockings are preferred. The use of adaptive systems is possible.

Table 29.2 Summary of the effects of CT demonstrated in studies

- Reduction of the venous cross-section both at rest and under muscle contraction
- Increase in venous return flow
- Restoration of the functionality of relatively insufficient venous valves in dilated veins
- Reduction of oedema
- Improvement of macro- and microcirculation
- Improvement of venous refill time
- Pain relief and volume reduction
- Increase of the reabsorption of tissue fluid in the venous thigh of the microcirculation
- Acceleration of blood flow in dilated capillary loops
- Reduction of capillary filtration and increase in resorption
- Modification of the paracellular barrier and reduction of oedema formation
- Increase in cellular blood flow
- Reduction of the minimum epidermis thickness
- Decrease in inflammatory activity
- Intracutaneous improvement of flow velocity and vascular muscle activity
- Reduction of the progression of CVI
- Accelerated healing of venous ulcerations

range of materials available today for CT is vast and enables individualised care.

29.4.1 Bandages

A distinction must be made between short- and long-stretch bandages and padding materials (cotton wool, foam rubber, cotton tube, gauze bandages). These components can be used individually or in combination (➤ Fig. 29.1).

A combination, e. g. padding and short-stretch bandage, increases material strength, the resulting working pressure, as well as reducing skin damage and making the short-stretch material slip less. Dressings have proven themselves, especially in the initial phase of decongestion. Unfortunately, they are often used much longer in clinical practice than necessary and without padding materials, which could be the reason for the negative attitude of many patients towards CT. Dressings can be differentiated as those with light (< 20 mmHg), medium (20–40 mmHg) and strong (40–60 mmHg) compression. The use of pressure sensors,

Table 29.3 Indications and contraindications for CT

Indications	Relative contraindications	Absolute contraindications
Therapy of venous diseases – CVI, deep vein thrombosis, postthrombotic syndrome, venous leg ulcer	Heavy weeping dermatoses	Primary chronic polyarthritis
After venous interventions	Severe sensitivity disorders of the extremities/advanced neuropathy	Advanced peripheral artery disease (critical ischaemia)
Thrombosis prophylaxis	Compensated peripheral artery disease (ABI > 0.5 absolute systolic ankle artery pressure > 60 mmHg)	Decompensated heart failure
Therapy of lipoedema	Compensated heart failure	Septic phlebitis
Lymphoedema therapy	Incompatibility/allergies to the compression material	Phlegmasia cerulea dolens
Therapy and prevention of oedema of other causes (e. g. pregnancy)		

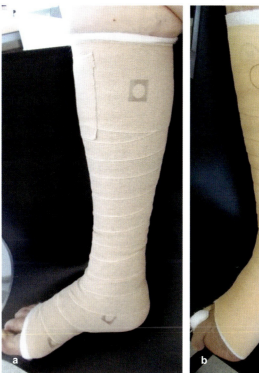
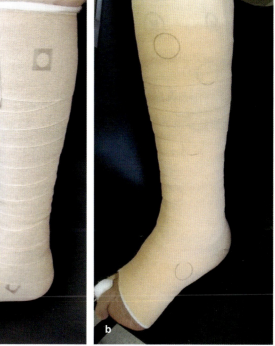

Fig. 29.1 Different types of compression bandages from single components (**a**) or multi components (**b**) [P586]

29

such as Kikuhime® or PicoPress®, is recommended during training for the correct application technique.

As an alternative to the individual combination of individual components, ready-made multi-component systems are available on the market. They usually consist of short-stretch and padding materials, but some are also made with short-stretch, padding and long-stretch materials. If they are applied correctly, they maintain the target contact pressure very reliably and can be left on the leg for up to seven days. They therefore offer practical advantages, especially in the outpatient decongestion phase. In the case of multi-component systems, those with full contact pressure (approx. 40–50 mmHg according to the manufacturer) are to be distinguished from so-called 'Lite' versions with reduced contact pressure (approx. 20–30 mmHg according to the manufacturer). The latter were designed for patients with a combination of CVI and compensated PAD (ABI 0.5–0.8, systolic ankle artery pressure > 60 mmHg, NOT in critical ischaemia!). Here they have proven to be safe. In practical everyday use, the use of these lite systems has also proven itself in decongestion therapy for patients who were previously very critical of CT and had reservations about high compression pressures. It has been shown that lower pressure values are also useful in the treatment of lymphatic diseases, CVI and leg ulcers. Some of the multi-component systems offer optical orientation aids for the assessment of the correct contact pressure in the applied state.

For the optimal application of compression bandages, the use of pads in this area of fluctuating circumference has proven successful to ensure uniform contact pressure and to avoid ridge formation. The use of pads with uneven surfaces can also accelerate decongestion. (➤ Table 29.4).

Table 29.4 Overview of practical tips for CT with bandages

- Apply padding to protect against skin and nerve damage, especially in the ankle region, the front edge of the tibia or at the head of the fibula.
- If necessary, use pads to cushion depressions.
- If necessary, incorporation of uneven surfaces to optimise and accelerate decongestion.
- The CT should be worn all day during the decongestion phase. During the maintenance phase, the compression can be discarded overnight if necessary.
- Adhesion of the compression bandage is with adhesive bandages or adhesive tapes – NOT with the often enclosed clamps (**warning:** injuries).
- Start off with the compression bandage on the metatarsophalangeal joint of the big toe, if necessary wrapping individual toes in the decongestion phase with existing oedema on the forefoot.
- Functional position of the foot (= right angle in the ankle joint or dorsiflexion) when applying the compression bandage.
- Always include the heel.
- Create a decreasing pressure drop from distal to proximal.
- Feed (do not pull) the bandage onto the skin with the bandage roller under permanent tension so that the bandage stays smooth and even (**warning:** constrictions).

29.4.2 Medical compression stockings

Medical compression stockings (MCS) are available in various classes of compression, knitting, material strengths and types. It is an aid that can be prescribed so that it does not affect the budget.

According to the RAL regulation RAL-GZ 387/1, four different types of knitting are available in Germany.

The compression classes (CCL) are defined differently in different countries (➤ Table 29.5). The classification is made according to the resting pressure at the anatomical point B. Starting from point B, the pressure significantly decreases proximally. Here the standard requires residual pressure ratios of 70–100% at measuring point B1, 50–70% (CCL III–IV) or 50–80% (CCL I–II) at measuring point C as well as 20–60% (CCL I), 20–50% (CCL II) and 20–40% (CCL III–IV) at measuring point F or G. If a high-pressure value at the thigh is required, e. g. in severe postthrombotic syndrome or proximal lymphoedema, this must be noted on the prescription.

Concerning the type of knitting, a distinction is made between finer, round and coarser, flat knitted materials with very different properties (➤ Table 29.6; ➤ Fig. 29.2). About 90% of the materials used in the supply system are circular knitted fabrics. While circular knitting materials can be produced as a series and made to measure, flat knit materials are always individual productions. Flat knit materials are also more complex to produce and are therefore understandably more expensive. Accordingly, indicating the selection of a flat knit material should be made very carefully and purposefully.

Table 29.5 Compression classes of medical compression stockings compared in different countries

	Class I	Class II	Class III	Class IV
British standard	14–17	18–24	25–35	N/A
German standard	18–21	23–32	34–46	> 49
French standard	10–15	15–20	20–36	> 36
Draft European standard	15–21	23–32	34–46	> 49
USA standard	15–20	20–30	30–40	N/A

Table 29.6 Comparison of circular and flat knit properties

	Circular knitting	Flat knitting
Type of knitting/production	• On a cylinder • Largely mechanical	• Flat on a knitting machine • More manual work required
Needlework	Low proportion	High proportion
Mesh number	Same number per row from top to bottom	In each row a different number of meshes possible
Contour/size	Changes due to pre-tensioning of the weft thread and stitch size	Contour and size are controlled by a variation of the number of meshes
Material	• Thin, highly elastic • Close-meshed • Single surface – less transverse elastic – 20 stitches per inch	• Approx. 30–40% coarser mesh size • Correspondingly thicker knitted fabric • Wide-meshed • Two-surface – accordion effect, more transverse elastic, 14 stitches per inch
Seam	Seamless	Usually a seam on the back of the stocking
Strength/Stiffness	Partly different within a compression class	Strong, less elastic material
Form stability	Low → Risk of ridge formation from overstretching	High → low risk of cord furrows and overstretching
Variability	A large variety of colours and patterns possible	Reduced range of colours and patterns possible
Compression classes	I–III	I–IV
Variants	Series and made-to-measure production	Made to measure only
Additions	Only the adhesive edge	Wide range of different additions possible, e.g. function zones, diagonal terminations, hold functions
'Massage effect' of the CT	Flat massage	Also punctiform massage between the meshes

29

Although there is no fixed assignment for circular or flat knit materials, the indication for flat knit compression has proven itself in the following situations:
- Significant volume differences
- Deep skin wrinkles
- Severe oedema of the toes (despite sufficient decongestion)
- Reduced perfusion or sensitivity as the risk of constriction and consequential damage is lower under the dimensionally stable flat-knit compression
- All other body regions except extremities

While virtually every area and circumference of the body can be supplied at any pressure using flat knit material, the circular knit supply is limited by the knitting technique. The largest circumference on the thigh can be a maximum of 2.5 times larger than the smallest circumference on the ankle. Besides, the circular knitting technique allows a maximum circumference change of 1 cm within a length change of 1 cm. Accordingly, extreme differences in handling (e.g. the so-called 'bottleneck bone') or variations in the shape of a leg cannot be treated with circular knitting.

However, it should be noted that there can also be very different material strengths within a circular knit supply and a CCL which result from the manufacture of the MCS. Depending on the weft thread and pretension as well as the choice of material, elastic or rather inelastic (= short) materials can be produced. In the case of a leg of greater circumference, a rather firm stocking material should be chosen for sufficient therapy. A largely slender leg can be well treated with elastic MCS. The selection of the MCS suitable for the individual patient can be based on the compression logic of Kröger et al. (➤ Fig. 29.3). Here, too, the decisive factor is not the assignment of a specific MCS according to a diagnosis, but a selection of materials

29

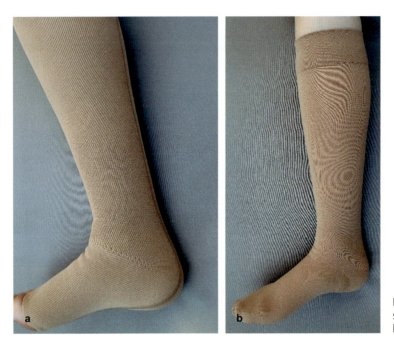

Fig. 29.2 Medical compression stockings in flat knit (**a**) and round knit (**b**). [P586]

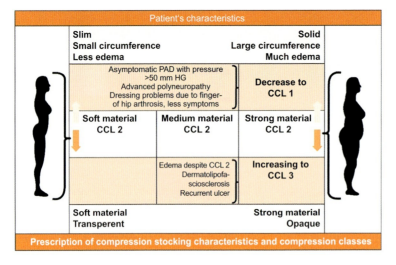

Fig. 29.3 Compression logic, according to Kröger et al.: corresponding to the usual regulation, the primary assumption is compression class 2. The selection of the right knit material, depending on the physique, is paramount. Possible comorbidities, cofactors and the course of therapy may require a variation of the compression class. [O1089]

which are adapted to the symptoms and individual considerations of the patient, such as concomitant diseases, habitus, etc.

As a special feature, since autumn 2017, there has been an MCS specially designed for patients with CVI and (compensated) PAD, similar to the so-called 'Lite' bandages (➤ Fig. 29.4). Although this stocking also follows the RAL standard for MCS, it offers a resting pressure of the CCL I and a working pressure similar to a CCL III because of the changed knit tech-nique. The stocking is available as a calf-length stocking with a reinforced back of the foot and padded sole, and exclusively as made-to-measure to reduce the risk of ridge formation with this sensitive group of patients.

Finally, the type of CT must be determined. For leg care, MCS for calf, thigh and half leg, as well as tights are available in different variants (single- or double-legged). There are very few medical products that require the mandatory selection of a particular type.

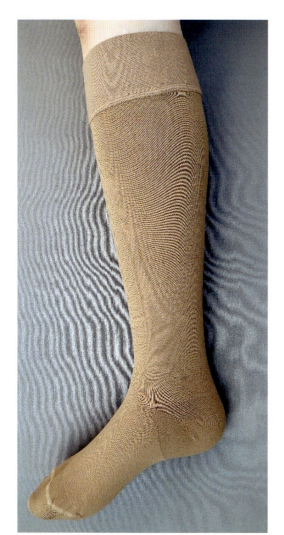

Fig. 29.4 First medical compression stocking specially designed for patients with venous disorders and incipient arterial occlusive disease (mixed leg ulcers): low resting pressure, high working pressure. [P586]

the problem area. All other conditions can usually be treated with calf stockings.

In the case of considerable obesity, pronounced lymph-oedema or lipoedema, the use of separate garments (cropped trousers + calf stockings, or cycling pants + thigh stockings) has also proved to be effective, as they significantly facilitate getting dressed and going to the toilet during the day. However, these product variants, as well as the incorporation of functional zones for individual complaints (e. g. in the knee region), are only possible in the flat knit area.

The decision for a series of products or a fitted supply is based on the deviations of the circumferential dimensions at one or more measuring points. However, all MCS – including series supplies – are appropriate! The only difference is the type of production!

29.4.3 Ulcer compression stocking systems

The ulcer compression stocking systems (UCS) available on the market consist of two components – an inner and an outer stocking (➤ Fig. 29.5). The inner stocking predominantly consists of low contact pressure and serves above all to protect the skin and as a gliding or tightening aid for the outer stocking. The outer stocking largely corresponds to a normal MCS with a contact pressure of CCL II. Together, the inner and outer stockings then achieve a resting pressure value corresponding to CCL III. By pulling the one stocking over the other, the overall system achieves a higher material strength and can generate a high working pressure. Following initial decongestion, the UCS is indicated for therapy and (initial) prevention of recurrence of the venous leg ulcer. Currently available on the international markets are systems from various companies, some of which are only available as a series of products, others as both a series and as customised products, which are therefore also suitable for difficult leg shapes.

29.4.4 Medical thrombosis prophylaxis stockings

Medical thrombosis prophylaxis stockings (MTPS) are **not** MCS according to the German RAL regulation and are only listed here to be comprehensive. They follow

Instead, the choice should be based on the patient's preferences. Someone who only wears knee-high socks will find it difficult to be enthusiastic about wearing compression tights for long periods. Compromises are therefore often necessary. As much as medically necessary, but also as little as possible.

Indications necessitating a high level of care (tights or thigh stockings) are above all thromboses or oedema in the thigh or groin area, as well as excessive obesity with overhanging tissue flaps in the knee region. In this case, the compression should go beyond

29

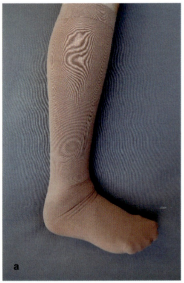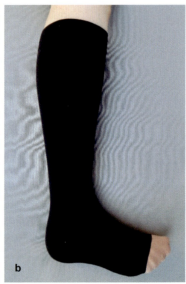

Fig. 29.5 Ulcer compression stocking system consisting of inner (**b**) and outer (**a**) stockings. [P586]

their own regulations. They are designed only for bedridden patients. They are exclusively round knitted and seamless stockings for the thigh or lower leg. The pressure curve corresponds to that of the MCS, but the pressure values are usually found below the level of CCL I. The pressure values are not available in CCL I. Depending on the manufacturer, the MTPS is available in various sizes as standard products. A customised supply as with the MCS is not possible here.

29.4.5 Medical adaptive systems

Medical adaptive systems (MAS) for compression therapy, also known as Velcro or wrap bandages, offer an alternative to conventional bandages (➤ Fig. 29.6). MAS are used internationally for the treatment of chronic wounds and oedema. Currently, the various systems differ in the type of materials, application and care of the products.

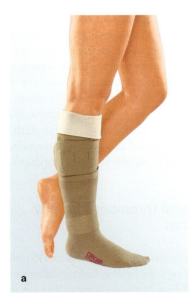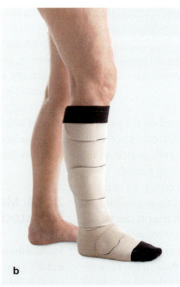

Fig. 29.6 Various medical adaptive systems of compression therapy are available; **a** circaid juxtacures [V481], **b** Juzo calf compression wrap. [V600]

The indication for MAS is, in particular, the active venous leg ulcer with moderate to severe oedema. Here it can be used in the decongestion and maintenance phase. With some MAS there is also the possibility of visual pressure control using a supplied template and markings on the bandages. With appropriate guidance, MAS can also be applied by relatives or the patient themselves and readjusted during the day. There are limitations in the use of MAS for severely overweight patients or difficult leg formations. Also, being comfortable to wear and being compatible with footwear mean they have a better rating than conventional bandages.

29.4.6 Intermittent pneumatic compression therapy

Intermittent pneumatic compression (IPC) therapy is an application of pneumatic alternating pressures for thromboembolism prophylaxis, decongestion therapy for oedema diseases and the positive influence of arterial and venous blood circulation with improvement of clinical symptoms and faster ulcer healing in the outpatient and inpatient area. The devices used differ depending on their indication and target area. They consist of a generator or control unit (group IIa medical device) and cuffs (foot, lower leg, whole leg, trousers, etc.; ➤ Fig. 29.7) to be selected according to the target area. The control unit is decisive for the course of treatment – pressure build-up, pressure maintenance phase, release phase, pause times and cycle repetition. As a rule, the pressure values of 12–200 mmHg are built up. Depending on requirements, the pressure build-up can be intermittent or sequential. The individually required pressure is built up and released at defined intervals.

Also, but never as a replacement for CT with bandages or stockings, IPC can be used as an in-patient, out-patient and home therapy.

According to the recommendations of the newly revised guideline, the following applies to the therapy of patients with chronic wounds:
- Therapy with IPC should be used for venous leg ulcers with no tendency to heal despite consistent CT using stocking systems or compression bandages.
- The IPC for legs should be used in patients whose venous leg ulcer shows no healing tendency under standard therapy with multi-stage cuffs (sequential pressure build-up, target pressure 40–50 mmHg, for at least one hour per day, at least three times per week) to promote wound-healing.
- In the case of PAD with stable intermittent claudication or critical ischaemia, the indication for IPC should be examined. A prerequisite for therapy with IPC, however, is that an interventional or

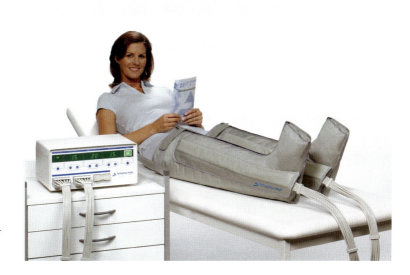

Fig. 29.7 Example of a device for intermittent pneumatic compression therapy consisting of a generator and leg cuffs. [V858]

29

Table 29.7 Contraindications of IPC

Relative contraindications	Absolute contraindications
Extended, possibly open soft-tissue trauma of the extremities	Acute erysipelas
Pronounced neuropathy of the extremities	Acute cellulitis
Blistering autoimmune dermatoses such as linear IgA dermatosis or bullous pemphigoid	Compartment syndrome
Decompensated heart failure	Severe, untreated hypertension
Extensive thrombophlebitis, thrombosis or suspected thrombosis	At the same time, no IPC should be performed with occluding processes in the lymphatic flow area, in which congestion in the groin or genital area has developed under IPC

surgical reconstruction is out of the question and a guided exercise programme is not possible.

- IPC in PAD should be performed with foot and calf cuff, target pressure of 85–120 mmHg, short inflation time, three cycles per minute and daily use.
- To reduce postoperative oedema, IPC can be used after an operative reconstructive procedure for PAD.

IPC is an effective and safe therapeutic measure if the indication is carefully defined, the contraindications (➤ Table 29.7) are observed, and the devices are used correctly. To avoid skin damage, textile skin protection should be applied under the plastic cuff, and regular inspection and care of the skin should be carried out. Padding over disposition points should be used, especially for slim or cachectic patients, to prevent nerve damage and pressure-induced necrosis. Genital oedema has not been described or explicitly denied in any study since 1998; however, care should be taken. If there is an increase in oedema in the pelvic or genital area during lymphoedema under IPC, no further IPC should be performed, and a diagnosis pertaining to a drainage obstruction should be extended or repeated.

29.5 Choosing the right material

The current guidelines and the list of aids purposefully do not include a fixed assignment of specific indications for different compression materials or related contact pressure. Everyday clinical experience has shown that it makes much more sense to select the CT in a symptom-oriented manner. The following questions should be asked:

- **What is the indication for compression therapy?**
  CT has proven itself in the treatment and prophylaxis of a large number of diseases (➤ Table 29.3). The more severe the venous or lymphatic drainage disorder or the tendency to oedema (e. g. postthrombotic syndrome, leg ulcer), the higher the selected contact pressure and the firmer the chosen compression material should be.

- **Is there still active congestion, or should CT be used for prophylaxis or maintenance?**
  If congestion exists, adaptive systems or padded compression bandages should be used until sufficient decongestion is achieved. Adapted compression stockings or adaptive systems have proven effective for prevention and maintenance in medium and long-term therapy. In contrast to the bandages, which depend on the experience and skill of the user, the stockings provide constant contact pressure.

- **Which concomitant illnesses does the patient have?**
  If the patient suffers from concomitant illnesses that restrict the use of CT or are among the relative contraindications, special care should be taken in the selection of the compression material. ➤ Table 29.8 provides some indications for appropriate adaptation concerning possible limitations. In the case of concomitant PAD and neuropathy, close medical and nursing checks should be carried out, and the patient should be

Table 29.8 Tips for the individual adaptation of CT, depending on existing concomitant diseases or limitations

Disease or limitation	Possible measures
Obesity	• Prevention of ridge formation in flexed joints • Material with high strength, if necessary adhesion aids
Anorexia	• Prevention of pressure sores • Underpadding
Painful changes in hands, hips, or knees	• Reduction of contact pressure • Aids for dressing and undressing
Joint deformity/extremity deformity	• Individualised adaptation • Flat knit material
Skin diseases/eczema	• Use of inner stockings • Intensified skincare
Neuropathy	• Reduction of contact pressure, e.g. 20–30 mmHg • Prevention of ridge formation, high strength material • Regular checks, in particular during initiation of therapy
PAD with ABI > 0.5 or absolute systolic ankle contact pressure > 60 mmHg	• Reduction of contact pressure, e.g. 20–30 mmHg • Prevention of ridge formation, high strength material • Regular checks, in particular when starting therapy
Excessive body hair, MCS slips	• Shave, if possible • CT with supporting aids, such as tights, hip brace, adhesives

29

informed in detail about potential signs of danger (skin changes, discolouration).

• **What are the patient's preferences for compression therapy?**
Compliance or adherence is an essential factor for the therapeutic success of CT. It is effective only if worn regularly. Accordingly, the patient should be informed extensively about the purpose, benefit and type of application. At the same time, however, the patient should also be included in the choice of therapy. In most cases, calf-length medical care is completely sufficient. Compression tights or thigh-length products often represent a particular obstacle or annoyance for the patient in everyday life, e.g. when putting on and taking off clothes, going to the toilet, choosing clothes, doing sports or while at work. Here, compromises should be found between what is medically necessary and the individual wishes and needs. Particularly in the area of flat knitting for patients with lipoedema and lymphoedema of the entire leg, the incorporation of functional zones or, if necessary, divided treatments (instead of tights) should also be considered, which can make everyday life with CT significantly easier.

29.6 Side effects, risks and their avoidance

Real side effects of CT are rare. In most cases, however, risks and side effects result from an incorrect choice of material or application. Possible side effects of CT are:
• Allergic contact reactions, e.g. through the adhesive edge
• Itching
• Skin reddening
• Skin dryness
• Sweating
• Constriction
• Blistering
• Thromboses
• From skin, soft tissue and nerve damage to ulcerations

The patient should always be informed about these potential risks. If problems or pain occur during compression, the patient should immediately remove the dressing or stocking and contact their doctor or nurse. In particular, warnings should be given to the patient: blue or white discolouration of the toes, abnormal sensations or numbness in the leg or foot, increasing pain under compression, shortness of breath or outbreaks of sweating as well as acute movement restrictions in compression.

Typically, with all patients and all types of CT, dehydration and irritation of the skin is a problem at some point. This phenomenon is not to be classified as intolerance of CT, but an expected side effect, which can be counteracted by regular moisturising skincare (e.g. in the evening after removal of the compression).

Genuine intolerances in the sense of an allergy to modern CT materials are rare today. Only a few bandage systems still use latex. MCS no longer contain latex fibres but are made of advanced elastic textile fibres. Therefore, latex allergies no longer play a role in CT regulations. Occasionally, incompatibilities with dark dyes or the silicone adhesive edges of the compression materials can be observed. Epicutaneous tests can be carried out to confirm the diagnosis of type IV sensibilisation. To solve the problem, materials without dark dyes and adhesive margins can be chosen.

Many patients, especially the elderly, find it challenging to apply and remove CT on their own. A distinction must be made between bandages and stockings. With the appropriate practise and mobility,

patients can possibly apply their own arm or leg compression bandages, but it requires great skill and is not recommended for everyday use. On the other hand, they can easily put on stocking systems and MAS by themselves. Prescribing aids to help with putting on and taking off stocking systems (separate prescription) should possibly be considered. The market offers a variety of different systems. Here the patient should select a suitable and practicable system after appropriate consultation with a medical supply store.

REFERENCES

Protz K, Heyer K, Dörler M, et al. Compression therapy: scientific background and practical applications. J Dtsch Dermatol Ges 2014; 12: 794–801.

Protz K, Reich-Schupke S, Müller K, Augustin M, Hagenström K. [Compression bandages with and without padding: Observational controlled survey of pressure and comfort]. Hautarzt 2018; 69: 653–661.

Reich-Schupke S, Protz K, Kröger K, Dissemond J. Erhebung zur Kompressionstherapie bei Ärzten, Therapeuten und medizinischem sowie pflegerischem Fachpersonal. Vasomed 2017; 29: 6–12.

Reich-Schupke S, Stücker M. Moderne Kompressionstherapie – ein praktischer Leitfaden. 1. Auflage, Köln: Viavital-Verlag; 2013.

30

Dirk Hochlenert, Gerald Engels, Jan Kottner

Systematics of pressure relief

30.1 Pressure relief in diabetic foot syndrome

Dirk Hochlenert, Gerald Engels

─────────────── **Key notes** ───────────────

- The causal treatment of pressure related damage to areas of the foot is to offload them. Treatment can also include infection control and further treatment of causes, such as revascularisation.
- Offloading can be achieved by reducing steps and by redistributing load. The limitation of the number of steps is easy to prescribe and popular, but it is not beneficial to patients in the long run and is unsuitable outside of inpatient facilities. Load redistribution is achieved by performing operations (internal offloading) or by devices (external offloading). Stan-

dardisation is possible depending on the anatomical localisation (entity concept). External offloading is achieved by spacers, by tilting the foot (eversion/inversion) and by immobilising joints.
- Offloading is underestimated. Patients underestimate its importance and the practitioner underestimates it to the extent of omission. Any offloading devices which are seen as indispensable, must not be removable. Offloading must allow the patient's everyday mobility.
- Offloading should be absolutely dependable when treating ulcers whilst in prophylaxis, compromises are possible and often necessary.

30.1.1 Introduction

Loss of protective sensation (LOPS) is the main characteristic of diabetic foot syndrome (DFS). LOPS is irreversible and so, the diabetic foot persists for the entire life. It will switch back and forth between active phases (ulcers and active Charcot's foot) and inactive phases (prophylaxis). The basic measure is therefore to restore protection by offloading ulcers and immobilising the Charcot feet. In the prophylactic phase, the aim is to reduce the likelihood of overloading and to thereby make a renewed active phase less likely.

Overloaded areas of the foot are found on the sole, side areas of the foot, on toes, back of the heel and sometimes in other areas, such as amputation stumps. Areas which are not under pressure physiologically, but which become a contact or support area due to pathological changes in the biomechanics (plantarisation), occupy a unique position. These plantarisa-

tions often only occur when the foot is loaded and are therefore overlooked when at rest. A biomechanical examination is therefore necessary to achieve effective offloading. It helps to identify the causes of overloading and to determine which areas are suitable for increased loadbearing.

The immobilisation of joints and offloading are two different treatment concepts. Immobilisations are achieved by using cross-joint aids which also contribute to offloading. They are decisive in the treatment of the Charcot foot and are also highly effective in offloading ulcers and ulcer-endangered areas. However, they are also associated with disadvantages. For example, the muscles which should have been used to move the immobilised joints atrophy, and the risk of falling will increase with bulkier, heavier devices. A combination of different load redistribution methods can avoid the need for immobilisation.

30.1.2 No overloading without bone prominence

Overloading occurs above a bone protrusion area. The superficial tissue layers, including the skin, are pulled, stretched, and thinned out over these bony lumps or spurs. External pressure from the environment also squeezes these layers. The number of bony protrusions is limited. It is also not by accident that certain bony protrusions are overloaded, as the biomechanical characteristics of the individuals walking cycle determine the location. It is possible to determine its biomechanical background by looking at the wound location and to normalise the offloading accordingly. The lesion site characterises a subgroup of the DFS, the entity ➤ Fig. 30.1). According to the entity concept, each entity has a typical biomechanical relationship between overloading and possible offloading techniques.

It is easy for a therapist to recommend offloading by advising patients not to walk or reduce walking. However, this advice has many flaws. It limits mobility, independence and working ability. Reduced mobility also causes other health issues.

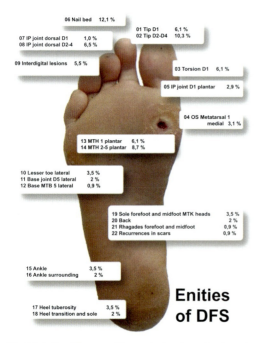

Fig. 30.1 The different entities on the foot (overview image). [P587]

Offloading measures should redistribute load instead, be nonremovable and allow everyday mobility without putting the ulcer under stress. Surgical procedures help to relieve pressure internally and have a decisive advantage over conservative procedures, as they cannot be forgotten or not complied with for any other reasons.

Since the offloading measures might have an impact on the patient's everyday life, they must be discussed extensively with the patients. Patients are the experts in their everyday lives and know best what they can and cannot do. The focus of offloading measures should be as effortless as possible and not require the patient to pay too much attention. The focus should also not be dependent on their pain perception from overloading as their nervous system can no longer detect any pain due to the impairment; this is called LOPS. Other sensations can remain unimpaired and neurological tests can appear normal, or sensations such as tickling can even be perceived as exaggerated, which makes diagnosis difficult. It is primarily based on the ease with which the patient uses his injured foot, rather than on neurological tests.

Communicating and selecting recommendations are also based on the patient's felt body (loss of sensation, ➤ Chap. 43.5). The patient becomes alienated from their foot, which is only perceived as part of the surrounding environment. The practitioner must be aware that removable devices will be disregarded, at least for parts of everyday life.

The goal is to combine the protection of the foot and everyday mobility. If this is successful, wound closure is secured and recurrence can be prevented.

30.1.3 Load redistribution through adhesive pads

There are materials available which can relieve the bony protrusion under the wound by supporting the associated bone at a certain distance from the wound itself. They are made of a semi-solid material and are positioned at least about 3 mm from the margin of the wound. Soft pads applied directly on the wound on the other hand have disadvantages. They increase the contact surface of the caved-in bone protrusion by including the immediate surroundings in loadbearing tasks. This pressure at the wound margin would be counterproductive. Similarly, circular relief rings are harmful at the plantar surface and cause window oedema. The bone protrusion also sinks through the wound into this recess, stretching the wound and traumatising the wound margin. In most cases, the ring is not completely able to prevent the sinking bone projection colliding with the contact surface.

Spacer pads can not only support the foot in the area of the wound but can also tilt it so that the walking cycle uses the plantar surface distant from the wound. A raising of the outer margin thus relieves the outer margin because more of the load is placed on the inner margin during the walking cycle.

30.1.4 Insole

In the manufacture of an insole, the same principles apply as with adhesive pads. However, since the foot shifts on the insole, the support cannot be planned so precisely. The adhesive pads are constantly attached to the foot, while the patient can simply disregard the shoe with its insole. An advantage of the insole is that there is no need for a replacement after every dressing change. With an existing ulcer, the advantages of adhesive pads outweigh the advantages of the insole. On the other hand, if there is no existing wound, the insole is the preferred choice. Both can be combined.

30.1.5 Shoes

A shoe (➤ Fig. 30.2) not only protects against adverse environmental influences, but it can also change the pressure on the sole of the foot during the walking process. Most of all shoes are used for walking, and the patient must be able to walk well in them. For this purpose, the properties of the sole are decisive. The sole is slightly curved, with the tip of the sole curving upwards towards the toe. The heel area should be higher than the ball of the foot.

This curved sole is also called 'roller' or 'rocker bottom sole'. The toes need to be extended less in the metatarsophalangeal joint, since the curvature of the sole already takes over part of this necessity imposed by the gait cycle. This reduces the pressure on the metatarsal heads. The foot can stand in a relaxed position on the curved sole by adjusting the thickness of the sole. The curvature is flatter on the surface in touch with the foot than on the outside. The extent of the curvature, its apex, position, and rotation are crucial for load redistribution and smooth walking. Since every person walks differently, the demands made are different. People with neuropathy can provide limited information which makes it challenging to design the shoe. Stiffening the sole can further increase the offloading effect of the rocker bottom sole. The toes can then no longer be dorsally extended in the metatarsophalangeal joints, and the function of this joint movement is taken over by the rolling sole. The shoe however becomes thicker, heavier, and clumsier which counteracts mobility. It should therefore be considered whether the affected person needs this stiffening.

If customised shoes are not based on the patient's individual needs, but according to the motto 'the more, the better', there will be a risk of non-compliance on wearing the shoe. In these cases, a patient may wear any shoe considered to fit. Objections made by patients such as 'But I can walk better with this' should therefore be taken seriously as they will point out that changes to the shoe are necessary. These compromises may also bring about an increase in comfort while reducing relieving properties.

In prophylactic therapy, these shoes are classified as comfort shoes (not covered by insurances in many countries), protective shoes or custom-made shoes. When treating ulcers, therapy shoes are used. They also accommodate thick layers of bandage. Many therapeutic shoes, so-called forefoot-offloading shoes or hindfoot-offloading shoes, are **not** endorsed by many including the authors, because it is possible that they can generate new high-pressure areas or reinforce existing overloading.

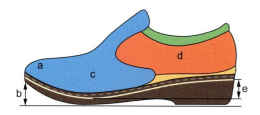

Fig. 30.2 Illustration of a shoe from the side with **a** toe box, **b** toe spring, **c** vamp, **d** quarter, **e** heel seat. The shoe has a ball roller and a sole stiffener (light yellow). The firm hold is generated between instep, sole and heel. The shoe has lacing or Velcro fasteners on the instep. [V864/L231]

30.1.6 Knee-high, non-removable casts

These are given the highest recommendation in the international guidelines, according to current evidence as well as being the most traditionally used. With the introduction of wound treatment for diabetic feet as a continuation of the treatment of leprosy patients by Paul Brand at the end of the 1970s, the leg was plastered in Total Contact Cast (TCC) after wound care, and left until the next dressing change. Attempts at using 'windows' in the plaster were not successful.

With the introduction of plastic materials and the possibility of sawing the plaster into two shells or even using it as a prefabricated, ready-made orthoses, this practice was abandoned by many. Treatment of the wounds became possible, and the procedures could be used also by non-specialised clinics. However, the results are worse. Hidden pedometers prove that even under study conditions, 870 out of an average of 1,220 steps per day were taken without these aids. Attempts are being made to address this with disciplinary measures such as cable ties, which met with understandable resistance and failed to gain general acceptance. The superior standard method which has been used for centuries, is now broadly ignored. On the contrary, there are discussions about whether this

standard should be adapted to current practices and to amend the guidelines, despite poor compliance from the patient. The authors support a TCC with two shells, of which the ventral, front part is divided again, and the proximal part is attached again so that the TCC becomes 'non-removable'. A large window is created in the ventral part of the TCC, through which the foot can be pulled out of the TCC and treated. This is a Ventral Windowed TCC or VW-TCC (➤ Fig. 30.3).

30.1.7 Further procedures

When discussing the individual lesion sites on the following pages, a concern is a particularly increased risk of peripheral arterial disease (PAD). In principle, a PAD can play a role in wounds in all locations. This circulatory disorder reduces the patient's defence against infection as well as the proliferation of new tissue layers for repair. It contributes to tissue destruction, which maybe later becomes an unavoidable indication for amputation. Therefore, the timely improvement of circulation is crucial. When a relevant PAD exists, and there is no progress in ulcer closure, improvement of blood circulation should be discussed. In the case of an indication of blood circulation-related disorder as the causal factor for a non-healing wound, actions

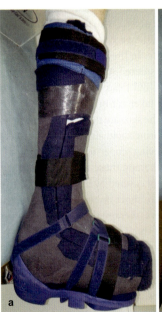
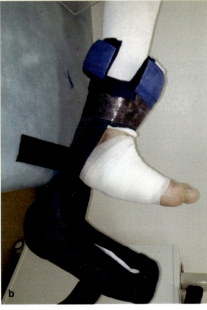

Fig. 30.3 VW-TCC (Ventral Windowed Total Contact Cast): **a** closed state, **b** open state. One advantage is the possibility of responding to individual needs. In this case, an additional flap was attached to the calf. [P587]

must take place without delay. Typically, neuropathy does not cause pain and other typical symptoms such as intermittent claudication. The widely used pain-based Fontaine-Classification must not be applied in DFS. Lack of pain should not be the reason for delayed follow-up or to delay revascularisation indications.

30.1.8 Entities in detail

➤ Table 30.1

Entity 1 – the tips of the hallux and Entity 2 – the 2nd to 4th toe The leading cause is a plantarisation

Table 30.1 The entities of the diabetic foot

Nr.	Entity	%	Special features
1	Tip D1	6.1	Before attributing the cause to shoes, clawing has to be excluded (push-up test, claw test and standing). Tenotomy of the FHL tendon is a low-complication permanent solution. Additional nail bed involvement is an indicator of revascularisation needs (18.1%) and high risk (4.9% major amputation).
2	Tip D2–D4	10.3	Tenotomy of the FDL tendon is low-complication and permanently effective, a spacer in the flexion fold is a short-term solution.
3	Torsional lesion D1 medial	6.1	Protracted, high risk of recurrence, provocation tests for functional plantarisation and good chance with tenotomy of the FHL tendon.
4	Medial 1st MTH	3.1	Rare opening of the joint, even if it appears so.
5	IP joint D1 plantar	2.9	High recurrence rate (50.5% in the subsequent year), hallux rigidus can be functional: test!
6	Nail bed	12.1	90% of D1, prognosis good, nail extractions usually not useful.
7	IP joint D1 dorsal	1	Frequent bone involvement. This is not a necessarily an indication for amputation! Combined tendon surgery to reduce zigzag deformity is a permanently effective alternative in many situations.
8	IP joint D2–D4 dorsal	6.5	Short-term: spacer pads, long-term: toe straightening through soft tissue intervention, effective and low risk of complication.
9	Interdigital	5.5	Often bone involvement, fewer relapses.
10	Small toe	3.5	Often bone involvement, rotation treatable with tenotomy.
11	MP-joint D5 lateral	2	High bone involvement, high revascularisation frequency (17.7%) and major amputation frequency (2.9%)
12	Base MT bone 5 lateral	0.9	High frequency of revascularisation and major amputation.
13	MTH1 plantar	6.7	Recurrences very frequent (over 50% in the subsequent year), many possibilities for internal relief.
14	MTH2–5 plantar	8.7	Internal offloading with high potential.
15	Ankle tip	1.9	Lesions with an exacerbation just above the bony prominence often caused by PAD with a high risk of major amputation.
16	Ankle area	2.1	Compression therapy concerning PAD and malleoli (perimalleolar pads), lengthy.
17	Calcaneal tuberosity	3.2	Prophylaxis is essential, also perioperative, high frequency of major amputations (4.3%) and long courses of treatment.
18	Heel: Sole and edge (rhagades)	5.6	PAD important, even a narrow necrosis margin is an alarm signal, major amputations.
19	Sole in unstressed areas	1.7	Prognosis generally good.
20	Back of the foot	2.2	Average forecast.
21	Rhagades on fore-/midfoot	1.3	Prognosis generally good.
22	Scars	5.7	Re-ulcerations in the scar area expand rapidly into the depths and often have serious consequences.

30

of the tip of the toe by a muscle imbalance that turns the toe into a claw. The force of the long flexor tendons predominates. They have their muscle in the calf and pull the toes towards the plantar side. The straight alignment of the proximal phalanx by muscles in the foot (Mm. interossei) is weakened by distal motor neuropathy to such an extent that each pull on the distal phalanx automatically leads to a zig-zag-deformity. It can also cause lesions on the back of the interphalangeal joints and under the metatarsal heads. Since the clawing movement may become apparent only under stress, it needs to be provoked. Without such a provocation, the cause may be seen erroneously in a shoe, since suspected shoes are common and can obscure the actual cause, the clawing of the toes, when viewed cursorily. These provocation tests are:

- Push-up test: in a patient lying down with a relaxed foot posture, by exerting pressure at the level of the metatarsal heads, the foot is brought into a 90° position in the ankle joint.
- Claw test: the patient is asked to turn their toes into a claw while lying down.
- Stand: observation of the patient getting up.

A second, rarer cause is the tip of the toe pressing against the inner lining of the toecap within the shoe.

Conservative measures can be: a pad in the flexion fold of the affected toe relieves the tip (➤ Fig. 30.4c). The materials used to make this pad vary and range from simple felt to orthosis individually made by po-diatrists. In shoe manufacturing, the padding under the toes can be softened. But in the end, shoe design is relatively powerless in the long run against the strong muscular force that continues to turn the toe into a claw.

The surgical procedures include:
1. Cutting the long flexor tendon
2. Loosening the joint capsules of the proximal interphalangeal joint (PIP) and the metatarso-phalangeal joint (MTP)
3. Lengthening or cutting the long extensor tendon

On this occasion, avital bones will also be removed. These procedures show excellent results with rare complications and are also possible with restricted blood circulation and anticoagulation or with platelet aggregation inhibition.

Entity 3: torsion of the hallux   The medial side of the hallux can rotate in plantar direction (downwards), involving the joints of the metatarsal bone. As another factor allowing rotation, the foot can deviate into a pronated and outwardly turned (abducted) position. In the last phase of the gate cycle, the medial side of the distal phalanx takes much of the load and is not provided with sufficient protection for this effort. There, two bone protrusions dominate: the IP joint and the medial edge of the distal phalanx.

Conservatively, a condylar pad is used for offloading (➤ Fig. 30.5b). It relieves the medial condyle and puts

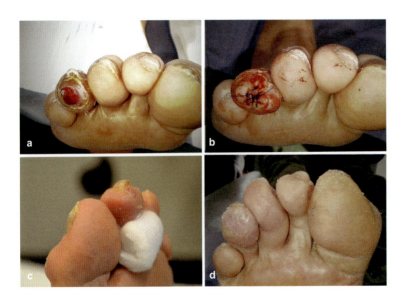

Fig. 30.4 Toe tip lesion: **a** ulcer on the tip of the 4th toe before debridement; **b** treated ulcer supplied, closed with a primary suture; **c** hollow moulded pad; **d** toe from **a** and **b** after wound closure, offloading here through tenotomy of the long flexor tendon. [P587]

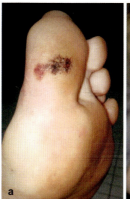
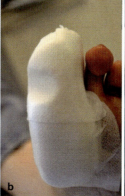
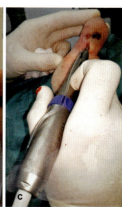

Fig. 30.5 Ulcer of the 1st toe due to torsion and overstretching in hallux rigidus: **a** visual appearance, **b** with condylar pad, **c** medial condylectomy in minimally invasive technique. [P587]

the stress on the tip and metatarsal head (MTH) 1 and 2. This is more difficult to reproduce in an insole than with adhesive felt in the acute phase, but still possible. The shoe can also help to offload a little with a sole stiffener and a rocker-bottom sole.

With a tenotomy, the surgeon can sever the tendons causing the rotation.

Entity 4: hallux valgus Hallux valgus is described as the combination of a medially deviating metatarsal head with a laterally pointing 1st toe. In this deformity, there is an exposure of the head of the 1st metatarsal bone to medial pressure. An injury here does not lead to bone contact as frequently as might be assumed since fibrous structures such as the tendon of the abductor hallucis muscle between the skin and the MTH provide a certain degree of protection.

Offloading is the domain of conservative treatment with sufficiently broad footwear and padding in front of and behind the metatarsal head. A reduction of the wound surface can be achieved by minimally invasive surgery with a transcutaneous 'lateral release'. This is not one of the established procedures of hallux valgus surgery. These procedures should be considered after wound closure because of the need to introduce foreign material such as screws.

Entity 5: IP joint of the hallux The plantar side of the hallux's IP joint, centrally or slightly medially, comes under pressure due to a hallux limitus or rigidus ($\succ$ Fig. 30.5). In these two deformities, the 1st toe's metatarsophalangeal (MTP) joint is partially (limitus) or completely (rigidus) stiffened. However, the dorsal extension of the 1st toe is necessary during the gate cycle.

If this dorsal extension in the MTP joint is no longer possible, there will be overstretching of the IP joint instead. This joint is physiologically not intended for a dorsal extension, and the skin on the plantar side of the joint is not prepared to be subjected to pressure. In case of stress from overstretching, the plantarised skin may express an ulcer under the medial condyle of the joint.

Conservatively, offloading with condylar padding is possible. In the shoe, the stiffening of the sole prevents further overstretching when attempting dorsal extension in the IP joint. Slipping in the heel area should be prevented to avoid increased pressure under the hallux.

The surgical procedures range from resection of the medial condyle, which is the least invasive procedure ($\succ$ Fig. 30.5c), to the Valenti procedure with a dorsal V-shaped partial resection of the metatarsophalangeal joint of the hallux.

Entity 6: nail bed injuries Nail bed injuries are frequent. Causes vary from structural changes of the nail in nail pathologies such as onychomycoses or psoriasis to traumatic injuries and ingrown toenails. An appearance like an ingrown toenail needs a meticulous analysis of the underlying cause of inflammation. Repeated lingering traumas in the nail fold (sulcus) lead to a state of irritation as well as infections and errors in care resulting in an ingrown nail. The causes are trauma from extrinsic factors (footwear or neighbouring toe) or pressure of the soft tissue against the nail as a consequence of malpositioning of the toes.

Conservative treatment consists in podological care and therapy of nail problems. Nail mycosis can be eradicated with medication but tends to recur. Nails

30

which were previously damaged by pressure are pre-disposed to fungal infection. Selecting broader shoes, especially at the toe box, avoids pressure on the nail. The toe box should not contain any stiffening materials.

Ingrown toenails are also treated surgically, e. g. by phenolisation (partial nail avulsion), or other destruction of the nail matrix of the nail part close to the sulcus. The cause of the situation is particularly well treatable when repeated pressure from the side or plantar causes irritation of the sulcus, which can easily be misinterpreted as an 'ingrown nail'. The pressure can be removed permanently by a tenotomy.

Entity 7 and 8: dorsum of the 1st toe (7) and the lesser toes (8) at the IP joints

These are affected by the typical zigzag malposition. At the hallux (entity 7) and the proximal interphalangeal joints (PIP joints) of the toes 2–4 (entity 8), bony tips are formed by overbending and pressing against the inner lining of the toes box.

Pyramid-shaped spacers, which are attached to the back of the foot above the MP joint, i. e. as distally as possible, have proven successful in ulcers (➤ Fig. 30.6). After the wound has closed, a spacious toe box without stiffening material is recommended.

Severing or lengthening both the tendons of the plantar flexors and those of the dorsal extensors can permanently reduce the zigzag deformity. The capsules of the MTP joint and PIP joint have often shrunk if the deformity has existed for many years; it makes sense to perform a capsule release. In the context of the wound situation, the joint can be removed

if it has been opened widely. Since the wound surface will be reduced with the removal of the overbending in the context of tendon-surgical procedures, the wound can often be closed (sutured) in one or two steps.

Entity 9: interdigital lesions

Interdigital lesions occur when toes are pressed against each other. The IP joints are enlargements of the toe's diameter that can cause pressure on the skin above the joint itself and on the opposite side. The shoe must be broad enough so that the front portion does not exert pressure on the sides of the toes. The width is expressed in letters and describes the height and broadness of the ball of the foot. Broadness alone describes only one dimension and is less suitable. A certain degree of tightness is necessary for the shoe to give the foot a firm hold. However, the shoe must not be so tight that the toes are crushed against each other. It is difficult to find the correct measure if the patient can no longer provide meaningful information, due to reduced sensitivity. Therefore, it makes sense to fix the foot within the shoe between the instep, sole and heel cap, and to be broad in the area at the front.

Spacers between the toes are problematic because they further restrict the available space. In any case, the authors use a distally doubled-up wound dressing made of flexible foam. Additionally, a small plantar support in the zone between the metatarsal heads can be helpful, reducing the load, slightly distancing the toes from each other.

Surgically, a lateral release in the hallux valgus or removal of the IP joint can be helpful. Resection of the

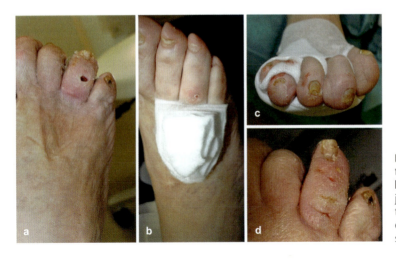

Fig. 30.6 Ulcer on the back of the PIP joint: **a** visual appearance, **b** spacer pads, **c** after sparing joint resection, **d** after combination intervention with tenotomies of the tendons and capsule-splitting. [P587]

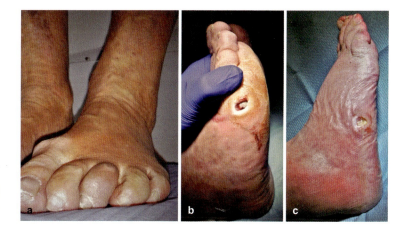

Fig. 30.7 Lateral side of the foot: **a** Quadratus plantae insufficiency with a rotation of the small toe, **b** ulcer at the head of MTH 5 lateral and **c** ulcer at the base of MTH 5. [P587]

joint is simple and should not be confused with the indication of amputation.

Entity 10–12: foot The foot shows five bone protrusions **laterally:** three at the small toe (entity 10) which are very close to each other, at the 5th MTP joint laterally (entity 11), and at the base of the 5th metatarsal bone (entity 12).

The bone protrusions on the 5th toe are very close to each other and are practically impossible to differentiate. They are put under pressure if the small toe twists so that its lateral side becomes the contact surface with the ground (➤ Fig. 30.7a). This rotation, caused by a muscle imbalance, is called 'quadratus plantae insufficiency'. It is corrected by a tenotomy of the long flexor tendon of the small toe. Conservative treatment is possible using spacers on the metatarsal bones. If the cause of pressure against the lateral side of the foot is a deviation of the foot within the shoe, raising the outer edge might limit this deviation.

If the lesion on the 5th metatarsophalangeal joint is strictly lateral, limited blood supply is often involved. Spacers, wide shoes and a resection of the head are possible treatments.

Strictly separated from this is a position at the limit between the lateral and the plantar face of the joint. Tilting of the foot with its lateral margin in plantar direction (inversion/supination), and overloading of the lateral side causes these lesions. The lateral condyle of the 5th metatarsal head is the internal pressure point and can be removed with relatively little effort. Increased tension on the Achilles tendon can maintain this inversion/supination. If this is the case the cause

can be corrected with a lengthening of the tendon. Additionally, the 1st ray can be lowered by a diagonal elevation of the outer edge. This is discussed in detail with the overloading on the 5th MTH's plantar tissue.

There is a protrusion at the base of the 5th MT bone at which the tendon of the fibularis brevis muscle (also known as peroneus brevis muscle) is attached. Lateral pressure will damage the skin and soft tissue above it. Removal of the prominence is not possible because then the whole foot supinates as a sickle foot, through the loss of the function of the fibularis brevis muscle. Surgical measures aim at restoring pronation by transferring the tendon of the tibialis anterior muscle to the lateral fibularis-tertius tendon. However, conservative measures and in particular spacer pads and recesses in the shoe are predominantly used. At this lesion site, too, circulatory disorders are described as clinically relevant with above-average frequency.

Entity 13 and 14: metatarsal heads These can exert pressure in **plantar** direction and cause skin damage. Usually, ulcers at this site are considered the typical lesions of the diabetic foot, although they occur far less frequently than toe lesions. Various mechanisms are involved in the high pressure under MTH:

1. These lesions are predominantly purely neuropathic. Vascular problems can also occur, but revascularisation is only performed in 5–8% of cases in specialised care.
2. Besides causing LOPS, neuropathy also causes muscle imbalance with the result of the typical zigzag deformity (see entity 1, 2 as well as 7 and 8). The constantly overextended MT-joint over-

stretches the protective padding structures under the MTH. These protective pads thin out and can even tear. The MTHs become palpable directly under the skin.

3. The fat padding of the sole, typically 1 cm thick beneath the MTHs and even 2 cm under the heel, decreases in people with neuropathy. It is not a direct consequence of overuse and also affects people with neuropathy but without diabetes mellitus. How exactly neuropathy is linked to the degradation of the fat cushion has not yet been clarified.

4. Repeated borderline pressure excess leads to a thickening of the skin (callous), which at the same time becomes less elastic. Due to autonomous neuropathy, the compromised nerves address sweat glands less effectively, which makes the skin drier. This thick, brittle horn plate is bent back and forth with every step and then tears. At the interface to the subcutaneous tissue, spot bleeding occurs. Patients with normal ability to sense pain will notice considerable pain before bleeding occurs, which leads to the interruption of the load. These spot bleedings are the first clear evidence of a limited pain sensation and an urgent warning signal in a patient with neuropathy. A blood-filled blister may develop underneath skin if left unattended, and bacteria will migrate when there are cracks on the surface which come into contact with them. A callous abscess will develop. The liquids will no longer be drained when the cracks become encrusted. If the patient continues to walk, the pus is pushed deeper into the abscess and a defect develops, creating an opening which resembles a borehole, also known in some countries as malum perforans.

5. Additional overloading of the entire forefoot occurs if the Achilles tendon pulls too early and too strongly. It is often referred to as Achilles tendon shortening, even though not the tendon but the muscles (triceps surae) usually constitute the shrinking structure. Sometimes it is only shortened to a certain extent, which on its own would still make walking possible, but together with an increased muscle tone, it works just like a shortening. During the examination, it is essential that the examiner holds the heel with one hand and aligns it just below the lower leg before testing the dorsal extension of the foot.

6. At the 1st metatarsal head, it is usually the medial sesamoid bone that represents the inner pressure point. The 1st metatarsal bone of the hallux valgus deviates medially from the straight alignment. The sesamoid bones are attached to the other metatarsal heads by ligaments and cannot participate in this movement. While the lateral sesamoid bone slips between the 1st and 2nd metatarsal heads and is harmless, the medial sesamoid bone slips out of its mould in the head of the 1st metatarsal bone, and ends up on top of a ridge between both moulds exerting an excessive pressure. At the same time, the oblique metatarsal bone also turns towards plantar with its medial side.

7. While walking, mostly one foot only is loaded at a time. Thus, balancing can be achieved by ensuring that the 1st and 5th metatarsal bones are mobile and operated with muscle power, and not fixed firmly in the tarsal bones. This mobility can be very pronounced, and the muscles can get exhausted. In this case, the two outer metatarsal bones carry less of a load. In contrast, the central metatarsal bones 2, 3 and 4, which are anchored firmly in the tarsus, cannot move. They end up being situated at a lower level with respect to the outer metatarsals and exposed to excessive pressure.

8. Overloading of the 5th MTH occurs when the foot rolls mainly over to the outside. There can be various reasons for this. For targeted therapy, it is essential to recognise when a low 1st metatarsal tilts the forefoot outwards. The Coleman block test serves this purpose: if the heel is viewed from behind while standing, the longitudinal axis is turned inwards through the heel (varus). If the 1st metatarsal is tilted downwards by placing the foot on a block, the edge of which supports the heel and the 5th ray and the 1st metatarsal drops. If this is the case, insoles are effective to reproduce this correction in the shoe. If the heel does not straighten in this position, other – usually operative – measures must be considered. If, however, the heel can basically be aligned with the lower leg and is not aligned in the block test, a shortening of the triceps surae can be the trigger. An extension of the Achilles tendon is then often helpful.

For lesions below the 1st MTH, offloading devices can be attached underneath the foot to ensure full offloading (➤ Fig. 30.8). Retrocapital support, a recess

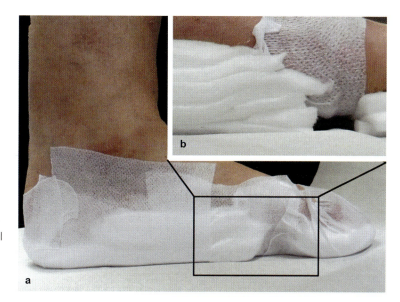

Fig. 30.8 Offloading of an ulcer under MTH 1: **a** seen from medial side with fixation, **b** detail without fixation. Seven layers of felt can be observed retrocapitally. [P587]

under the 1st MTH, a toe balcony, and support of the medial arch with the redistribution of the load to the lateral part of the foot are used. A similar approach can be applied to the insole. The shoe can also be equipped with a curved sole and maybe a sole stiffener.

Surgically, there are many possibilities to achieve permanent offloading, which is also useful during remission (➤ Fig. 30.9). It largely eliminates the zigzag deformity with tendon interventions and capsule release. Additionally, a wedge can be removed from the metatarsal

30

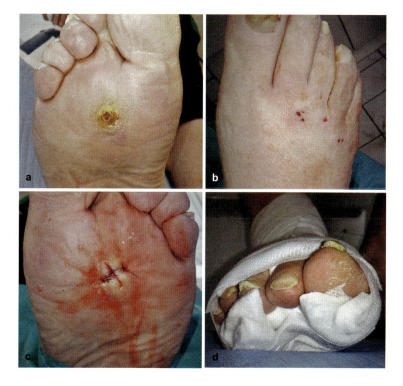

Fig. 30.9 Straightening of various toe deformities and thus relieving a plantar wound. [P587]

bone immediately retrocapitally, which allows the head to be tilted slightly upwards. Alternatively, a few millimetres are removed from the shaft, after which the head adjusts slightly further dorsally and proximally. A resection of the entire head is only necessary if parts of the bone or cartilage are necrotic or if the joint is exposed within the wound. It often leads to a bacterial invasion and destruction of the joint surface. However, toe amputation, which is performed in about 10% of cases, can often be avoided if alternative concepts are used consistently and in good time.

For lesions below the 2nd MTH, a toe balcony and support of the neighbouring MTHs, as well as retrocapital support and local recess, also help. The adhesive supports are usually less bulky than for the 1st metatarsal bone. Rocker-bottom soles and maybe sole stiffeners in the shoe additionally relieve pressure. Among the surgical measures, the straightening of the zigzag deformity by needle tenotomy and percutaneous capsule release is often and surprisingly useful for first-time users.

The conservative relief of ulcers under the 5th MTH depends on the simultaneous influence of the 1st MTH. If the 1st MTH is lowered and the inversion of the heel resulting from this can be corrected, the principal offloading technique is to lower the first metatarsal in relation to the entire foot. If not, a simple raising of the outer edge together with a retrocapital support is sufficient.

Removing the lateral condyle of the metatarsal head, a wedge resection or microsurgically removing a small part of the metatarsal bone can correct the internal pressure and relieve stress.

Offloading of the 4th MTH is similar to the 5th MTH.

Beneath the 3rd MTH, involvement of neighbouring MTHs, retrocapital support, as well as a curved sole and maybe sole stiffening are useful. Zigzag deformity can be surgically corrected by needle tenotomy and capsule release. The head can be moved dorsally after a wedge resection, or a piece of the distal, subcapital metatarsal bone can be removed by minimally invasive surgery to achieve dorsal displacement.

Entity 15: ankle and Entity 16: area of the ankle

These are therapeutically compressed in chronic congestion conditions. The compression of the ankle area is desired, but not that of the malleolae. Pads are lined in order not to overdo the compression on the tips

and to allow it to become effective as much as possible in the depressions. Ankle tips are also susceptible to acute trauma. Accordingly, critical PAD can usually be found in wounds on the tips and not in wounds in the area.

Conservative offloading consists of perimalleolar pads, which fill out the depressed area between the malleolae, Achilles heel and the sole. Surgical procedures to relieve the pressure are not useful here, but plastic surgery procedures to close the wound can be useful, just as with other foot ulcers.

Entity 17 and 18: heel

The heel has three areas where ulcers can occur: the tuberosity, the sole and the transition area between them (➤ Fig. 30.10). On the tuberosity, pressure ulcers occur in people who have difficulty in spontaneously changing their contact area with the supporting surface. These are not only people in nursing homes; often these ulcers develop postoperatively. Therefore, prophylaxis must be well organised and not limited to the operating theatre itself. Until the patients have overcome possible somnolence and general postoperative weakness, prophylaxis of the heel must be ensured uninterruptedly in patients with neuropathy, especially in patients with accompanying PAD. The transition area often shows considerable hyperkeratosis and rhagades. In contrast, plantar ulcers rarely develop because of permanent pressure, as can occur in heel runners when the Achilles tendon function has failed. More often, an ulcer occurs after trauma and it is important to remove any foreign bodies which may have entered the ulcer.

Relieving pressure on the heel can be achieved with conservative measures. In ulcers at the tuberosity, these are mainly devices that offload the heel. Pressure on the sole of the heel can be relieved most effectively with orthoses or a TCC, which allow epicondylar support in the area of the tibial head. If the Achilles tendon is functioning, a slight dorsal extension of the foot can help to relieve the heel.

Entity 19–22: atypical areas

Atypical areas are areas without a typical bone protrusion and include the sole apart from the heel and the metatarsal heads, the back of the foot, rhagades outside the heel and scars after previous procedures. There is no standardised relief from pressure here. Lesions on scars have a particularly poor prognosis as re-ulceration in previously damaged areas.

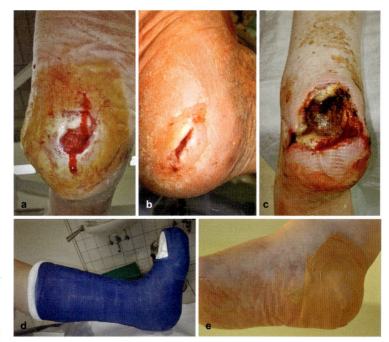

Fig. 30.10 Heel lesions: **a** plantar heel, **b** rhagade in a marginal area, **c** pressure of tuberosity, **d** relief of pressure in a flex-cast, **e** tape dressing of a rhagade. [P587]

REFERENCES
Brand P, Yancey P. The gift of pain. Grand Rapids: Zondervan; 1994.
Bus SA, Armstrong DG, van Deursen RW, et al. IWGDF guidance on footwear and offloading interventions to prevent and heal foot ulcers in patients with diabetes. Diabetes Metab Res Rev 2016; 32 (Suppl. 1): 25–36.

Hochlenert D, Engels G, Morbach S, Schliewa Sgame FL. Diabetic foot syndrome – from entity to therapy. Basel: Springer International Publishing; 2018.
Risse A. Phänomenologische und psychopathologische Aspekte in der Diabetologie. Berlin, New York: Walter de Gruyter; 1997.

30.2 Pressure relief for pressure ulcers
Jan Kottner

Key notes

- Existing pressure ulcers must be offloaded.
- If permanent offloading is not possible, the wound must be relieved regularly.

- Specialised mattresses and overlays should be used, rather than standard mattresses.

30.2.1 Introduction

Consistent relief and off-loading of existing pressure ulcers are the cornerstones of any successful pressure treatment. This concerns both early clinical signs such as persistent erythema or dark livid discolourations with intact skin as well as existing wounds (Section 13). Patients should not be positioned on areas of existing or suspected pressure ulcers.

In the case of several pressure ulcers, other health restrictions, or competing therapy priorities, achieving prolonged or even temporary offloading may not be possible. Soft positioning on special mattresses should be an additional consideration. Putting pressure on the ulcers must be kept to a minimum. In the case of device-related ulcers, e. g. through cannulae or wires, the wound must also not be exposed to any further mechanical influences, i. e. the devices must be removed or arranged differently.

30.2.2 Proper positioning

Pressure ulcers located at typical predilection sites such as the sacral area, trochanter, back of the head or heels can be relieved by traditional positioning techniques which includes 30° to 40° lateral positioning and 135° (abdominal) positioning. Sufficiently large and soft positioning aids such as cushions and rollers should be used. Positioning pads can keep pressure ulcers contact- and pressure free. Patients with pressure ulcers in the buttock area should never directly sit on that area at any time. It is important to do positioning professionally so that the wound is truly and sustainably relieved.

The presence of a pressure ulcer is the strongest predictor that further pressure ulcers can develop. It is therefore imperative that patients do not develop new pressure ulcers, both during the positioning procedure and during the positioning period. All principles of evidence-based pressure prevention must be followed during pressure ulcer treatment, which includes close inspection of all pressure predilection sites.

30.2.3 Special devices for proper positioning

There are several special devices for the positioning or offloading of certain parts of the body.

Heels

For pressure ulcers on the heels, there are many products available on the market for heel off-loading. They are designed so that the lower leg and foot are in a kind of shoe or splint, and the heels are free (➤ Fig. 30.11, ➤ Fig. 30.12, ➤ Fig. 30.13). The type of materials used, the construction, the cost and also the user-friendliness vary greatly. In principle, the aids must ensure that the contact area of the lower leg is considerable and that the Achilles tendon does not rest directly on the support, as this, in turn, represents a risk of a pressure ulcer. Also, the heels must be free,

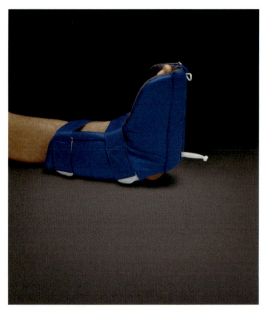

Fig. 30.11 Auxiliary aid for heel-free positioning I. [V860]

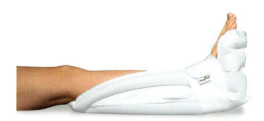

Fig. 30.12 Auxiliary aid for heel-free positioning II. [V861]

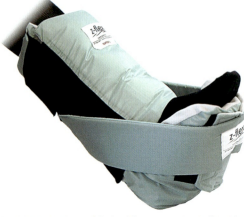

Fig. 30.13 Auxiliary aid for heel-free positioning III. [U349]

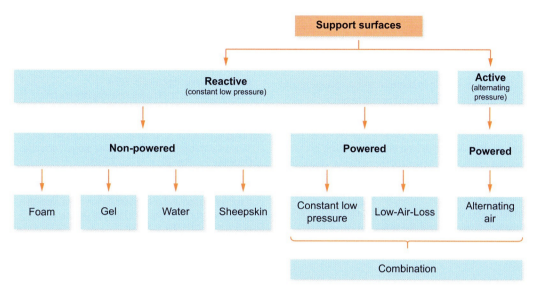

Fig. 30.14 Classification of mattresses and overlays. [P576/L231]

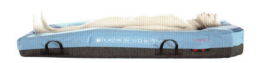

Fig. 30.15 Sinking of the body into a soft positioning mattress. [V863]

and the knees should bend slightly at 5–10°. Finally, the choice of materials and construction should cause as little occlusion as possible. There is currently no evidence to suggest that one device is superior to another for the treatment of heel ulcers. The heels (and feet) must be carefully observed when using aids for heel-free positioning.

Foams and gels

For the optimal positioning of particular body parts, there are numerous other aids such as air-filled cushions, or aids which can be individually shaped and adapted from suitable materials such as cuttable foams or formable gels. These can be useful for certain unique pressure points presenting challenges such as pressure ulcers at the back of the head or the ear or at the buttocks. However, specialised experience and

expertise are essential to ensure that this procedure is effective and does not produce undesirable effects, e. g. new pressure ulcers as a result of the use of the device. So-called ring pillows, water-filled bags or gloves should never be used.

Specialised mattresses, overlays and pillows

Pressure-relieving systems are classified into two groups: active and reactive systems (➤ Fig. 30.14). Active systems are effective in alternately aerating and ventilating mattress elements, whereby alternating aeration and relief of skin and tissues can be achieved. Reactive systems allow the body to sink into and become enclosed by the support (soft positioning), which reduces the surface pressure and thus the deformation of the underlying tissue (➤ Fig. 30.15). Many specialised mattresses consist of combinations of both elements.

Pressure-relieving systems are particularly suitable for the prevention of pressure ulcers. Whenever possible, pressure ulcers should not be in direct contact with these specialised support surfaces. Additionally, guidelines recommend that patients with grades 1 or 2 pressure injuries should at least lie on a reactive system, and patients with grades 3 or 4 pressure in-

30

juries on an active system. Although the scientific evidence is heterogeneous, it is assumed that healing of existing pressure ulcers on these specialised mattresses is promoted, in comparison to standard mattresses. Air fluidised beds enable maximum soft positioning and do not impede the healing of pressure ulcers.

The selection of special support surfaces should not only be dependent on its effect but also on its practical criteria. Motor-driven and alternating pressure systems can be very stressful for patients, due to the constant noise and movement. Structural conditions such as the size and weight of the system must be correct, and the operating and maintenance costs must be affordable, e. g. for informal caregivers.

REFERENCES

Haesler E (ed.); National Pressure Ulcer Advisory Panel, European Pressure Ulcer Advisory Panel, Pan Pacific Pressure Injury Alliance. Prevention and treatment of pressure ulcers: Clinical practice guideline. Osborne Park, Western Australia: Cambridge Media; 2014.

McGinnis E, Stubbs N. Pressure-relieving devices for treating heel pressure ulcers. Cochrane Database Syst Rev 2014; 2: CD005485.

McInnes E, Dumville JC, Jammali-Blasi A, Bell-Syer SE. Support surfaces for treating pressure ulcers. Cochrane Database Syst Rev 2011; 12: CD009490.

McNichol L, Watts C, Mackey D, Beitz JM, Gray M. Identifying the right surface for the right patient at the right time: generation and content validation of an algorithm for support surface selection. J Wound Ostomy Continence Nurs 2015 42; 1: 19–37.

30

31

Peter Engels, Knut Kröger, Joachim Dissemond

Systematics of oxygen therapy in wound treatment

Key notes

- Oxygen is an essential component in physiological wound-healing.
- Chronic wounds tend to have an oxygen deficit which makes them hypoxic.
- In addition to the treatment of the primary underlying disease to improve the blood

circulation situation, there are various adjuvant therapy approaches using oxygen.
- In addition to systemic approaches, such as hyperbaric oxygen therapy (HBOT), there are also increasing possibilities for supplying additional oxygen to wounds topically, which promotes wound-healing.

31.1 Role of oxygen in wound-healing

Most metabolic processes of the human body require oxygen, directly or indirectly. Oxygen is essential for wound-healing in many processes, such as angiogenesis, defence against infection, or collagen synthesis and cross-linking (➤ Fig. 31.1). Wound-healing requires an increased energy metabolism which requires considerably more oxygen than the normal metabolism of intact skin. Reactive oxygen species (ROS) are released to a considerable extent for defence against infection. It is produced, e. g. in neutrophilic granulocytes or macrophages, by the reduction of oxygen (O_2). The oxygen requirement increases by more than 50% in an infected wound, mainly because of the consumption of oxygen during aerobic respiration (cell respiration). In the successive phases of wound-healing, a large number of different biochemical and cellular processes are highly dependent on adequate oxygen supply. Fibroblasts, endothelial cells and keratinocytes also require a continuously sufficient oxygen supply to produce new tissue during granulation, angiogenesis and epithelialisation phases. Besides, oxygen is directly or indirectly involved in the chemotaxis of various cells via the release of messenger substances.

In addition to cellular processes, the formation of a new extracellular matrix (ECM) depends on the sufficiency of oxygen. It applies to collagen synthesis and later to the maturation of type III collagen – initially

formed in the early wound-healing phase – into more elastic type I collagen. It is therefore clear that the state of oxygen supply to a wound and the surrounding tissue is an essential parameter for its healing process.

The transcutaneous partial pressure of oxygen ($tcPO_2$) present in the tissue is a known indicator associated with wound-healing. Literature shows that $tcPO_2$ of approximately 30 mmHg is deemed as a critical limit value, as wound-healing will not take place below this value. This condition is called hypoxia. Such oxygen deficiency occurs when the demand for oxygen consumption exceeds the amount of oxygen delivered from the blood to the tissue. Transiently, cells can tolerate hypoxia and stimulate early wound-healing processes. However, tissue ischaemia may still occur if the oxygen supply to tissue remains poor, e. g. due to reduced blood flow in connection with peripheral artery disease (PAD) or chronic venous insufficiency (CVI). A persistent circulatory disorder leads to a permanently reduced $tcPO_2$ in the affected tissues and will result in hypoxia, which can lead to tissue destruction. If the hypoxia persists, wound-healing stagnates. If these pathological processes progress, necroses may occur increasingly.

31.2 Oxygen wound treatment

Very little of the oxygen reaches the cells in the wound bed and the underlying layers, despite having suf-

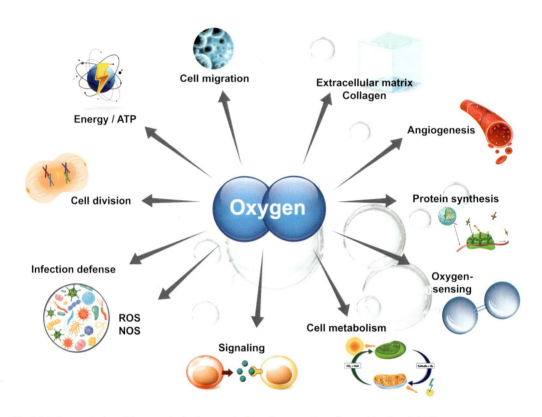

Fig. 31.1 Representation of the central role of oxygen in the various processes of wound-healing. [V862]

ficient oxygen in the ambient air because a film of moisture usually covers wounds. This film of moisture is essential for wound-healing and is promoted in modern moist wound therapy. However, there will be a significant reduction in the wound receiving oxygen through the film of moisture, as oxygen dissolves poorly in fluids.

One of the fundamental problems with most types of chronic wounds is hypoxia, as there is a significant increase in the diffusion distance of freely dissolved oxygen from the existing supplying blood vessels to the oxygen-consuming tissue. Various approaches in providing the hypoxic tissue of chronic wounds with additional oxygen have been developed, ranging from hyperbaric systemic oxygen therapy to local oxygen supply and local improvement of oxygen diffusion.

31.2.1 Hyperbaric oxygen therapy

With hyperbaric oxygen therapy (HBOT), additional oxygen is systemically supplied by making use of the possibility of physically dissolving more oxygen in the blood through the increased pressure in the oxygen chamber. The aim is to increase the partial pressure of oxygen, thereby also supplying the hypoxic areas with additional oxygen. HBOT has been in operation for more than 50 years for the treatment of chronic wounds, especially diabetic foot ulceration (DFU). HBOT is available in either mono-place or multi-place chambers which allow parallel treatment for several patients. In Europe, multi-place chambers are most commonly used.

In both systems, the entire body is exposed to pressure that is significantly higher than the normal atmospheric pressure of an absolute atmosphere (ATA). The patient inhales pure oxygen which in the single-user chamber will fill the entire chamber for the patient to inhale, whereas in the multi-user chamber, the patient will inhale the pure oxygen through a mask. At sufficiently high pressure, typically from 2 to 3 ATA, significantly more oxygen can dissolve in the blood. The oxygen additionally dissolved in the blood plasma diffuses from the capillaries into the surrounding tissue. If the capillaries or arteries are not entirely occluded, this oxygen can enter the less-perfused tissues of the wound and counteract the local hypoxia. During physiological respiration of air, about 97% of the oxygen in the blood is transported via haemoglobin; about 0.3 ml oxygen/dl is dissolved physically in the blood plasma. With HBOT, the physically dissolved proportion of oxygen can be increased to 2.1 ml oxygen/dl at 1 ATA; at 2.94 ATA (3 bar) it is then 6.8 ml oxygen/dl. A typical treatment regime for patients with chronic wounds, for example, provides for a 90-minute treatment, five days/week for six weeks.

There are numerous published studies which show that HBOT as adjuvant therapy in non-healing wounds of different genesis promotes wound-healing and may prevent amputations, in particular for patients with DFU. The clinical evidence is controversial, as there are both randomised controlled trials (RCTs) with a positive outcome for HBOT in terms of wound-healing and avoidance of amputation and study results that do not show significant benefits from HBOT. A Cochrane meta-analysis summarises the results of twelve clinical trials. A total of ten studies dealt with patients with DFU. The authors conclude that HBOT significantly promotes wound-healing and prevents amputations in patients with DFU, at least in the short term. The combined data from five studies involving 205 patients showed an increase in the healing rate after six weeks

for the HBOT group; however, this advantage was no longer evident after one year. Concerning major amputations, the analysis showed no statistically significant difference between the HBOT-treated group and the control group after one year.

In a study published in 2017, the effect of HBOT as a supplement to modern standard treatment in DFU patients was compared to a control group with analogous treatment without HBOT. There was an examination on their wound-healing, amputation risk and other parameters in a total of 38 patients over four weeks. In this RCT, which was admittedly performed without blinding, HBOT showed a positive effect on wound-healing and amputation risk. In contrast, another multicentre RCT (DAMO2CLES) for patients with diabetes and lower leg wounds, showed no improvement in wound-healing after treatment with HBOT compared with the control group over 12 months.

31.2.2 Local topical oxygen therapies

In systemic HBOT, oxygenation causes a more significant amount of oxygen to be dissolved in the blood and transported to the various tissues. In contrast, local topical oxygen therapy attempts to increase the oxygen concentration in the wound area by external means (➤ Fig. 31.2). Various therapeutic approaches

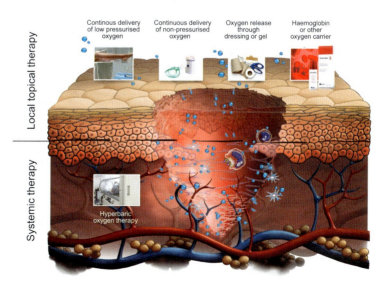

Fig. 31.2 Overview of oxygen therapies for wound-healing disorders. In addition to systemic hyperbaric oxygen therapy, various locally applied approaches are also available to expose a wound to additional oxygen. [V862]

31

have developed in recent years to achieve this goal (> Table 31.1):

1. Therapy with slight oxygen overpressure
2. Therapy with continuous oxygen therapy without overpressure
3. Oxygen-releasing wound dressings
4. Oxygen transporter

The first clinical trials of local oxygen therapy first started in the 1960s. Since then, there have been numerous publications on the clinical use of local therapy options with oxygen.

N O T I C E

In any case, in the case of chronic wounds, treatment of the primary underlying disease must be in parallel with adjuvant oxygen therapy to improve the blood supply to the affected areas.

Oxygen therapies do not replace moist modern wound care; they are **complementary** measures to accelerate/improve wound-healing.

Systemic or local oxygen therapies require proper wound-cleansing to reduce or avoid oxygen barriers to achieve optimum effect.

Table 31.1 Different therapeutic approaches for improving oxygen supply in chronic wounds (modified from Gottrup et al. 2017 and Dissemond et al. 2015)

Oxygen therapies for chronic wounds	Devices/ medical devices	Treatment details					Clinical evidence
	Product	Oxygen pressure	Treatment duration	Treatment frequency	Wound treatment		Grade level (adapted from Gottrup et al. 2017)
Systemic therapy							
HBOT	Single pressure chamber	2–3 ATA	60–120 min.	5 × per week	Patient lies in a 100% oxygen atmosphere		Grade 1B (1 RCT, controlled cohort studies and various case studies that showed positive effects on wound-healing)
HBOT	Multi-person pressure chamber	2–3 ATA	60–120 min.	5 × per week	Patients are surrounded by atmospheric air and breathe 100% oxygen through masks		
Local oxygen therapy approaches							
Local pressure chamber with cyclically intermittent oxygen overpressure	TWO2	5–50 mbar cycles	60–90 min.	3–7 × per week	Wound without support in pressure chamber or cuff		Grade 1B (1 RCT, controlled cohort studies and various case studies that showed positive effects on wound-healing)
Local pressure chamber with constant slight overpressure	O₂ Topi-Care-System	2–5 l/min.; < 50 mbar	60–90 min.	3–7 × per week	Wound without support in pressure chamber or cuff		
	TO₂	2–5 l/min.; < 50 bar	60–90 min.	3–7 × per week	Wound without support in pressure chamber or cuff		

31

Table 31.1 Different therapeutic approaches for improving oxygen supply in chronic wounds (modified from Gottrup et al. 2017 and Dissemond et al. 2015) *(cont'd)*

Oxygen therapies for chronic wounds	Devices/ medical devices	Treatment details					Clinical evidence
	Product	Oxygen pressure	Treatment duration	Treatment frequency	Wound treatment		Grade level (adapted from Gottrup et al. 2017)
Continuous normobaric oxygen supply (CDO)	EpiFLO	Continuous slow flow of pure oxygen (about 3 ml/h) for up to 15 days through a thin tube to the wound	24 h	Throughout	Occlusive wound cover		Grade 2C (only weak evidence, 1 interim report of an RCT showed no significant advantages over the control, cohort studies, case series)
	Natrox	Continuous slow flow of pure oxygen (about 12 ml/h) for several days via a thin tube to the diffuser directly on the wound	24 h		Occlusive wound cover		
Oxygen-releasing wound dressings	OxyBand	Release of oxygen over 5 days after contact with wound exudate from an occlusive dressing	24 h		Occlusive wound dressing		Grade 2B (1 RCT, cohort studies, various case series; only weak recommendation for oxyzyme by NICE)
	OxygeneSys Continous	Foam dressing; release of oxygen up to 5 days after contact with wound exudate	24 h		Occlusive wound dressing		
	OxygeneSys on Demand	Release of oxygen over 5 days after contact with wound exudate from an occlusive dressing	24 h		Occlusive wound dressing		
	Oxyzyme	Release of oxygen when the two components of the primary dressing are combined	24 h		Semipermeable wound dressing		
Oxygen transporter	Granulox	10% purified haemoglobin is applied thinly to the wound bed; then cover with a non-occlusive layer	24 h	1 ×/day–2 ×/ week, as a supplement in the regular wound treatment regime	Aqueous spray		Grade 1B, (1 RCT. 1 controlled open-label study, 3 controlled cohort studies, numerous case series). Positive effect is statistically proven, clearly positive benefit/ risk assessment

31

In the following, there will be explanations on some of the systems for local oxygen therapy available today for wound treatment.

Therapy with slight oxygen overpressure

For local topical oxygen therapy, smaller chambers or cuffs or bags have been developed to take the place of the large HBOT hyperbaric chambers. In addition, there are two treatment variants using a constant slight positive pressure or intermittent pressure. In both cases, these mobile units make it easier to use in daily practice. In addition to the goal of improved flexibility, some of the known side effects of HBOT are eliminated, such as fatigue, dizziness, middle ear problems, etc. In all cases, delivery of the overpressure oxygen is exclusive to the area of the wound and the wound environment. A cuff or small pressure chamber with a tightly fitting connection is placed around the wound or leg. They connect to an oxygen concentrator which generates almost pure oxygen from the air. Pure oxygen is pumped with a slight overpressure into the cuff or pressure box. In the devices with a constant increase in pressure, the treatment is carried out at about 35 mbar inside the chamber, which is usually a simple cuff or plastic bag. In contrast, the devices with intermittent pressure work with wave-like cycles of 5–50 mbar, whereby the moistened oxygen is introduced into the chamber. These devices also generate a continuous compression of the lower leg without direct contact with the leg, which reduces oedema and also supports perfusion of the wound.

There is a publication of case reports and uncontrolled clinical studies for devices that work with constant pressure. A 1988 RCT study reported evidence of the ineffectiveness of these devices. However, this study was underpowered with only 28 patients and with a total of four treatments in two weeks, which was far too small to provide precise results. In another study by Gordillo et al., the use of topical oxygen therapy using slight positive pressure had a significantly positive effect on the reduction in wound size and also an increase in the expression of the vascular endothelial growth factor (VEGF) at the wound margins.

The scientific evidence for the effectiveness of cyclically intermittent oxygen therapy devices is also mostly dependent on case reports and several prospective clinical studies. Several authors report improved healing in various wound types, particularly DFU. However, most of the studies are not randomised or controlled, and mostly include patients with refractory therapy. For example, some studies show that in a group of patients with DFU, treated with this topical oxygen therapy, wounds healed significantly more frequently and in a shorter time than wounds in patients in the control group.

Therapy with continuous oxygenation without overpressure

In a small portable device, almost pure oxygen (> 95%) is generated from the circulating air. In contrast to the therapy approach with slight oxygen overpressure, pure oxygen flows directly and continuously through a thin tube or through a diffuser, onto the wound surface without additional pressure. The therapy unit is attached to a part of the patient's body near the wound so that the patient remains mobile. In both cases, the system is used in combination with an airtight occlusive dressing. The continuous oxygen supply can be used for 24 hours a day for several days or weeks. This therapy is particularly suitable for small and medium-sized wounds that do not have excessive depressions or cavities which are too large.

To date, two RCTs studying these systems have been published. One of these studies involving 122 patients with DFU, investigated and compared the wound-healing time and the proportion of wounds healed over 12 weeks with a control group. Although there were no significant differences in wound-healing between the two groups, there was a subgroup analysis of patients over 65 years of age, showing a clear trend in favour of oxygen therapy. In the second multicentre RCT with 100 patients with DFU, it showed that a more significant number of wounds healed in the active study arm than in the control group. Similarly, the difference became clearer with a consideration of a subgroup analysis of 'particularly severe chronic wounds'. The patients in the oxygen therapy arm showed significantly faster wound closure in comparison with the control group.

Oxygen-releasing wound dressings

Various products are available which either directly release pure oxygen incorporated in the wound dressing, or release oxygen after a biochemical reaction in a hydrogel. In wound dressings which release oxygen directly, the oxygen depots are enclosed in the wound dressing as membrane vesicles (> 2,800 ppm O_2). However, the oxygen is only released when the wound dressing comes into contact with wound exudate. These continuously oxygen-releasing wound dressings can be used as a primary wound dressing.

There are two approaches to hydrogel wound dressings, which generate oxygen through chemical or biochemical reactions. One approach is an occlusive wound dressing which uses the chemical reactivity of hydrogen peroxide (H_2O_2) to water (H_2O) and dissolved oxygen (O_2). The oxygen can then diffuse to the wound bed via a permeable separator. The hydrogel serves as the primary wound dressing. The other alternative is a two-component system. Here, two dressings must be applied together to initiate a biochemical reaction. One component is a hydrogel dressing containing glucose and iodide ions in low concentrations. The second component contains the enzyme glucose oxidase, which catalyses the oxidation of glucose to gluconic acid and H_2O_2 in the presence of oxygen. Through the diffusion of the H_2O_2 to the wound bed, there is a rerelease of free oxygen by metabolisation. However, part of the H_2O_2 can also react with the iodine ions contained in the first component, resulting in free iodine and oxygen. Free iodine has an antimicrobial effect.

Apart from a few case descriptions, no further clinical data are available for wound dressings which release oxygen directly. For the hydrogel wound dressings and here in particular for the two-component system, however, there are various case studies which demonstrate an improvement in wound-healing. For example, this wound dressing was tested in a non-controlled multicentre study with 51 patients with chronic wounds. After a six-week test phase, six wounds showed complete wound closure, and 37 wounds at least showed improvement. A monocentric RCT (n = 100) with the two-component system showed no significant difference from the control group in terms of speed of wound-healing, pain or other measured parameters.

Oxygen transporter

Biofilm on wounds constitutes a diffusion barrier for oxygen. A spray with haemoglobin as an oxygen transporter was developed to enable oxygen to diffuse more effectively through this barrier. It is well-known that purified haemoglobin can significantly improve diffusion in liquids compared to normal diffusion. The binding and release of oxygen by the haemoglobin depends on the surrounding oxygen concentration. In this way, at high oxygen concentrations, oxygen is bound to haemoglobin, while low oxygen concentrations lead to the release of oxygen. Haemoglobin is therefore an ideal molecule to bridge the gap between the wound surface with a high oxygen concentration and the wound bed with a low oxygen concentration by binding oxygen from the environment and transporting it by diffusion to the wound bed. Thus a more significant amount of oxygen can be provided locally to the wound and rereleased by the haemoglobin in areas with low oxygen concentration. In a clinical study, it was demonstrated by photoacoustic tomography that a significant increase in oxygenated haemoglobin was detectable within 20 minutes after application of the haemoglobin spray to venous ulcers, thus confirming the *in vitro* data. Occlusive dressings are not advisable, since haemoglobin depends on the accessibility of atmospheric oxygen.

A monocentric RCT examined the influence of haemoglobin spray on wound-healing in patients with therapy-refractory venous leg ulcers for 13 weeks. The haemoglobin spray group showed a significant reduction in wound size of 53% on average, whereas the wounds in the control group did not improve. Other clinical studies with various chronic wound types (DFU, venous leg ulcer, arterial ulcers and mixed) also showed a significant benefit in wound-healing through the adjuvant use of haemoglobin spray. In three cohort studies, they examine the influence of haemoglobin spray on wound-healing and other parameters such as pain in patients with various chronic wounds. Retrospectively collected data served as a control for the prospectively treated haemoglobin spray group. In the study with DFU patients, groups of 20 patients each were included; in the study of patients with chronic wounds, groups of 50 patients each were included; and for the study of patients with chronic wounds with coatings, groups of 100 patients each

31

were included. All three studies showed that the use of haemoglobin spray led to significantly better healing results and less pain compared to the control groups. In the study with wound coatings, the wounds in the haemoglobin group were free of coatings within a significantly shorter time. In all cases, wounds were cleansed or debrided if necessary before application of the haemoglobin spray, so that the aim was rather the formation of new wound coatings.

31.3 Conclusion

Oxygen is essential in wound-healing. Tissue under-supplied with oxygen is called hypoxic. Transient hypoxia in tissue injury is initially physiological and promotes wound-healing. Persistent hypoxia due to a permanent oxygen deficiency in the tissue leads to stagnation of wound-healing. In addition to the treatment of the primary underlying disease to improve the blood circulation situation, there are already various adjuvant therapy approaches with oxygen in wound treatment. Systemic therapies such as hyperbaric oxygen therapy is distinguished from other treatment approaches with topical application of oxygen.

As in many areas of wound treatment, the evidence for oxygen therapies in wound treatment is still insufficient to make concrete recommendations. Nevertheless, there is increasing scientific evidence that oxygen therapies support wound-healing in the long term. These therapy options can be considered in the future, particularly in therapy-refractory processes.

REFERENCES
Dissemond J, Kröger K, Storck M, Risse A, Engels P. Topical oxygen wound therapies for chronic wounds: a review. J Wound Care 2015; 24: 53–63.
Eisenbud DE. Oxygen in wound-healing: nutrient, antibiotic, signaling molecule, and therapeutic agent. Clin Plast Surg 2012; 39: 293–310.
Gottrup F, Dissemond J, Baines C, et al. use of oxygen therapies in wound-healing. J Wound Care 2017; 26 (Suppl. 5): 1–43.
Kimmel HM, Grant A, Ditata J. The presence of oxygen in wound-healing. Wounds 2016; 28: 264–270.
Kranke P, Bennett MH, Martyn-St James M, et al. Hyperbaric oxygen therapy for chronic wounds. Cochrane Database Syst Rev 2015; 6: CD004123.
Schreml S, Szeimies RM, Prantl L, Karrer S, Landthaler M, Babilas P. Oxygen in acute and chronic wound-healing. Br J Dermatol 2010; 163: 257–268.
Sen CK. Wound-healing essentials: let there be oxygen. Wound Repair Regen 2009; 17: 1–18.

31

32 André Glod
Systematics of physiotherapy

Key notes

- Manual lymphatic drainage (MLD) is a specialised massage technique for the treatment of lymphoedema. MLD is only one mainstay of complete (or complex) decongestive therapy (CDT) and has no lasting effect without subsequent compression treatment.
- Wound margin drainage promotes wound-healing in chronic wounds associated with lymphoedema by loosening the wound edge fibrosis and reducing wound-surrounding oedema.

- Decongestive therapy improves venous return transport and activates lymphangiomotor functions.
- Structured gait training in PAD is used as a conservative primary therapy for intermittent claudication in the aftercare of interventional or surgical revascularisations and as secondary cardiovascular prevention.
- Intermittent pneumatic compression (IPC) is an additional therapy option in the decongestive treatment of oedema, but cannot replace compression treatment and CDT.

32.1 Introduction

This chapter deals with oedema and vascular diseases. Treatment methods of physical therapy are presented in particular, they are mostly carried out by specially trained physiotherapists.

32.2 Complete decongestive therapy (CDT)

Complete decongestive therapy (CDT; ➤ Table 32.1) is the standard conservative treatment for primary and secondary lymphoedema (➤ Chap. 19.2). These are chronic diseases which require long-term treatment. However, there is a short-term to medium-term treatment indication for oedema diseases such as posttraumatic oedema, postoperative oedema, reperfusion oedema and inflammatory oedema. Cardiac oedema and oedema due to protein loss or protein synthesis disorders are not indications for CDT and require drug therapy.

The compression treatment described in ➤ Chap. 29 makes particular reference to lymphological compression bandages and flat knitted compression textiles. Skin restoration and skincare are described in ➤ Chap. 38.

In addition to the four recognised mainstays of CDT, patient education is regarded as the fifth mainstay of CDT and an important component of self-management with lymphoedema:

1. Manual lymphatic drainage
2. Compression treatment
3. Skincare and skin restoration
4. Decongestion-promoting movement therapy
5. In addition: education and training for individual self-therapy (patient education)

Effect of CDT:
- Mobilisation and reduction of pathologically interstitial fluid increase and removal of lymph dependent substances
- Improvement of disturbed homeostasis in the interstitium
- Reduction of stasis-induced inflammatory processes
- Reduction of fibrotic alteration of the connective tissue

Table 32.1 Phases of CDT

Phase I	Phase II
Intensified acute tissue decongestion	Conservation and optimisation of the therapy result
Objective: normalisation of tissue homeostasis*	Objective: stabilisation of the decongestion situation
Treatment frequency: 1–2 ×/day	Treatment frequency: findings-oriented
Inpatient treatment Outpatient treatment in specialised practices	Outpatient treatment
* Self-regulation of a biological system in dynamic physiological equilibrium	

The goal of CDT:
- Reduction of oedema-induced swelling of the extremities
- Reduction of congestion-related complaints
- Improved mobility
- Improvement of stasis-related skin conditions
- Reduction of erysipelas relapses

32.3 Manual lymph drainage (MLD)

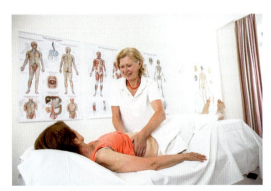

Fig. 32.1 MLD – central pretreatment. [T1054]

32.3.1 The MLD technique

Manual lymph drainage is a decongestive massage technique developed by the philologist and physiotherapist Emil Vodder around 1932. It was later scientifically supported and propagated by the physicians Johannes Asdonk and Michael Földi.

It consists of four basic techniques: standing circle, pump technique, scoop technique, twist technique as well as additional oedema techniques and fibrosis-loosening techniques.

As a specialised treatment technique, the MLD exerts a stretch stimulus on the skin and subcutis. The execution of a lymph drainage technique is divided into a thrust phase to stimulate the lymphangiomotoric system and a relaxation phase, which causes the lymph capillaries to refill distally by suction.

MLD begins with a central pretreatment to activate the healthy lymphatic drainage pathways and achieve a central suction effect (➤ Fig. 32.1). There is an activation of the cervical lymph nodes and the confluence region of the left thoracic duct and the right lymphatic duct in the respective subclavicular venous angle for this purpose. MLD is always combined with breathing exercises for central lymphatic stimulation.

Deep abdominal drainage additionally stimulates the cisterna chyli and the lymphatic trunks of the abdominal and pelvic regions.

As well as the local damage to the lymphatic transport system of an extremity, there is a chance of the alteration or removal of the associated groups of lymph nodes (lymphatic tributaries), for example, as part of oncological surgery. The corresponding body quadrant is also often oedematously altered as part of the lymphatic drainage disorder. The trained lymph therapist will draw up a therapy plan. They will drain the free tissue fluid from oedema-rich regions to oedema-free regions to allow uptake of fluid into undamaged lymph capillaries. When there is an alteration in the lymphatic tributaries or relevant lymph collectors, manual lymph drainage will stimulate the anatomically preformed anastomotic pathways (axillo-axillary, axillo-inguinal, inguino-inguinal) and deviate the lymph flow accordingly.

Only then the lymphatic drainage of the limb is carried out with direction from distal to proximal, respecting the lymphatic tributaries of the limb and central lymph drainage pathways.

32.3.2 Effect of MLD

MLD leads to the increased pulse frequency of the individual lymphangions of a lymph collector via an stretch stimulus of the lymph vessel walls. An increase in the pulse frequency of the lymphangions leads to an increased lymph time volume.

> **Lymphangion:** Section between two valves of a lymph collector. Since the lymphatic vascular system has no direct connection to the heart, the spontaneous rhythmic contractions of the regional lymphatic walls determine the relapsing lymph flow centrally.

The initial lymph vessels or lymph capillaries are connected upstream to the lymph collectors. At increased interstitial pressure, the free interstitial fluid enters the initial lymph vessels via raised endothelial margins. This is called the 'lymph fluid formation' and triggered by manual lymph drainage.

The post-inflammatory fibrosclerosis is broken up by a fibrotic tissue-loosening massage technique. This leads to an improved mobilisation of the free liquid in the interstitium and the uptake in the lymph vessel system (➤ Fig. 32.2).

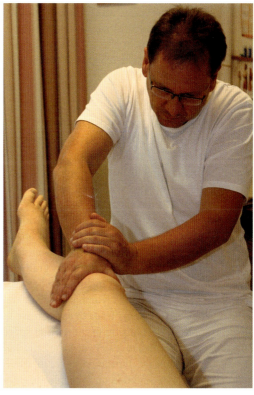

Fig. 32.2 MLD – pump technique. [P588]

32.3.3 Indications for MLD

- Lymphoedema (primary and secondary)
- Phlebolymphoedema, oedema due to venous congestion
- Posttraumatic and postoperative oedema
- Reperfusion oedema
- Inflammatory oedema (inflammation)
- Immobility oedema (paralysis)
- Lipoedema

32.3.4 Contraindications for MLD

Absolute contraindications:
- Decompensated heart failure
- Acute deep vein thrombosis
- Erosive dermatosis
- Acute erysipelas
- PAD (not revascularised)

Relative contraindications:
- Malignant lymphoedema
- Skin infections
- Skin diseases (blister-forming dermatoses)

Local contraindications:
- **Neck treatment:** hyperthyroidism, carotid sinus hypersensitivity, cardiac arrhythmia (vagus irritation), atherosclerosis of the carotids
- **Abdominal deep drainage:** after abdominal surgery, inflammatory intestinal diseases, abdominal aortic aneurysm, atherosclerosis of the abdominal aorta, pregnancy, menstruation, postoperative abdominal adhesions, radiation cystitis, radiation colitis, pelvic vein thrombosis

32.3.5 MLD – treatment of lymphatic fibrosis

With lymphatic fibrosis in lymphoedema stages II and III, special fibrotic tissue-loosening techniques must supplement the classic MLD. These techniques are stronger, slower and must not cause any pain. To achieve a lasting treatment effect, foam inserts partially containing profiles are integrated into the subsequent lymphological compression bandage.

32.3.6 Oedema and wounds – influence of MLD on wound-healing

Wound formation and disorders of wound-healing are caused by disturbances of the cellular nutrition or following an inflammatory process.

The most important form of cell nutrition is diffusion, a passive exchange mechanism of nutrients and waste products between intra- and extracellular fluids along a concentration gradient. Other transport mechanisms include capillary filtration and reabsorption via lymph capillaries and venous capillaries. Oedema leads to an increase in tissue volume and expansion of interstitial space which expands the distance between the cells and the capillaries. Thus, the diffusion distance increases and affects the skin condition up to cell death, since the keratinocytes are fed mainly by diffusion.

Fluid overload, the lymphoedema-typical accumulation of protein molecules and other lymph-dependent substances in the interstitium, are leading to extensive immune reactions. These inflammatory processes cause increased incorporation of collagen fibres in the extracellular space with the participation of profibrotic cytokines. The fibrotic alteration makes the access of the interstitial fluid to the lymph capillaries more difficult. The increased tissue pressure and the post-inflammatory fibrosis lead to disturbances of the microcirculation and lymph fluid transport. The thickening of the skin, typical of lymphoedema, is also a consequence of oedema, inflammation and fibrosis. The skin is increasingly interspersed with collagen and loses its elasticity.

Acute wounds and wound-healing disorders can occur accompanied by inflammatory, posttraumatic or postoperative oedema and are usually of limited duration. Here, decongestion therapy through compression is often sufficient.

Chronic wounds are frequently associated with lymphoedema, whereby Michael Földi rightly rejects the existence of a 'lymphogenic' ulcer. Primary and conco-

mitant diseases cause these wounds. Some examples of such conditions are CVI, diabetes mellitus, infections (erysipelas), PAD, and autoimmune vasculitis. On the other hand, delayed wound-healing is closely related to lymphoedema, because of a safety valve insufficiency of the lymphatic system. There is a combination of mechanical damage to the lymphatic transport pathways by inflammation and fibrosis and on the other hand volume overloading, due to inflammation-induced oedema enhancement with further lymphatic loads, e.g. protein molecules and detritus. The discharge of the excess interstitial fluid is possibly visible in the form of wound exudation.

In the case of oedema-associated wounds, the primary treatment objective is decongestion. The method of choice is CDT, with its four coordinated therapy mainstays. The compression treatment is indispensable for the long-term preservation of the decongestion result and the prevention of tissue fibrosis (➤ Chap. 29).

In postoperative and posttraumatic oedema, the temporary use of manual lymph drainage can be useful. By reducing the oedema volume, the healing process accelerates and reduces the frequency of postoperative complications (lymphocele, seroma, keloids). MLD also relieves pain by accelerating the removal of inflammatory mediators. MLD is considered as a significant therapy option for ulcerations of various origins. For venous ulcers, MLD, together with the other components of CDT, could be attributed a cure rate of 93% within a study collective, with a recurrence rate of 20%.

Effects of CDT on wound-healing:
- Decongestion by improving lymphatic and venous transport capacity
- Securing cell nutrition through enhanced diffusion
- Improved CO_2 removal, reduction of tissue acidosis
- Regulation of inflammatory processes by a decrease in inflammatory mediators, reactive oxygen species (ROS), leukocytes
- Reduction of factors which disturb wound-healing, such as MMPs and TNFα
- Sealing of the capillary wall (glycocalyx regeneration), reduction of filtration and oedema formation

Chronic lymphoedema-associated wounds show a longer development period; this concerns both the severity and extent of the lymphoedema as well as the wound findings. Lymphoedema in stage II or III describes a decompensated stasis with an accompanying stasis dermatitis. Massive lymphatic fibrosis indurates the tissue. The wounds are confluent and weeping, and often critical colonisation or infection are present. Fibrosis indurates the wound margins with wall-like edges, whereas the wound-surrounding environment is often macerated. Only a permanent oedema reduction can promote wound-healing, which requires long-term and high-frequency MLD therapy as part of CDT.

The treatment of chronic wounds in lymphoedema involves interprofessional cooperation of lymph and wound therapists. At the beginning of CDT, besides MLD and compression, skin rehabilitation is of primary importance. Antibiotic therapy must often be used in addition to local disinfection to prevent erysipelas. Wound-healing only takes place with sufficient decongestion. However, increased wound exudation remains until the achievement of the first decongestion result. Because of healthcare costs, wound therapists should limit themselves to highly absorbent wound dressings, until they see first effects of the CDT, such as reduction of wound exudation.

32.3.7 Wound margin drainage

Wound margin drainage is a specialised massage technique used to treat fibrotic induration and oedema around the wound (➤ Fig. 32.3). Since wound-healing takes place from the wound margin to centripetal, the migration and proliferation of keratinocytes must not impede. The drainage of the wound margin is guided from the healthy tissue into the fibrosis with individual fingers in circular movements. The treatment takes place in direct contact with the wound, which is why the strictest hygiene criteria apply. Disinfec-

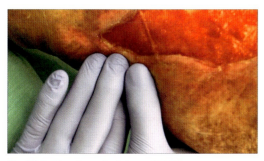

Fig. 32.3 Wound margin drainage. [P588]

tion of the wound and its surroundings, as well as the wearing of protective gloves, are mandatory; it is also possible to work directly on the wound with sterile gloves or to cover the wound area with a sterile wound film. The wound margin drainage flattens the wound margin, reduces the wound surrounding oedema and improves tissue shifting. Micro- and macrocirculation of the wound area and after all the diffusion to the skin cells are improved. The effectiveness of wound margin drainage in the treatment of chronic wounds with lymphoedema is confirmed in daily clinical practice. Unfortunately, there is no scientific evidence for this method due to a lack of publications.

32.3.8 No MLD without compression

CDT, with its four mainstays of therapy, is a coordinated concept for the treatment of lymphoedema. Numerous publications prove that isolated MLD is not suitable for long-term decongestive therapy and complication prevention. Reduction in volume can be measured immediately after performing MLD, but it can reverse within hours without subsequent lymphological compression treatment.

32.3.9 MLD as part of inpatient treatment

Stage II and stage III lymphoedema require regular intervals of active phase I decongestion therapy to avoid a worsening in the condition and lymphoedema-enhancing complications (erysipelas). Patients with decompensated lymphoedema and lymphoedema in combination with immobility or multiple co-morbidity are also indicative of this treatment. It is recommended that patients with lymphoedema-associated chronic wounds are treated as inpatients. In Europe, many lymphological specialist clinics are classified as rehabilitation clinics, so that inpatient admission can only take place after application and approval by the pension or health insurance. The core activity of these clinics is high-frequency and differentiated Phase I decongestion therapy. An additional qualification in the treatment of chronic wounds is required for these facilities before treating lymphoedema patients with a wound. Those clinics should have an interdisciplinary and interprofessional therapy qualification, that guarantees a good scheduling for stage-appropriate wound treatment in combination with CDT. The practitioners should be able to treat concomitant diseases.

32.3.10 MLD as part of outpatient treatment

After preliminary planning, intensive outpatient decongestion of phase I is even possible in well-structured, lymphologically-oriented physiotherapy practice. However, the core activity of these practices is the maintenance therapy of phase II. The frequency of the MLD and the other CDT elements depends on the findings.

A coordinated interprofessional treatment of lymph-oedema-associated chronic wounds is challenging in an outpatient setting. It requires communication and appointment coordination between the lymph therapist, outpatient nursing service or wound therapist and the prescribing physician.

Wound treatment must be carried out first and dressings fixed provisionally. MLD should be performed in a prompt timing, subsequently the wound dressings will be fixed by the lymphological bandage or by combining an inner stocking with a flat-knit compression stocking (phase II).

Lymph therapists have the opportunity to undergo additional training as wound assistants. However, in most countries, there is so far no incentive relevant to remuneration to compensate the extra expense of wound care in addition to MLD. Most physiotherapists do not practice wound margin drainage for hygienic reasons.

Since the frequency of wound care and CDT appointments do not necessarily correlate in the outpatient situation, compression treatment must be guaranteed on MLD-free days.

32.4 Decongestive respiratory and exercise therapy

32.4.1 Respiratory therapy

Intensive respiratory therapy causes an increase in venous blood flow and an increase in lymph flow.

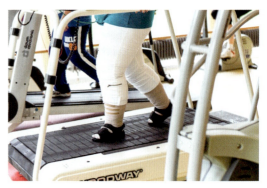

Fig. 32.4 Decongestive exercise therapy for lymphoedema. [T1054]

32.4.2 Decongestive exercise therapy in lymphoedema

Exercise therapy and sports activity are useful components of complete decongestive therapy (CDT). A targeted exercise programme stimulates lymphangio-motor activity in the sense of increased pulsation of the lymphangions and increases interstitial pressure, especially in combination with compression treatment (➤ Fig. 32.4). It leads to increased uptake of tissue fluid into the initial lymph vessels (lymph formation) and thus supports decongestion. In addition to the decongestive lymphatic therapy exercises, sports such as (Nordic) walking and (indoor) cycling have proven themselves in oedema therapy. Swimming and water gymnastics are only possible with skin conditions without a wound, good hygiene criteria and moderate water temperatures are required.

32.4.3 Exercise therapy for CVI and venous leg ulcers

The development and severity of CVI correlate with a reduced functional capacity of the leg muscle pump and a restriction of ankle mobility. It is also illustrated by the so-called dependency (obesity-associated) syndrome and arthrogenic congestion syndrome. Patients with venous leg ulcers show a significantly lower number of steps for the same period of movement. In the primary therapy of CVI, therefore, improving movement restrictions and the increase of self-mobility play a fundamental role. Compression and movement therapy should always be combined to optimise the effect. By optimal utilisation of the muscle pump, this combination leads to an improvement of venous reflux and increased lymphatic drainage in the area of the lower extremity. The effectiveness of the calf muscles largely depends on the improvement of ankle mobility. A specific venous exercise programme includes gait training, ankle activation and repeated elevation of the lower extremities. The venous exercise programme can be carried out in a group or individually.

In cases of paralysis or extensive immobility, an active exercise programme is only possible to a limited extent or not at all. Physiotherapeutic treatment implements passive movement of the joints with the aim of contracture prevention and to improve venous return flow and lymphangiomotoric function.

A regular exercise programme can improve the ulcer-healing rate and reduce the recurrence rate. The cutaneous microcirculation will be optimised and the tcpO$_2$ value increases. In addition to improved ankle mobility, patients also report a reduction in wound pain.

32.4.4 Structured gait training as conservative therapy for PAD

In peripheral artery disease (PAD), physical activity and an exercise programme lead not only to a significant improvement in the walking distance but also to an improvement in the maximum oxygen uptake in the tissue. The positive effects of an exercise programme on glucose and fat metabolism are well known. Stimulation of the local production of VEGF (vascular endothelial growth factor) favours the formation of collaterals and the improvement of endothelial function. There will be a restriction of the inflammatory reactions, stimulation of mitochondrial metabolism and local muscle function. Targeted vascular training for patients with chronic wounds after revascularisation of arterial circulatory disorders leads to a higher healing tendency.

Structured gait training is indicated in the conservative and drug therapy of PAD, in the aftercare of interventional and surgical treatment procedures as well as in the sense of secondary cardiovascular prevention. In this context, monitored gait training, e. g. in a rehabilitation group, is superior to unmonitored gait training. Patients with PAD and chronic wounds should also be admitted to structured gait training after revascularisation, as far as wound conditions permit.

An exercise programme with structured gait training is effective if followed for at least 3×/week for 30–60 minutes. This program within a vascular sports group includes not only walking phases but also warm-up phases, stretching and coordination exercises as well as games. There is a recommendation to have an independent daily exercise program of over 60 minutes with 5- to 15-minute load intervals; the intensity should only be increased until the onset of stress pain. It makes more sense to determine the walking distance, this is 70% of the maximum walking distance (time at which claudication-related pain occurs) under standardised testing conditions. In addition to simple walking, Nordic walking is particularly effective in the context of arterial gait training. Exercising the arm muscles promotes the cardiovascular effect. If structured gait training is not possible due to paralysis or other functional reasons, regular arm ergometer training is recommended as an alternative.

32.5 Intermittent pneumatic compression (IPC)

32.5.1 Effects of IPC

Intermittent pneumatic compression (IPC) is a dynamic compression system which is characterised by the constant alternation of pressure build-up and pressure relief (➤ Fig. 32.5). IPC is an instrumental, processor-controlled method; the devices used vary according to indication and localisation. IPC reduces oedema in the treated limb area and improves venous and lymphatic return flow. It demonstrates an improvement in micro- and macro-perfusion; the method is also used under defined conditions as a conservative measure for arterial circulatory disorders. Thromboembolism prophylaxis is an important indication of IPC as it has been proven as an activation of fibrinolysis. The effect of pressure and shear forces on the vascular endothelium during IPC leads to the release of tissue plasminogen and vasodilating nitric oxide (NO).

32

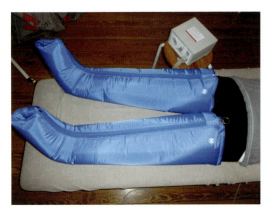

Fig. 32.5 IPC with leg cuffs – 3-chamber system. [M291]

32.5.2 IPC equipment

Control unit:

The setting of the following treatment parameters can be adjusted via the control unit: pressure build-up, pressure maintenance phase, pause time and cycle repetition. The therapeutic pressure values vary between 12 and 200 mmHg. Pressure build-up is intermittent or sequential, i. e. continuous from distal to proximal. Similar to the principle of compression therapy, some intermittent compression devices use a pressure gradient, i. e. the pressure decreases from distal to proximal. The intermittent compression imitates the effect of the muscle pump.

Multi-stage devices make it possible to set different pressure levels according to the tissue condition and localisation. Their use is preferable for lymphological findings.

Cuffs:

The double-walled, inflatable cuffs vary according to the area needing decongestion. There are foot and lower leg cuffs, extremity cuffs (legs, arms) as well as trouser or jacket cuffs. The cuffs can have one or more chambers. Only multi-chamber cuffs are suitable for intermittent and sequential pressure build-up. The air chambers lie next to each other or overlap.

32.5.3 Indications and contraindications of IPC

N O T E

Even if IPC shows very positive effects in some areas, there is nothing to indicate that it would be the only and essential therapeutic measure.

Indications:

- Thromboembolism prophylaxis
- Postthrombotic syndrome, if no drug prophylaxis possible
- Venous leg ulcers without a healing tendency despite adequate compression treatment
- Pronounced CVI, CEAP C4b-C6
- Lymphoedema of one extremity, only as additive! (in the absence of compensation under CDT)
- PAD with stable intermittent claudication or critical ischaemia, when structured gait training and revascularisation are not possible

Conditional indications:

- Posttraumatic oedema
- Therapy-resistant venous oedema
- Lipoedema
- Lymphoedema of the extremities additive to CDT
- Hemiplegia with sensory disorder and oedema
- Thromboembolism prophylaxis in addition to drug prophylaxis

Absolute contraindications:

- Decompensated heart failure
- Thrombosis, extensive thrombophlebitis
- Erysipelas and cellulitis
- Compartment syndrome
- Severe hypertension without drug treatment
- Occluding processes in the lymph vessel system, in which IPC has led to congestion in the groin or genital area

Conditional contraindications:

- Extended, possibly open soft-tissue trauma
- Extended polyneuropathy
- Blister-forming dermatosis

IPC cannot be performed in the case of absolute contraindications. Where oedema is combined with cardiac issues, drug recompensation is of primary importance. In the case of conditional contraindications, IPC is possible under close clinical control.

Intermittent pneumatic compression cannot replace CDT and is an adjuvant therapy in regard to decongestion therapy of lymphoedema. It is suitable for distal oedema localisation of the extremities without the involvement of the ipsilateral trunk quadrant and for patients with limited mobility. Above all a mobilisation of free fluid in the interstitial space has been described for IPC. Thus far, central lymph drainage and an essential protein mobilisation from the interstitial space could not be proven. Therefore, there is a recommendation to always precede a central and peripheral decongestion treatment with CDT before starting the IPC treatment. IPC can be used as a home therapy for patients with lymphoedema and thus represents a self-managed therapy supplement on MLD-free days.

IPC is recognised as an adjuvant decongestive measure, but cannot replace either compression therapy or complex physical decongestion for cases of phlebological and lymphological findings. Good results of oedema reduction can be found in revascularisation oedema, postoperative and inflammatory oedema. The positive side effect of thromboembolism prophylaxis can be exploited perioperatively.

IPC seems to be a useful method for the passive activation of the missing muscle pump function in immobile patients or patients with mobility limitations. In hemiplegic patients, IPC is used to improve sensory disturbance.

It is advisable to protect the extremity with fabric skin protection to prevent skin and nerve damage caused by cuff pressure. Additional padding is recommended for high-risk patients.

A careful indication and regular follow-up is required to detect complications such as genital oedema at an early stage.

32.5.4 IPC and wound-healing

An improved healing rate, accelerated healing time, optimised skin circulation and pain reduction are described in several studies for the application of IPC in venous leg ulcers. There is evidence that IPC, in addition to compression therapy, improves the healing of venous ulcers. For the treatment of chronic wounds with CVI, the use of multi-stage cuffs with sequential pressure build-up from distal to proximal is recommended. A clean, liquid-tight dressing must cover existing wounds before the application of the compression cuff to the affected extremity. If a cuff is used for more than one patient, wipe disinfection is required after each application.

32.5.5 IPC in practice

Intermittent pneumatic compression (IPC) is not limited to inpatient or outpatient treatment in a medical institution. It is suitable for long-term use in the home as part of self-treatment.

REFERENCES

AWMF. S2k-Leitlinie: Diagnostik und Therapie der Lymphödeme. 05/2017. AWMF Reg.-Nr. 058–001. Aus: www.awmf.org/uploads/tx_szleitlinien/058-001l_S2k_Diagnostik_und_Therapie_der_Lymphoedeme_2017-05.pdf (last accessed 12 October 2020).

AWMF. S3-Leitlinie: Diagnostik und Therapie des Ulcus cruris venosum. 2008. AWMF Reg.-Nr. 037–009. Aktuelle Dermatologie 2009; 35 (06): 221–224.

AWMF. S3-Leitlinie zur Diagnostik, Therapie und Nachsorge der peripheren arteriellen Verschlusskrankheit. 2015. AWMF Reg.-Nr. 065/003. Aus: www.awmf.org/uploads/tx_szleitlinien/065-003m_S3_PAVK_periphere_arterielle_Verschlusskrankheitfinal-2015-11.pdf (last accessed 12 October 2020).

Chen AH, Frangos SG, Kilaru S, Sumpio BE. Intermittend pneumatic compression devices – physiological mechanisms of action. Eur J Vasc Endovasc Surg 2001; 21: 383–392.

Clarke-Moloney M, Godfrey A, O'Connor V, et al. Mobility in patients with venous leg ulceration. Eur J Vasc Endovasc Surg 2007; 4: 488–493.

Cornelsen H. Komplexe Lymphdrainage – Wundtherapie in der Therapiepraxis. LymphForsch 2015; 19: 28–32.

Düppers P, Floros N, Garabet W, et al. Strukturiertes Gehtraining zur Behandlung der Claudicatio intermittens. Ein wichtiger Schritt in der Gefäßmedizin. Gefässchirurgie 2017; 22: 572–579.

Földi M, Földi E. Lehrbuch Lymphologie. 7. A. München: Elsevier/Urban&Fischer 2010; 477–495.

Földi M, Strößenreuther R. Grundlagen der manuellen Lymphdrainage. 5. A. München: Elsevier 2011.

Glod A, Oberlin M, Földi E. Lymphödem und chronische Wunde. Vasomed 2016; 4: 184–195.

Glod A. Das Ulcus cruris venosum beim Lymphödem – eine besondere interdisziplinäre Herausforderung. Medizin&Praxis Spezial: Venenerkrankungen und Ulcus cruris 2015; 8: 2–13.

Häfner HM, Steins A. Ulcus cruris und die apparative intermittierende Kompression. In: Rabe E (Hrsg): Apparative intermittierende Kompressionstherapie. Köln: Viavital, 2003: 76–94.

Heinig B, Florek HJ. Physiotherapeutische Möglichkeiten bei postoperativen Ödemen nach arterieller Gefäßrekonstruktion. In: Hepp W, Brunner UV, Gußmann A. Lymphologische Gesichtspunkte in der Gefäßchirurgie. Darmstadt: Steinkopff, 2006; 45–55.

Hutzschenreuter P, Kunze KU, Hermann H, Walcher AM. Beinulzera – chronische Wunden. LymphForsch 2000; 4: 6–10.

Klimaschewski H. Entstauungstherapie – ihr Stellenwert bei Ulzerationen verschiedener Genese an den unteren Extremitäten. Lymph Forsch 2000; 4: 28–30.

Kröger K, Fahrig C, Nüllen H. Gehtraining bei pAVK: Ausbau der Angebote notwendig. Dtsch Ärztebl 2013; 110 (13): A-606/B-538/C-538.

32

Lymphologischer Informationsdienst. Aktuelle Regelung für die Verschreibung von Lymphdrainage. Lymphe & Gesundheit 2017; 2: 1–9.

Rabe E. (Hrsg.). Grundlagen der Phlebologie. Köln: Viavital, 2003: 189–190.

Schwahn-Schreiber C, Reich-Schupke S, Breu FX, et al. S1-Leitlinie: Intermittierende pneumatische Kompression (IPK, AIK). 01/2018; AWMF Reg.-Nr. 037–007. Aus: www.awmf.org/uploads/tx_szleitlinien/037-007l_S1_Intermittierende-pneumatische-Kompression-IPK-AIK_2018-07.pdf (last accessed 12 October 2020).

Schwahn-Schreiber C, Reich-Schupke S. Leitlinie intermittierende pneumatische Kompressionstherapie – eine Zusammenfassung. Vasomed 2018; 2: 72–73.

Weissleder H, Schuchhardt Ch. Erkrankungen des Lymphgefäßsystems. Köln: Viavital 2015.

33

Theresa Hauck, Raymund E. Horch

Skin substitutes

Key notes

- Cultured skin substitutes are used both in the treatment of severely burned patients and increasingly in the treatment of patients with chronic wounds.
- The combination of cultured autologous keratinocytes on alloplastic or mixed synthetic-

  biological carriers is already being used successfully in clinical applications.
- Currently available skin substitutes cannot entirely replace a split- or full-thickness skin graft.

33.1 Introduction

Wound-healing of the skin as a natural biological process with successful reepithelialisation of the wound surface is a fundamental process in tissue regeneration and the primary defence against environmental influences. Particularly in the treatment of a severely burned patient, the extent of the burned skin potentially exceeds possible donor areas for autologous skin graft coverage. Thus the use of skin substitutes becomes necessary. These should replace the properties of both the epidermis and the dermis. They must perform a protective function against infection and dehydration. Further, the dermal matrix should be permeable to transport essential metabolites to optimise wound-healing. Through the effective use of skin substitutes, it is possible to reduce the amount of skin grafting and to shorten the recovery time of severely burned patients. Cultured skin substitutes are not only essential for severely burned patients, but they are also increasingly used in the treatment of patients with chronic and complex wounds. Despite decades of intensive research, there is still no skin substitute product that could permanently replace classic autologous split skin transplants for the treatment of deep wounds in a single-stage procedure. It will continue to be the subject of current research, which includes a wide variety of approaches to tissue engineering.

33.2 Classification of available skin substitutes

Skin substitutes can be divided into different groups according to the primary application. On the one hand, the tissue can be applied to the fresh wound and can remain there until healing (temporary skin substitute). On the other hand, the tissue can be administered to the wound and replaced by autologous skin grafts (semi-permanent). Dermal and/or epidermal analogues are assigned to the group of permanent skin substitutes if they have been used as the final skin substitute in the first place. Besides synthetic and biological, epidermal and dermal, as well as cell-free and cell-populated tissue can be differentiated.

33.3 Special features of the burn wound

Success in the treatment of patients with burn wounds depends on the rapid debridement of the burn eschar, as well as rapid wound closure. Early surgical interventions lead to a higher survival rate and reduced length of hospital stay compared to conservative therapy, in which antimicrobial dressings are used initially for several weeks until the separation of the necrotic tissue.

This can be attributed to a lower release of inflammatory mediators and reduced bacterial colonisation of the wound, which lead to a lower probability of the occurrence of SIRS (Systemic Inflammatory Response Syndrome) and multiorgan failure. Autologous split skin transplantation is an established standard surgical procedure for restoring the damaged body surface. However, this gold standard of autologous skin transplantation is limited in severely burned patients as the unburned skin areas available for transplantation are minimised due to the extensiveness of the burn. Alternatives for an autologous split skin transplantation are therefore required.

Over the last few decades, doctors specialising in burns have increasingly made use of the clinical application of skin grafts obtained by cell cultivation. In contrast to allogeneic skin substitute products or allogeneic skin grafts, which can only serve as temporary soft tissue cover due to a probable later rejection reaction, cultured autologous skin substitutes are intended as a long-term and final solution in reconstructive surgery. The demand for skin grafts obtained by cell cultivation is growing continually and includes a short cultivation period with rapid and sufficient availability of the cultured skin.

33.4 Development of keratinocyte cultures

The basis for the large-scale clinical application of keratinocyte cultures was influenced by the reports of Rheinwald and Green in 1975, who succeeded in serial subcultivation of keratinocytes with multiplication intervals of less than 24 hours in defined media on lethally irradiated mouse fibroblasts as feeder layers. In 1977, the epidermal growth factor (EGF) was described as enabling the rapid growth of epidermal cell cultures, independent of hormonal influences. The combination of perfectly matched media was then the subject of research in numerous working groups, so that keratinocytes could subsequently be produced without a feeder layer. This discovery also created the basis for covering extensive wounds after debridement and temporary skin substitutes within about 3–4 weeks.

In principle, the further development of in vitro cultured skin substitutes can be divided into two different pathways. One pathway is to encourage the formation of multi-layered epithelial grafts, or so-called sheet grafts. A second pathway is the development of composite epidermal and dermal analogues.

33.5 Cultured epidermal autografts (CEA)

Due to its many disadvantages, the use of cultured epidermal skin equivalents from autologous keratinocytes (cultured epidermal autografts, CEA) is under discussion. It has been shown to require a longer hospital stay, a higher rate of necessary corrective operations due to scar contractures, and also incurs significantly higher costs compared to classical autologous split skin transplantation. The healing rate of CEA and the corresponding necessity of repeated transplantations varies considerably in the literature. At a healing rate which is sometimes less than 50%, it is below the healing rate of split skin transplants. Bacterial infections are considered to be the main cause. As a rule, applied cultured epidermal transplants consist of 3–5 cell layers, which can lead to problems in handling during and after transplantation. The transplants also show a lack of adherence and a tendency to form blisters, even months after transplantation, particularly under mechanical stress. It is observed especially in chronic wounds and severely burned patients with third-degree burns, lacking in dermal component. The junctional attachment structures are missing, without which increased blister formation occurs. Therefore the development of dermis substitute products or combination preparations of dermal analogues of different composition was therefore a goal and had clinically already been applied successfully.

Alternatively, surgical approaches were combined with keratinocyte culture to allow temporary covering of debrided wounds with allogenic or xenogenic skin to integrate dermal components. Due to the initial immunosuppressive component, these heal initially to allow time for the availability of CEA to be bridged. The allograft serves as protection against infection. After removal of the immunocompetent allo-epidermis, the remaining allo-dermis required as the attachment structure is covered with cultured epidermal transplants. In the treatment of severely burned patients, allografts are used for stable temporary wound coverage until donor areas for split skin are available again. The split skin can be expanded accordingly for this application.

33.6 Cell suspensions

As early as 1895, Mangoldt described scraping off of skin cell clusters from the forearm to make a suspension in an autologous wound serum with blood components. He administered them to wounds in order to close large wound areas. Mangoldt described how individual cells or cell clusters adhere better to the wound bed than pieces of skin. Injections into the wound bed containing the scraped cells suspended in serum were performed. However, due to the risk of epithelial cysts, it was not widely used.

Fibrin plays a crucial role in wound-healing and is also used to fix split skin grafts to the wound bed. Keratinocytes suspended in fibrin glue were a promising approach. In 1988, Hunyadi et al. reported the successful use of uncultured, trypsinised human keratinocytes suspended in a fibrin matrix in patients with a venous leg ulcer. Further working groups embraced this idea and were able to show reproducible healing of keratinocytes suspended in fibrin glue or fibrin gel. The keratinocyte-fibrin suspension is available after ten days. Compared to CEA, which is only available after three weeks, this method is available in a shorter period of time. It is evident that reepithelialisation could be achieved about one week after the application of keratinocytes suspended in fibrin to a wound surface. However, mechanical instability was also observed, similarly to CEA. The latter is achieved by transplantation of a meshed allogeneic skin graft onto the keratinocyte-fibrin bandage. Observation found that the initial healing of the allogeneic skin graft was similar to an autologous split skin graft, but that a rejection reaction took place after about two weeks.

The use of allogeneic cells, which can shorten the reepithelialisation time in superficial injuries, also plays a role in the treatment of severely burned patients. Even with third-degree burns, which are temporarily covered with a skin substitute, their use can lead to faster re-availability.

33.7 Cultured cells and biological or mixed synthetic-biological carriers

Mature, differentiated cells cannot continue to divide. Therefore, it is assumed that these cells cannot contribute to the reepithelialisation process. Instead, proliferating basal cells are required for wound closure as they are responsible for the initial reconstruction of the epithelium.

A concept developed from experimental and clinical studies to shorten the time required for the production of skin substitutes in the laboratory and to rapidly integrate the cultured epidermal cells into a natural medium. Experimentally and clinically, the combination of cultured autologous keratinocytes on alloplastic or mixed synthetic-biological carriers has been shown to be successful.

The cultured keratinocytes must be applied sustainably and evenly to a carrier substance to treat wounds of a larger surface, for which spray techniques were developed. The cultured cells could be distributed evenly over a large area using a fibrin matrix technique. The fact that the cultured keratinocytes survive this process has been demonstrated both experimentally and clinically. In 2000, Ronfard et al. succeeded in optimising the growth of cultured keratinocytes by applying the keratinocytes to a stabilised fibrin matrix. After sufficient proliferation on the fibrin matrix, the keratinocytes could then be transplanted together with the fibrin matrix onto the recipient. Thus it was possible to transfer keratinocytes simply and reliably.

The enzymatic detachment of the cultured keratinocytes from their culture dishes can be harmful to the cells and is regarded as the main reason for the sheets to not adhere to wound surfaces. Transplanting the dermal matrix to which the cultured keratinocytes have been applied would give a distinct advantage. It could avoid enzymatic treatment and provide a dermis replacement at the same time. Several groups have already investigated the production of dermal

33

regeneration matrices. In 1981, Yannas produced a skin equivalent by centrifugation of primarily trypsinised keratinocytes and fibroblasts into a collagen-glycosaminoglycan matrix (C-GAG), showing success in transplantation to guinea pigs. This approach was not successful due to the difficulty in production. Today, synthetic materials such as Biobrane® or Integra® are used clinically for the treatment of burn injuries which serve as temporary bandages and will be replaced after removal by the transplantation of thin split skin or CEA. Use in the context of third-degree burns is currently under discussion. Suprathel® is used for second-degree burns. It does not have to be removed from the wound bed again but detaches itself automatically during the reepithelialisation progresses (➤ Fig. 33.1, ➤ Fig. 33.2).

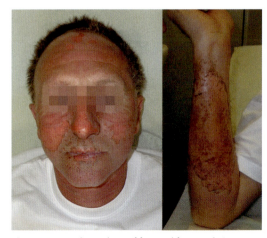

Fig. 33.1 A 2a degree burn of face and forearm during an explosion of a petrol drum. [P607]

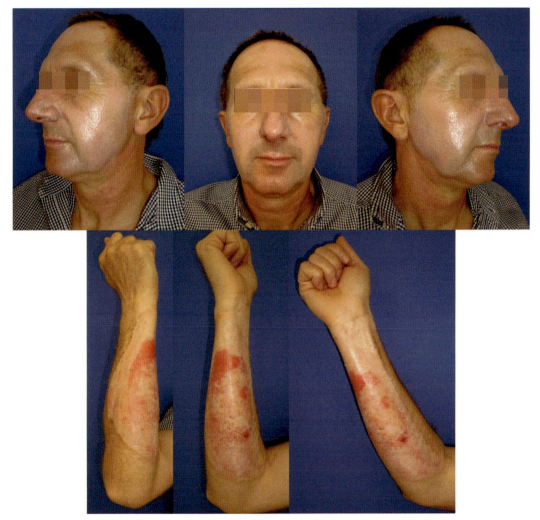

Fig. 33.2 Results 17 days after blister ablation and application of Suprathel® to face and forearm. [P607]

In recent years, the collagen elastin matrix Matriderm® has been used as a significant representative of the biological matrices. Matriderm® is used as a dermal substitute and can cover large areas. Colonisation with keratinocytes and fibroblasts as well as adipose-derived stromal cells (ADSC) could serve as a replacement for the epidermis, dermis and subcutis.

33.8 Outlook

In the future, tissue engineering will continue to play a decisive role in the field of skin substitutes for patients with different types of wounds. Another promising therapy is stem cell therapy. Human epidermal and mesenchymal stem cells are a promising option for the treatment of patients with burns or chronic wounds in the future. Growth factors and cytokines are also of great importance. These bioactive molecules, bound to a corresponding matrix, are to be released in a targeted sequence and concentration and thus have a positive influence on wound-healing.

In addition to further developments at the cellular level, technical developments can also contribute to the healing of skin substitute products. Negative pressure wound therapy is an option for the preparation of the wound bed and to fix temporary skin substitute products. Further developments in this area can contribute to a continuous improvement of the results. However, further progress is necessary both in basic research and in the clinical area to achieve a complete, functional replacement for split- or full-thickness skin transplantation with skin substitutes.

REFERENCES

Atiyeh BS, Costagliola M. Cultured epithelial autograft (CEA) in burn treatment: three decades later. Burns 2007; 33: 405–413.

Burd A, Ahmed K, Lam S, Ayyappan T, Huang L. Stem cell strategies in burns care. Burns 2007; 33: 282–291.

Horch RE, Kopp J, Kneser U, Beier J, Bach AD. Tissue engineering of cultured skin substitutes. J Cell Mol Med 2005; 9: 592–608.

Nguyen D Q, Potokar T S, Price P. An objective long-term evaluation of Integra (a dermal skin substitute) and split thickness skin grafts, in acute burns and reconstructive surgery. Burns 2010; 36: 23–28.

Ter Horst B, Chouhan G, Moiemen N S, Grover LM. Advances in keratinocyte delivery in burn wound care. Adv Drug Deliv Rev 2018; 123: 18–32.

Uhlig C, Rapp M, Hartmann B, Hierlemann H, Planck H, Dittel KK. Suprathel – an innovative, resorbable skin substitute for the treatment of burn victims. Burns 2007; 33: 221–229.

33

34 Systematics of drug therapy

Knut Kröger, Joachim Dissemond

──────── Key notes ────────

- In patients with chronic wounds caused by PAD, diabetes mellitus or CVI, the administration of acetylsalicylic acid (ASA) or low-molecular-weight heparin may be advisable on an experimental basis.
- In patients with chronic wounds and concomitant immunosuppression, the administration of a calcium antagonist may be advisable on a trial basis.
- There is currently no reason to discontinue certain drugs to promote wound-healing. Experimentally, ACE inhibitors can be replaced with calcium antagonists if the healing tendency is disturbed.
- A conversion of medicines should always take place in consultation with the family doctor or specialist.

34.1 Introduction

There is currently no sufficient scientific evidence that drugs effectively promote the healing of various chronic wounds. Drug therapy in the context of wound-healing is usually limited to antibiotic treatment of soft tissue infections. However, it can make sense to pause proliferation-inhibiting drugs such as chemotherapeutics, glucocorticoids and other immunosuppressive drugs until the desired wound-healing has been achieved if possible. Many elderly patients with multimorbidity take a variety of medications that are necessary from an intrinsic aspect, irrespective of the wound treatment. These include above all preparations that reduce the cardiovascular risk or drugs that alleviate the symptoms of chronic diseases of the cardiovascular system and the supporting apparatus. Antidiabetics have an indirect influence on wound-healing by improving glucose metabolism; however, there are not many studies about the effect of these drugs on wound-healing. Do antihypertensives or antiaggregants have a neutral impact on wound-healing or should some of these drugs be avoided, replaced or even explicitly used? The following will point out and discuss the effects of selected, widely used preparations on wound-healing.

34.2 Calcium channel blockers

Calcium channel blockers are synonymously referred to as calcium antagonists and are clinically used either as antihypertensives or antiarrhythmics. Research has used rats to test the effect of the calcium antagonists (i.e. nifedipine and amlodipine) on wound-healing. Two straight cuts were inflicted paravertebrally on them and the resilience of the scar was tested after ten days. The firmness of the wounds was significantly higher in animals treated with calcium antagonists than in animals without this drug. Contraction of the wound on the 4th and 16th postoperative day was also more pronounced. However, the epithelialisation phase was not affected. The authors concluded that calcium antagonists improve wound-healing and should be used in a particular group of patients who are undergoing glucocorticoid therapy. Better maturation and cross-linking of collagen fibres was found and discussed as the cause of the more stable wounds.

Another study analysed the effect of amlodipine on wound-healing in hares. They had their skin cut out in a 20 × 20 mm area of the back so that the subcutaneous fat tissue was exposed. They divided the animals into five groups of five animals each and, in addition to a dressing on the wound, received either no local treatment or, depending on the group, topical treatment with Eucerin 1%, with phenytoin 1% in

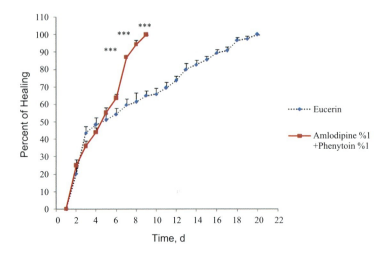

Fig. 34.1 The proportion of healed wounds as a function of time for the control group (no treatment) and the animals treated with Eucerin, amlodipine, phenytoin or with amlodipine and phenytoin (modified after Hemmati et al. 2014). [F1034-001]

Eucerin, with amlodipine 1% in Eucerin, or with amlodipine 1% and phenytoin 1% in Eucerin. All treatments were performed once a day until complete healing was achieved. ➤ Fig. 34.1 shows that wound-healing was significantly faster with the combination of amlodipine and phenytoin than with the comparative therapy with Eucerin, which had no effect.

34.3 Beta receptor blockers

Beta receptor blockers, which are synonymous with β blockers or beta-blockers, have a clinical indication for lowering blood pressure and regulating the heart rhythm. They are mainly used in wound-healing on patients with burns. In severely burnt patients, a pro-inflammatory stress reaction occurs after a few days. Cortisone and catecholamine levels rise and lead to a catabolic metabolism with reduction of muscle mass and disruption of wound-healing. The administration of β blockers can reduce the stress reaction. The exact mechanisms are unclear, but β blockers seem to stabilise muscle breakdown by increasing protein synthesis.

The keratinocytes, which are responsible for epithelialisation at the end of wound-healing, also have β receptors on their surface. These receptors seem to play a significant role in wound-healing, as disturbances in the function or number of these β receptors are found to be associated with several skin diseases. In a model

for the simulation of chronic wound-healing disorders of human skin, β blockers promote the migration of keratinocytes into the wound and accelerate re-epithelialisation.

34.4 Angiotensin-converting enzyme (ACE) inhibitors

Angiotensin II plays a role in inflammatory and fibrogenic processes throughout the body and accelerates wound-healing, among other things. It induces gene expression for collagen type I and influences the proliferation and migration of fibroblasts. Angiotensin-converting enzyme (ACE) inhibitors have an anti-fibrogenic effect.

In a study in 45 rats, they investigated the effect of ACE inhibitors on wound-healing after simulated small intestine surgery. The rats received either lisinopril in two different concentrations (50 and 5 mg/l, respectively) or placebo in drinking water for seven days postoperatively. On the 8th postoperative day, a relaparotomy was performed and inflated the intestine. The pressure required to burst the intestinal suture was measured and the result showed that lisinopril in the high dose hindered wound-healing. All the criteria of wound-healing such as the pressure at which the intestinal suture ruptured, tissue levels of hydroxyproline and collagen and epithelialisation were significantly worse than in the control group without lisinopril. The lower dose of lisinopril had no measurable negative effect on scar stability.

34.5 Antiaggregants, e. g. acetylsalicylic acid, clopidogrel

Antiaggregants such as acetylsalicylic acid (ASA) and clopidogrel inhibit the aggregation of platelets which plays a crucial role in the antiatherosclerotic therapy of patients with coronary heart disease (CHD), carotid stenosis or peripheral artery disease (PAD). Patients should take anti-aggregates in low doses for life to slow the progression of atherosclerosis.

There was a test in 1994 on the effect of ASA on the healing of chronic venous ulcers in a prospective placebo-controlled, double-blind, randomised study of 20 patients. These patients received either 300 mg ASA daily, or a placebo and standardised compression therapy. After four months, 38% of patients in the ASA group achieved ulcer-healing, but none in the placebo group. A total of 52% of patients in the ASA group showed a significant reduction in ulcer size, but only 26% in the placebo group. The ulcer size was significantly smaller in the ASA group after two and four months than in the placebo group.

Another study from 2012 confirms the effect. A total of 78 patients with venous leg ulcers with a diameter > 2 cm were randomised prospectively and either treated with 300 mg ASA or not. There was complete epithelialisation achieved in 21 (73%) of 28 patients with ASA and 17 (75%) of 23 patients in the control group. The mean healing time was significantly shorter with ASA. It was 12 weeks in the ASA group and 22 weeks in the control group.

34.6 Non-steroidal anti-inflammatory drugs, e. g. diclofenac, ibuprofen

The non-steroidal anti-inflammatory drug (NSAID) ibuprofen does not selectively inhibit cyclooxygenases

I and II, which are responsible for the formation of inflammatory prostaglandins in the body. Ibuprofen thus has analgesic, anti-inflammatory and antipyretic effects. Diclofenac is a non-selective inhibitor of cyclooxygenases with similar consequences.

There are no clinical studies that have directly investigated the effect of these drugs on wound-healing. However, there is a wound dressing that contains ibuprofen as a painkiller, intended to provide less painful wound care. In a randomised, double-blind study of 122 patients who received either the ibuprofen-containing dressing or an ibuprofen-free control dressing, wound-healing was neither improved nor delayed. In ophthalmology, NSAIDs were used to treat painful superficial corneal abrasion. An extensive analysis of several publications concludes that NSAIDs effectively relieve the pain without slowing the healing of the corneal injury.

34.7 Anticoagulants, e. g. heparins, vitamin K antagonists

The anticoagulant heparin influences the proliferation of the fibroblasts as well as the collagen formation via a change of the basal fibroblast growth factor (bFGF), as well as via the transforming growth factor beta 1 (TGF-β1) and thus modulates wound-healing. Thrombin additionally plays a central role in the initiation of wound-healing. Since all heparins act via the activation of antithrombin, they should also influence wound-healing via this mechanism; however, there are no useful clinical data on this topic so far. A meta-analysis of the influence of heparin on wound-healing after burns concludes that heparin has a beneficial effect on mortality, wound-healing and healing of skin grafts. However, the results are interpreted as incidental as the studies were not designed to analyse this question.

There is a randomised study for venous leg ulcers dating from 2015, in which a total of 284 patients were recruited over four years. All patients received optimal therapy and were randomised to either a control group or a therapy group. Over 12 months, the latter received nadroparin s. c. once daily, in addition to the standard 2,850 IU therapy. Wound-healing was measured plani-

34

Table 34.1 Development of ulcer size in 85 patients with diabetes mellitus and/or PAD who received either dalteparin or placebo at random. The absolute number is provided and the % shown in brackets

	Dalteparin n = 43	Placebo n = 42
Healed (intact skin)	14 (33)	9 (21)
Improved (reduction of ulcer size ≥ 50 %)	15 (35)	11 (26)
Unchanged (decrease in ulcer size < 50 %)	7 (16)	9 (21)
Worsened (increase in ulcer size ≥ 50 %)	5 (12)	5 (12)
Amputation	2 (5)	8 (19)

metrically. The nadroparin group showed a healing rate of 83.0% after 12 months, while the healing rate in the control group was 60.6%. Further analysis of the results by age group showed that the group of elderly patients benefited most from the long-term treatment with heparin. This group also had the lowest recurrence rate.

There was a prospective, randomised, double-blind study which investigated the effect of low molecular weight heparin dalteparin on the healing of chronic foot ulceration in 87 patients with diabetes mellitus and/or PAD. Patients received either a placebo or 5,000 IU of Dalteparin s.c. for six months or until complete ulcer-healing. The dalteparin group showed a significantly better course of the disease (➤ Table 34.1). A total of 29 patients in this group healed completely or achieved a reduction in ulcer size of at least 50%. There were only 20 patients in the control group. In both groups, five patients showed an increase in ulcer size. Amputation was necessary for two patients with dalteparin and in eight patients in the control group. Interestingly, the time to ulcer-healing showed no differences (17 ± 8 weeks vs. 16 ± 7 weeks).

The results are consistent with a Spanish triple-blind, randomised and placebo-controlled study. This study investigated the healing of foot lesions that existed for more than three months in patients who suffered from diabetes mellitus for at least three years. Patients received either 3,500 IU/day s.c. bemiparin for ten days in addition to standard therapy, followed by 2,500 IU/day for up to three months or placebo. The primary efficacy endpoint was the reduction of the ulcer size by ≥ 50% and/or a decrease by one degree in the Wagner classification. Ulcer size decreased in the bemiparin group in 70.3% (26 of 37 patients) and the placebo group in 45.5% (15 of 33 patients). The absolute difference was 24.8%. The proportion of completely healed ulcers after three months was similar in both groups, with 35.1% and 33.3%.

No comparable studies are available for vitamin K antagonists.

34.8 Doxycyclin

Chronic wounds, like many other chronic inflammatory processes, contain elevated concentrations of proinflammatory cytokines, such as tumour necrosis factor (TNF)-α and interleukin (IL)-1β, as well as matrix metalloproteinases (MMPs), which potentially impair wound-healing. In animal models and clinical studies in ulcer patients, doxycycline showed an inhibitory effect on MMPs and the TNF-α converting enzyme. A study of 64 patients with venous leg ulcers analysed the effect of low-dose oral doxycycline and ulcer-healing over 22 months. All patients received optimal standard therapy. A total of 32 patients received an additional 20 mg of doxycycline p.o. twice daily for three months, while the other 32 patients served as control groups. The planimetric evaluation of wound size showed a higher healing rate in the doxycycline group than in the control group. The MMP-9 content in wound exudate was lower in the doxycycline group than in the placebo group, and in the ulcers that healed rapidly (≥ 1 cm²/week), lower than in the ulcers that healed slowly (≥ 1 cm²/week). ➤ Fig. 34.2 shows the concentration of the vascular endothelial growth factor (VEGF) in the plasma level and wound exudate of both groups, depending on the healing process.

In 2012, ten patients each with chronic leg ulcers of different genesis were treated in Australia for four

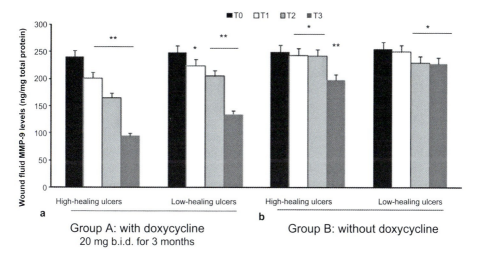

Fig. 34.2 Concentration of vascular endothelial growth factor (VEGF) in plasma (top) and wound exudate (bottom) in the ELISA test, both in the doxycycline group (A) and in the control group (B), depending on the rate of ulcer-healing. The results are provided. Mean ± SEM; T0 = study inclusion, T1 = 4 weeks, T2 = 3 months, T3 = 5 months, **p<0.01; *p<0.05 (taken from Serra et al. 2015). [F1035-001]

weeks with either 2 × 20 mg or 2 × 100 mg doxy-cycline p.o. in addition to their wound therapy. In the higher dose group, ulcers were reduced by 48%, and MMP-1 was reduced significantly in wound exudate. The group with the lower doxycycline dose does not show the same effect. In both groups, no effects were found on the concentrations of TNF-α or the number of bacteria in wound exudate.

Doxycycline has been successfully used for many years, locally or systemically, in the treatment of various diseases such as periodontitis, acne or rosacea. For example, the usual dosage is 2 × 100 mg/day. In recent years, successes with low doses such as 50 mg/day p.o. have been reported. Here, the immunomodulating effects are at the forefront, in particular the inhibition of MMPs, and less the antibiotic effects. The current data suggest that similar results can be expected in wound treatment. However, dose, duration of treatment, etc. have not yet been sufficiently investigated to recommend systematic use in patients with chronic wounds. Besides, the high contact-sensitising potential and the increasing development of bacterial resistance must be kept in mind, especially in topical applications.

34.9 Simvastatin

Simvastatin belongs to the group of statins and is mostly used therapeutically as a cholesterol-lowering agent. Approved indications include patients with serologically elevated LDL levels, acute coronary syndrome, unstable angina pectoris and myocardial infarction. Simvastatin inhibits HMG-CoA reductase, which otherwise acts as a catalyst in hepatic cholesterol synthesis. Simvastatin is additionally described as having antioxidative, anti-inflammatory and immunomodulatory effects, which can be of great importance for wound-healing.

Three groups of 36 rats each were all given a standardised skin wound and for 12 days received either a gel with 2% simvastatin, an identical gel without an active ingredient or no gel, but all received daily wound-cleansing with physiological saline solution. In the group treated with the simvastatin gel, there was a significantly faster wound closure of almost 100% compared to the group treated with the gel without the active ingredient (65%) and the control group (55%). These results were confirmed in the histopathological examinations, which investigated the following parameters: inflammation, fibroblast proliferation and vascularisation.

In a mouse model, the topical application of simvastatin (62.5 µg/ml in 0.5% DMSO) was shown to also make skin wounds, which had previously been treated with *Staphylococcus aureus*, heal faster than in the controls (0,5% DMSO in PBS). As potentially relevant effects, it could be shown here that simvastatin acts bacteriostatically as well as inhibiting the biofilm formation of *Staphylococcus aureus*.

In a randomised, double-blind clinical study, 66 patients with a chronic venous leg ulcer were investigated. In addition to standard treatment with modern wound care and compression therapy, 32 patients received systemic 40 mg/day simvastatin. In the group of patients with ulcerations ≤ 5 cm, 100% healed in the simvastatin group and 50% in the control group after an average of 7–8 weeks. In the group of patients with ulcerations > 5 cm, the simvastatin group was found to have healing rates of 67% after an average of nine weeks, with 0% in the control group. The authors were also able to correlate the improvement in wound-healing with an increase in quality of life measured by DLQI. Within this study, it was documented that simvastatin therapy had no relevant side effects.

Although these first, awe-inspiring results motivated an off-label use of simvastatin in wound treatment, some aspects have to be considered, especially in systemic therapy with this drug. Simvastatin is metabolised via cytochrome P450 3A4. This degradation pathway can be inhibited, for example, by taking ketoconazole, itraconazole, clarithromycin or grapefruit juice, which increases the risk of side effects. Toxic myopathies and rhabdomyolysis are feared as complications, besides various rather harmless side effects such as head or gastrointestinal complaints. Future scientific studies will be necessary to weigh up the usage of this drug across the board for patients with chronic wounds.

34.10 Conclusion

The systematic literature search shows how scant our current knowledge is about the effect of systemic therapies of various diseases on wound-healing. However, we then find that the influence of individual drugs on wound-healing is not entirely unexplored. If there is a continuation on this research, drug therapy could play an essential role in the future in addition to optimised local treatment and make it possible, for example, to control the collagen content or epithelialisation explicitly.

In addition, demand for future studies on wound-healing should always include careful documentation of all drugs, despite it not being directly related to wound-healing. This comedication could significantly influence the results of the studies.

REFERENCES

de Oliveira Carvalho PE, Magolbo NG, De Aquino RF, Weller CD. Oral aspirin for treating venous leg ulcers. Cochrane Database Syst Rev 2016; 18; 2: CD009432.

Dissemond J, Erfurt-Berge C, Goerge T, et al. Systemic therapies for leg ulcers. J Dtsch Dermatol Ges 2018; 16: 873–890.

Evangelista MT, Casintahan MF, Villafuerte LL. Simvastatin as a novel therapeutic agent for venous ulcers: a randomized, double-blind, placebo-controlled trial. Br J Dermatol 2014; 170: 1151–1157.

Hemmati AA, Mojiri Forushani H, Mohammad Asgari H. Wound-healing potential of topical amlodipine in full thickness wound of rabbit. Jundishapur J Nat Pharm Prod 2014; 9: 15638.

Serra R, Buffone G, Molinari V, et al. Low molecular weight heparin improves healing of chronic venous ulcers especially in the elderly. Int Wound J 2015; 12: 150–153.

Xu DH, Zhu Z, Fang Y. The effect of a common antibiotics doxycycline on non-healing chronic wound. Curr Pharm Biotechnol 2017; 18: 360–364.

35

Christian Münter

Special aspects of palliative medicine

Key notes

- In palliative medicine, quality of life comes before healing.
- 'Professional proximity' is better than 'professional distance'.

- Tumour-associated wounds and pressure ulcers are of particular importance in palliative medicine.
- The symptom-oriented treatment also includes unconventional methods in palliative medicine.

35.1 Introduction

The main goal of palliative medicine is to improve and maintain the subjectively perceived quality of life of the patients through comprehensive symptom relief so that patients can experience the most significant possible autonomy and dignity in their remaining time of life. Wound treatment is secondary to this goal. At the end of life, the curative goal – the healing of the wound – is no longer at the forefront. Instead, it is the symptoms of the non-healing wounds which frequently have a considerable impact on the patients and which often become very important due to their severity. They often represent the worst part of the suffering for those affected.

Of course, all types of chronic wounds can also occur in palliative medicine. In the palliative situation, venous ulcers or diabetic foot ulcers are treated according to the same principles as usual and avoid extensive surgical interventions if possible. Two entities have special significance in palliative medicine: tumour-associated wounds and pressure ulcers (➤ Fig. 35.1). Patients, relatives and health care professionals are confronted with the following problems in particular:

- Aches
- Odour
- Exudate
- Infection
- Bleedings
- Skincare

There are also psychological problems caused by the impairment of one's body image. Disfiguring wounds and inadequate unsightly dressings undermine self-

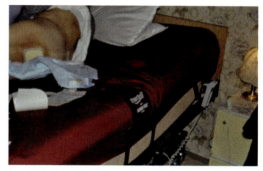

Fig. 35.1 Palliative patient with several pressure ulcers treated in a domestic environment. [P608]

confidence and are an obstacle to communication with the family and carers.

35.2 Situation of the health care professionals

The wound health care professionals (medical and nursing wound experts) must be aware of the unique situation in which they find themselves, together with the affected patients. Usually, the primary goals of wound treatment, such as reducing the wound area, cleaning the wound bed or reducing the wound depth, lose their significance in the palliative situation. Time-consuming attention to the patient in listening carefully and evaluating the patient's urgent needs are at the forefront. As justifiable as it is to monitor the profitability and efficiency of one's actions in a palliative situation, it is unacceptable to consider questions about the value of life and dignity, based on a cost-benefit analysis. Two-thirds of the hospital budget for statutory health insurance funds have been allocated to the care of people in their last year of life. This figure points to the need for the responsible use of social resources but does not serve as an appeal to make savings.

The often close contact with the dying person undoubtedly represents an enormous burden for the health care professionals. It is crucial to become aware of one's fears and feelings and to reflect on them regularly. Communication within the treatment team is indispensable. The psychological problems that can occur in the course of a – sometimes long – phase of being attended to by the therapist should be addressed openly. They are not an expression of weakness, but often evidence of empathy and reflection.

Death does not reflect the defeat and failure of medical efforts, but is the natural end of every life which can also be managed, while still prevailing in an otherwise 'healing-oriented' situation. The 'medicalisation' of dying focuses mainly on the extensive and intensive use of treatment; however, there is an inadequate level of humane attention to the patient. In reality, the shortage of staff means that medical professionals distance themselves from the suffering of those affected. However, the concept of 'professional distance' should give way to that of 'professional proximity', especially in palliative care. Given the existential experience of dying, allowing a connection or an attachment is acceptable. The emotions of practitioners are acknowledged, and they should be given the support they need. The practitioners can thus develop compassion for their patients without identifying with them.

The four general principles of action formulated in 1994 focus on the dying person:

- Beneficence: promoting the well-being of the patient
- Nonmaleficence: avoid damage to the patient
- Justice: Distribute existing resources fairly
- Autonomy: respecting the right of the dying to autonomy

Tumour-associated wounds

Tumour-associated wounds include primary skin tumours, metastases and tumours due to the longer

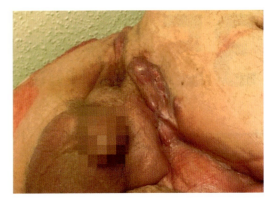

Fig. 35.2 Anal carcinoma metastasised to the groin. [P608]

existing wounds of another genesis. Relevant skin tumours include basal cell carcinomas, squamous cell carcinomas and malignant melanomas. All malignant tumours can develop skin metastases. The most common primary tumours are breast cancer and soft tissue sarcoma. Ovarian, caecum and rectal tumours also frequently metastasise into the abdominal wall area (➤ Fig. 35.2).

Tumours and wounds can develop as the number of malignant cells increases from small skin nodules. Tumour growth can damage the surrounding capillaries and lymph vessels, causing bleeding. The inferior tumour tissue itself cannot stop bleeding normally, but it does have very fragile capillaries, so even light contact can lead to bleeding. Anaerobes colonise necrotic tissue and produce fatty acids as metabolic end products. These acids contribute to the pungent and penetrating odour of wounds.

Every tenth person suffering from a metastatic disease develops skin metastases. The symptoms range from complete freedom from symptoms to itching and massive pain. The surrounding skin can thicken and harden.

35.3 Non-malignant wounds in palliative medicine

The most frequent non-malignant wounds in palliative medicine are pressure ulcers, in which chemical-toxic stimuli such as faeces or urine (incontinence-associated dermatitis) in the wound environment can also lead to a deterioration of the overall situation of the patient. The frequency of pressure ulcers varies greatly. A study conducted over two years in 2002 found pressure ulcers in 26.1% of patients admitted to a palliative care unit. During the study period, 12% also developed pressure sores during their stay. A total of 78.1% of pressure ulcers are found in the sacral area. A regular risk assessment is essential, given the speed at which skin changes can occur at the end of life. Palliative patients should classify as high-risk patients (➤ Chap. 13). Preventive measures naturally have a high priority here, but find their limits in palliative medicine, which is inclined towards the greatest possible comfort of the patient.

It is the role of the treating physician to provide complete information about realistic therapy options in a way that is easy to understand in their discussion with patients and their relatives and to determine the priority goal.

Important aspects here are:

- Pressure relief with adequate documentation, the selection of which depends on the patient's wishes
- Adapted pain therapy, e. g. international guidelines recommend the administration of pain medications 20–30 minutes before repositioning measures are taken
- Incontinence management (e. g. anal tampons, incontinence pants, etc.)

The discussion as to whether all pressure ulcers are avoidable in palliative medicine with good standard-compliant therapy is not over. In the phase shortly before death, the risk of pressure ulcers increases considerably, probably caused by reduced perfusion of the skin. On the other hand, healing rates of 50% with adequate wound therapy are also reported in the palliative situation, so that there is no justification for therapeutic or prophylactic nihilism.

35.4 Pain

In general, there is a distinction between neuropathic and nociceptive pain.

Neuropathic pain occurs when parts of the peripheral or central nervous system are directly damaged or irritated. An example in palliative medicine is pain caused by infiltrating tumours.

Neuropathic pain (burning, sharp, shooting) can lead to increased or decreased minus symptoms in the supply area of the affected nerves. **Increased symptoms include** allodynia, in which pain is triggered by an inadequate stimulus (touch), hyperesthesia (hypersensitivity) and hyperalgesia (increased sensitivity to pain). **Decreased symptoms** are hypaesthesia, hypalgesia, pallhypaesthesia (reduction of vibration sensation) and thermhypaesthesia.

Nociceptive pain is caused by the activation of nerve endings (nociceptors). Overacidification of the tissue leads to the release of messenger substances (e. g. bradykinin, prostaglandin). Afferent nerve pathways lead the impulses to the somatosensory cortex. Nociceptive pain is divided into somatic (easy to localise, penetrating, sharp) and visceral (difficult to localise, colicky, oppressive) pain.

Mixed pain is a combination of neuropathic and nociceptive pain caused by injury to both nerves and soft tissues in a wound.

The WHO grading scheme is a guide for the treatment of pain in palliative medicine. However, there are some unique features to consider. For example, the use of paracetamol is already problematic at the first stage if there is a poor nutritional condition or cachexia. Breaking down of paracetamol is mainly in the liver. Among others, it forms the highly reactive and hepatotoxic metabolite N-acetyl-p-benzoquinoneimine. It is inactivated by conjugation with glutathione. A glutathione deficiency thus leads to an increase in the metabolite.

About 40–80% of patients with tumour pain suffer from breakthrough pain. These is 'a transitory increase in pain that occurs against a background of constant pain that is otherwise adequately controlled by 24-hour opioid therapy'.

The EAPC (European Association for Palliative Care) recommends the timely administration of a non-retarded, fast-acting and short-acting opioid as a breakthrough medication in addition to the primary opioid medication. Morphine, hydromorphone and oxycodone are available in the non-retarded form. Their effect starts after 20–30 minutes and lasts for about four hours. Fentanyl is available as a nasal spray, and a sublingual and buccal tablet. The effect occurs after 7–20 minutes, and the effect lasts about 60–90 minutes.

Cannabinoids may be prescribed as a finished medicinal product, cannabis extract and dronabinol not approved as finished medicinal products, as well as cannabis flowers. Many patients with pain and their relatives have high hopes for this therapy after the massive media attention focusing on the permitted use of cannabis. However, there is not yet sufficient evidence for its use, and no recommendations are currently available for its use in palliative care.

Co-analgesics can complement and occasionally replace the effects of pain therapy.

In particular, the use of co-analgesics in:

- Anticonvulsants, e. g. gabapentin, pregabalin, carbamazepine, clonazepam
- Antidepressants
- Tricyclic antidepressants, such as doxepin, amitryptiline, clomipramine
- Serotonin reuptake inhibitors such as venlafaxine, duloxetine
- Mirtazapine
- Corticosteroids
- Muscle relaxants
- Bisphosphonates
- Spasmolytics
- Local anaesthetics

Co-analgesics can be used to supplement any level of the WHO scheme, but the sole administration is rarely useful.

A particular problem in wound treatment is the pain that occurs when a dressing is changed. Therefore, it makes sense to use non-adhesive dressings and advanced wound products which require minimal dressing change frequency. Scheduling of the dressing changes should be precise so that the administration of pain prophylaxis is possible. For example, administration of 40 drops of novaminsulfone approximately 40 minutes before the dressing change is usual. If this is not sufficient, there is a recommendation in the use of non-retarded opioids, as above-mentioned.

EMLA® cream is available for the local treatment of pain, e. g. during debridement. It contains 25 mg/g lidocaine and 25 mg/g prilocaine and should be applied at least 45 minutes before the planned procedure and covered with a film to be more effective.

Nociceptive pain responds well to non-steroidal anti-inflammatory drugs (NSAIDs), particularly.

35.5 Odour

A strong wound odour is very offensive to the patients, relatives and health care professionals, and presents a nursing and medical challenge. Since the odour cannot be measured objectively, the subjective impression of the patient is decisive here.

Possible treatment measures for unpleasant odours are:

- Thorough wound cleansing
- Debridement
- Deodorising agents (on the wound, air of the room)
- Antiseptics
- Wound dressings with activated carbon

In a systematic literature review, evidence level B was found on the grade scale for metronidazole, gauze with physiological saline solution, activated carbon and turmeric solution (ginger). For example clindamycin vaginal cream can be locally applied (warning: off label).

Irrespective of the antibiogram-resistogram, clindamycin or metronidazole have a systemic odour-reducing effect. This effect can be expected within two days for clindamycin and 4–5 days for metronidazole. Antibiotic doses typical for clindamycin are initially indicated, but with regard to the clinical effect during the rest of the course, the dose can often be reduced considerably, e. g. to 200 mg clindamycin twice a day.

Recommendations for local therapy which clinicians can try, are manuka honey, green tea, hydrogels and chlorophyll.

35.6 Exudate management

Increased capillary permeability, especially in tumour-associated wounds, and autolysis of the necrotic tissue by proteases are causes of increased exudate secretion. Periwound tissue is often edematous, so that even small wounds can produce considerable amounts of exudate.

Therapeutic measures of local therapy are:

- Topical antiseptics
- Absorbent dressings, e. g. superabsorbers

• Recording devices, e. g. stoma bags

The frequency of dressing changes depends on the degree of saturation of the dressings. Taking into account the palliative situation of the patients, one dressing change per day should be sufficient. Applying a stoma bag should be considered if one change of dressing a day is not sufficient due to a large amount of exudate. Attempts to absorb large amounts of exudate with the aid of vacuum therapy were promising for non-malignant wounds. In tumour-associated wounds, the risk of stimulating tumour growth with the use of vacuum therapy must be considered and discussed.

35.7 Infection management

As a rule, patients approaching the end of their lives only have reduced defences against pathogens. In the area of the skin, it is mainly bacteria and fungi that can lead to infections. Here, too, prophylaxis is of the utmost importance. Careful cleaning of the wounds at each dressing change should remove pathogens from the wound surface before they become adherent. If there are signs of a local infection (➤ Chap. 25), active antimicrobial substances such as octenidine, polihexanide, PVP iodine or silver should be used. Aggressive surgical debridement should only be performed under adequate pain therapy and is problematic due to the increased risk of bleeding (➤ Fig. 35.3).

In the palliative situation, there must be a strict indication for the use of systemic antibiotics. Expected benefits must be weighed up against possible side effects such as diarrhoea. The patient and their relatives should be involved in this decision.

35.8 Bleeding

The fragility of the capillaries can lead to spontaneous bleeding or to bleeding even after slight mechanical irritation. Atraumatic dressing changes are of particular importance. Non-adhesive wound dressings and spacers can minimise the traumatisation of the wound surface during dressing changes. Various wound dressings show haemostatic effects; e. g. alginates or pressure dressings with cool packs can bring bleeding to a standstill. In emergencies, topical adrenaline is applied in a dilution of 1:1,000. However, as serious local and systemic side effects may occur, only experienced centres should use this. Local nasal drops may be helpful for minor bleeding (warning: off label). Sucralfate has a good local haemostatic effect with and without subsequent compression in small to moderate bleeding, and without subsequent hyperemia. The suspension can remain on the wound surface. It also develops antipruritic efficacy (warning: off label). Oxidised regenerated cellulose and collagen wound dressings are further alternatives. If there is a risk of prolonged bleeding, discussions should take place in advance with the patient and any remaining therapeutic options should be clarified. In the case of (pre-)terminal bleeding, dark terry towels (to disguise the colour of the blood) should be used to cover the source of the bleeding, for psychological reasons.

35.9 Skincare

The wounds in palliative patients tend to maceration and develop eczema in the skin surrounding the wounds. An irritation-free, transparent skinprotection film, e. g. based on acrylate copolymer, has proved to be a good choice. The skin protection can last up to three days. Water-based moisturising products should be used to care for dry skin. They also increase the moisture level of the skin. Urea is used in the care of

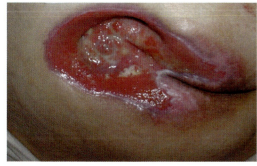

Fig. 35.3 Patient with a pressure ulcer after surgical debridement. [P608]

35

very dry skin and hyperkeratoses. Dexpanthenol, as well as silicone preparations, are often used for scar care.

35.10 Conclusion

Palliative medicine is medicine administered from a certain perspective. When healing is no longer the goal, symptomatic measures gain in importance. Implementing these expertly determines the patient's quality of life at the end.

REFERENCES

Aulbert E, Nauck F, Radbruch L (eds.). Lehrbuch der Palliativmedizin. Stuttgart: Schattauer; 2000.

Leitlinienprogramm Onkologie (Deutsche Krebsgesellschaft, Deutsche Krebshilfe, AWMF). S3-Leitlinie Palliativmedizin für Patienten mit einer nicht heilbaren Krebserkrankung. AWMF Register-Nummer: 128/001OL. http://leitlinien-programmonkologie.de/Palliativmedizin.80.0.html (last accessed 12 October 2020).

Haesler E (ed.); National Pressure Ulcer Advisory Panel, European Pressure Ulcer Advisory Panel and Pan Pacific Pressure Injury Alliance. Prevention and Treatment of Pressure Ulcers: Quick Reference Guide. Perth, Australia: Cambridge Media; 2014. www.npuap.org/wp-content/uploads/2014/08/Updated-10-16-14-Quick-Reference-Guide-DIGITAL-NPUAP-EPUAP-PPPIA-16Oct2014.pdf (last accessed 12 October 2020).

Ostgathe C, Rolke R (Hrsg.). Palliativmedizin. 2nd ed. Stuttgart: Thieme; 2018.

Panfil EM, Schröder G. Pflege von Menschen mit chronischen Wunden. Bern: Hans Huber; 2009.

36 Wound therapy for split skin grafts

Philipp Jansen, Joachim Dissemond

─────── Key notes ───────

- There are currently no guidelines on the care of split skin grafts and care of the donor sites.
- The donor area is usually the thigh, alternatively the capillitium.
- Currently, postoperative treatment of the donor site commonly uses foam dressings or impregnated gauze.
- Alginates and films are cost-effective alternatives.
- Alginates, in particular, can be left on the donor site until complete reepithelialisation. Secondary dressings can be changed if necessary.

36.1 Introduction

For the surgical treatment of primary non-closable or chronic non-healing wounds, an autologous split skin graft can be carried out following adequate wound bed preparation. Split skin grafts have been an established surgical procedure in various medical fields for many decades. Nevertheless, there are no guidelines on the care of split skin grafts and care of the donor sites. Various institutions therefore carry out practices according to their individual preferences and the practical experience of the experts involved.

36.2 Properties of split skin

Split skin grafts consist mostly of the epidermis as well as possible superficial parts of the dermis. Depending on the requirements of the recipient site, split skin grafts are taken with a thickness between 0.2 and 0.8 mm. Since the nutritive supply of a split skin graft takes place through diffusion, the recipient site must be healthy and sufficiently vascularised. Thinner split skin grafts adhere better to the wound; however, they are more susceptible to mechanical shearing forces. On the other hand, thicker split skin grafts tend to shrink in the course of wound-healing, and the resulting aesthetical concerns contradict the extensive use of split

skin on exposed body areas. For this reason, full skin grafts are preferred for areas such as the face.

Donor areas will need to resemble the recipient areas in structure and pigmentation. Since hypopigmentation of the donor site often occurs after removal of split skin, less exposed parts of the body normally covered by clothing are preferred, e.g. the thighs. An exception to this is the removal of split skin from the capillitium. The hair follicles deep in the dermis are not destroyed by the removal of split skin and hair can grow back and cover the removal site at the capillitium. Due to its exceptional vascularity, reepithelialisation at the capillitium will take place within a few days, and another split skin graft is possible shortly after complete healing of the donor site.

36.3 Practical implementation

The donor region is infused by injection with a local anaesthetic and can be sprayed with a silicone spray immediately before grafting to ensure smoother gliding of the dermatome. With the help of an electrodermatome, it is possible to remove parts of the skin evenly with a defined thickness and a variable width. Immediately after removal of the split skin, opening up the superficial vessels of the dermis usually leads to patchy bleeding.

A mesh device can enlarge the split skin from 1:1.5 to 1:3 for the treatment of chronic wounds. The result is a mesh skin graft. The split skin graft can also be enlarged by up to 1:6, particularly in the case of extensive burns. In most patients with chronic wounds, the mesh technique not only increases the surface area but also improves exudate and blood flow. With conventional split skin grafting, several stab incisions are made to enable exudate drainage. Otherwise, the graft transplant may fail.

Debridement on the recipient site must take place before the split skin graft to ensure induction of pinpoint bleeding. Consideration of a two-stage surgical procedure in the case of an extensive wound bed can minimise any differences in the tissue levels in the recipient area by promoting granulation postoperatively when preparing the wound bed. In principle, split skin grafts can however also be applied directly to deeper structures up to the muscles, after debridement or shave excision. Sutures, staple sutures and/or fibrin adhesive are used to anchor split skin grafts to the recipient sites, with an additional pressure dressing fixed onto the split skin for five days with a bolster technique. This guarantees sufficient contact between the split skin and the wound bed for adherence and growth, and prevents the formation of haematomas. Alternatively, adherence can take place with negative pressure wound therapy (NPWT) for 3–6 days with a negative pressure of 75–125 mmHg. A closed-pore polyvinyl alcohol (PVA) or an open-pore polyurethane (PU) foam with non-adhesive gauze must be applied directly to the split skin graft before the application of NPWT.

36.4 Postoperative wound care of the split skin donor site

The average time to complete postoperative re-epithelialisation of the split skin donor site is 14–21 days. Several factors which have significant influence on complete postoperative reepithelialisation includes the anatomical areas, the thickness of the split skin, the wound products used and the frequency of dressing changes. The grafting of a thin split skin causes a more superficial wound, which reepithelialises more quickly.

Likewise, increased capillarisation at the capillitium promotes faster reepithelialisation. Choosing a suitable wound dressing speeds up healing as it supports the reepithelialisation of the donor area by keeping the wound surface 'moist', and simultaneously maintaining drainage of the exudate. Bacterial superinfections as well as pain should be prevented, keeping costs low.

In German clinics, foam dressings and surgical gauze bandages are the materials most frequently used for postoperative treatment of the donor sites. These both help to keep donor sites moist in order to accelerate reepithelialisation. Alginates, hydrocolloids and films are also suitable for postoperative treatment of the split skin donor sites. In particular, alginates can absorb wound secretion or pass it on to a secondary dressing. An example of a wound dressing that is obsolete today is open-pored foams, as granulation tissue can grow into the wound dressings. Repetitive microtraumas can occur as a result of wound dressing changes, impeding reepithelialisation and causing avoidable pain.

There is no specific advice for any of the wound products on how often they need to be changed. The practice is therefore to change wound dressings daily until complete reepithelialisation of the primary wound. Especially alginates can be left on the split skin graft site until they drop off independently with complete reepithelialisation, with just the protective secondary dressing, which absorbs wound exudate, needing to be changed. Numerous clinical studies show the advantages of individual procedures (➤ Fig. 36.1).

Collectively, there is insufficient evidence for split skin graft adhesion recommendations. The choice of wound products used at the site of split skin removal will depend on the clinician's preference. Routine prophylactic disinfection of the wound is not necessary for any of the procedures. However, minimal dressing changes and interventions are beneficial for maintaining a moist wound environment to facilitate epithelialisation of split skin donor sites.

36.5 Conclusion

Currently, treatment of split skin donor sites involves a large number of wound care products, treatment strategies and dressing change intervals, the ap-

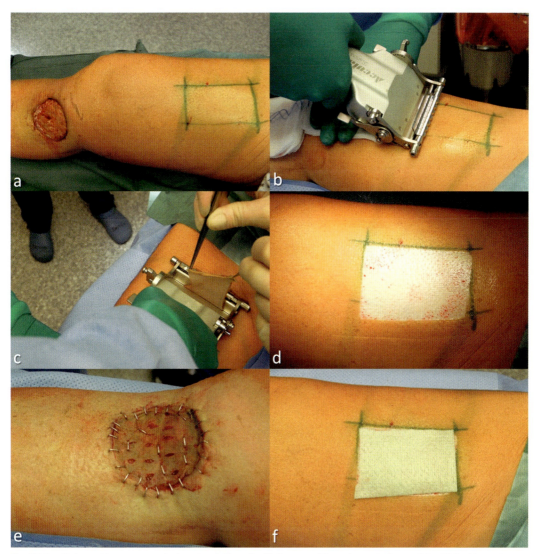

Fig. 36.1 a Patient with a postoperative leg ulcer. **b** The split skin is removed from the marked area of the thigh with an electro-dermatome. **c** The split skin removed here is 0.4 mm thick. **d** Postoperative presentation after split skin removal. **e** The split skin was applied to the ulcer and surgically fixed. **f** The split skin donor site is covered intraoperatively with an alginate dressing. This dressing remains directly on the wound until complete healing is achieved. The secondary dressing can be changed if necessary. [P580]

plication of which depends on individuals' preference and experience. Besides foam dressings and surgical gauzes, alginates are the commonly preferred choice as they can stay on the wound bed until complete re-epithelialisation of the split skin donor site.

REFERENCES

Ablove RH, Howell RM. The physiology and technique of skin grafting. Hand Clin 1997; 13: 163–173.

Geary PM, Tiernan E. Management of split skin graft donor sites – results of a national survey. J Plast Reconstr Aesthet Surg 2009; 62: 1677–1683.

Jansen P, Stoffels I, Klode J, et al. Postsurgical treatment of split skin graft donor sites in dermatological departments. Int J Low Extrem Wounds 2018; 17: 22–29.

Lyall PW, Sinclair SW. Australasian survey of split skin graft donor site dressings. Aust N Z J Surg 2000; 70: 114–116.

Ratner D. Skin grafting. Semin Cutan Med Surg 2003; 22: 295–305.

V

Prophylactic measures

37

Joachim Dissemond

Periwound skin

Key notes

- Changes in the periwound skin can indicate complications such as allergies or infections.
- Changes in the periwound skin can provide information on the cause(s) of the delay in wound-healing.
- Skin changes should be diagnosed, documented and treated in a differentiated manner.
- It is often sensible to obtain a dermatological co-evaluation on periwound skin changes.

37.1 Introduction

The skin has an approx. 2 m² surface area, and is the largest very complex organ of the human body. It is easily accessible for clinical inspection (➤ Fig. 37.1). Skin changes observed in a patient's periwound skin provides essential information on the wound conditions and/or the effectiveness of the current therapy. It is therefore necessary to assess and document the periwound skin condition adequately during the wound inspection and to include it in the treatment planning. Since the recognition and classification, as well as the treatment of skin changes, are often very difficult, a dermatological assessment should be included in the multidisciplinary management.

37.2 Symptoms

Some of the symptoms observed on the periwound skin are presented, described and explained with examples of wound treatment in ➤ Table 37.1.

37.3 Conclusion

In many patients with chronic wounds, there are skin changes in the periwound skin. These skin changes can give an indication of complications, inappropriate therapies and the underlying cause(s) of chronic wounds. Documentation, diagnosis and treatment of these skin changes are therefore necessary.

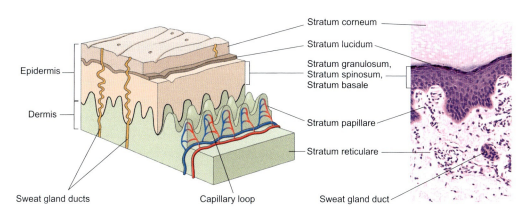

Fig. 37.1 Schematic structure of the skin. [L190/E645]

Table 37.1 Clinical presentations of the periwound skin, description and clinical examples

Clinical presentations	Description	Clinical examples
Erosion (abrasive wound)	Tissue defect that affects only the epidermis and heals scar-free	• Superficial trauma • Ruptured blister
Ulcer	Tissue defect that reaches at least into the dermis and heals with inevitable scarring	Almost any chronic wound
Bulla (blister, > 5 mm) Vesicle (blister, ≤ 5 mm)	Cavity raised above skin level and filled with liquid	• Pronounced oedema • Burning, frostbite • Blistering autoimmune dermatosis
Erythema (redness)	Occurs when there is increased blood circulation or dilation of skin vessels	• Inflammation • Infection • Hypodermitis (CVI)
Eczema (dermatitis)	Non-infectious inflammation of the skin	• Allergic contact dermatitis • Toxic contact dermatitis • Asteatotic eczema • Atopic dermatitis
Purpura (bleeding into the skin)	Multiple small spots of capillary bleeding under the skin	• Vasculitis • Haemorrhagic diathesis • Orthostatic purpura (CVI)
Squama (scale)	Parts of the stratum corneum detaching from the surface of the skin	• Tinea (mycosis) • Xerosis cutis (dry skin)
Hyperkeratosis	Thickened stratum corneum	• Areas subject to mechanical stress, e.g. DFS (often) • Squamous cell carcinoma (rare)
Maceration	Softening of the upper skin layers	Inadequate exudate management
Fissure	Mostly painful skin cracks	Areas subject to mechanical stress, hyperkeratosis
Excoriation	A substance defect of the skin that reaches at least into the dermis	• Trauma • Disease patterns with pruritus (itching), e.g. eczema, xerosis cutis, scabies
Pustule	Blisters filled with pus • Sterile: rare • Non-sterile: frequent	• Sterile: e.g. pyoderma gangrenosum, psoriasis pustulosa, Behcet's disease. • Non-sterile: mostly bacterial infection; less common in mycoses, e.g. candida intertrigo
Scar (cicatrix)	Irreversible replacement of connective tissue with the loss of deep tissue (ulcer)	• Healed trauma • Healed ulcer
Poikiloderma	Changes in the skin: • Atrophy • Erythema • Telangiectasias • Hyper- and depigmentation	• Primary (very rare): e.g. in progeroid syndromes (Rothmund-Thomson, Werner) • Secondary (rare): in chronic inflammatory dermatoses, e.g. dermatomyositis, mycosis fungoides, graft-versus-host
Skin tear	Extensive shearing of the skin from the underlying tissue	Trauma
Livedo	Usually symmetrical, lace-like, livid reddish skin pattern due to a focal slow-down of capillary blood flow	• Livedo reticularis (often): harmless skin change that disappears entirely after warming; especially on the inside of the thighs • Livedo racemosa (rare): persistent vascular pattern, e.g. in collagenosis, vasculitis

Table 37.1 Clinical presentations of the periwound skin, description and clinical examples *(cont'd)*

Clinical presentations	Description	Clinical examples
Crust (scab)	Dried liquid	• Dried wound exudate, blood, pus • Acute eczema
Atrophy	Acquired irreversible tissue degeneration	• Physiological age-related atrophy • Chronic steroid use • Vasculopathy → atrophie blanche • Chronic inflammatory reaction, e.g. necrobiosis lipoidica
Sclerosis	Hardening of tissue through multiplication of connective tissue	• Chronic inflammation, e.g. dermatoliposclerosis (CVI) • Collagenosis, e.g. scleroderma
Telangiectasia	Irreversibly dilated capillary vessels of the skin	• Collagenosis, e.g. CREST • Chronic sun damage • Neoplasia, e.g. basal cell carcinoma
Hyperpigmentation	Increased skin pigmentation	• Post-inflammation • Purpura, e.g. CVI
Hypopigmentation	Reduced pigmentation of the skin	• Atrophie blanche • Vitiligo • Scars

37

REFERENCES

Dissemond J, Körber A, Grabbe S. Differential diagnoses in leg ulcers. J Dtsch Dermatol Ges 2006; 4: 627–634.

Dissemond J. Blickdiagnose chronischer Wunden: Über die klinische Inspektion zur Diagnose. Köln: Viavital-Verlag; 2020.

Körber A, Dissemond J. Diagnostik und Therapie von Wundrandveränderungen bei Patienten mit Ulcus cruris. Pflege Z 2006; 5: 282–285.

Körber A, Dissemond J. Die Wundumgebung – Diagnostik und Therapie von pathologischen Veränderungen. Wundforum 2007; 1: 10–11.

Powers JG, Higham C, Broussard K, Phillips TJ. Woundhealing and treating wounds: Chronic wound care and management. J Am Acad Dermatol 2016; 74: 607–625.

38 Skincare

Johannes Wohlrab

Johannes Wohlrab

Key notes

- Periwound skin is exposed to many risk factors.
- Prophylactic measures should be used to protect the epidermal barrier.

- Identification and management of individual causal factors are required when periwound skin breaks down.

38.1 Introduction

Periwound skin surrounding the chronic wound has a higher risk of breakdown depending on the patient's age, comorbidities, comedication, which can all lead to a reduced vascular perfusion to the periwound skin, and be a causal factor in delayed wound-healing.

38.2 Basics of the epidermal barrier

The epidermal barrier is formed by physical, chemical and biological processes as well as structural conditions. The basic principle of 'adapted interaction' applies, i. e. the regulation of hydration, temperature and the invasion of microbes from outside and from inside out. The regulation processes involved are highly complex and dynamic. They are essential for the molecular order within the intercellular matrix in the stratum corneum, the resulting interaction of surfactant lipids (especially ceramides) with water and the resulting conditions for the formation and functionality of membranes. The metabolic functions, permeability and resistance of the system to toxic substances are determined by a multitude of molecule classes, such as protons (pH value), amino acids (natural humectant factor), antimicrobial peptides, structural proteins (e. g. filaggrin) or more complex structures (e. g. corneodesmosomes, cornified envelope).

38.3 Risk factors

Risk factors for the breaking down of periwound skin, which can affect clinical wound management (➤ Table 38.1).

Table 38.1 Risk factors for the breaking down of the skin barrier function

Change in the degree of hydration	With weeping wounds, application of a topical agent with high water content (e. g. hydrogels) or occlusion (reduction of transepidermal water flow) directly alter the conditions of membrane formation in the intercellular lipid matrix and influence its permeability.
Change in lipid composition of stratum corneum	Ceramides and other lipids are washed out of the stratum corneum by the application of ethanolic disinfectants or topical agents with ethanolic solvents as well as surfactant-rich cleaning preparations.
Changing the pH value	The use of alkaline soaps, water-containing topical agents with insufficient buffer capacity or occlusive dressings leads to the destruction of the protective acid mantle of the stratum corneum with impairment of the regeneration of the barrier or changes in the microbiome.
Stripping effect	As a result of the application of adhesive bandages (e. g. wound plasters) to the skin, the stratum corneum is partially torn off during the removal of the bandage, thus reducing the barrier.

38

38.4 Protection measures

To counteract the risk factors mentioned above, protective measures are recommended. It is especially important in older, immobile patients with comorbidities. These include barrier-protective basic therapy with water-containing care preparations (up to approx. 40% water content) of the W/O type (with approx. 5% glycerol and max. 5% urea) and cleaning with synthetic detergents (syndets) and low emulsifier content (i. e. **scant** foaming). Washing with antiseptic additives (e. g. polihexanide or octenidine HCl) 1–2×/week may additionally be useful to reduce pathogenic colonisation with bacteria and/or yeast fungi. Bandages with strong adhesive edges should be avoided for chronic wounds, and careful removal of the patch (slowly, tangentially and without turning over) should minimise the stripping effect. Thin hydrocolloids are known to be effective as subbandages for skin protection in the peristomal area. Silicone preparations (e. g. silicone gels) or, to a limited extent, water-free ointments (e. g. Vaseline) can also be used for skin protection to reduce the maceration of the stratum corneum in contact with heavy wound exudate.

38.5 Measures for regeneration

Analysis and identification of the influencing factors are required when desiccation, irritation or even erosion has occurred in the periwound skin. Only with consistent countermeasures and elimination of the causal factors, proper regeneration of the damaged barrier and recovery of the physiological compensatory capacity will be possible. The necessary measures for the regeneration of the wound environment are not identical with those for the actual wound care! Exoserosis will be minimised through the use of antiseptic (**not** antibiotic) preparations if there is a pathological colonisation of the affected areas. The application of topical anti-inflammatory agents can be useful for a limited time, but only if the application surface is mostly dry (warning: glucocorticoids and calcineurin inhibitors are lipophilic active agents). Avoiding the use of emulsifier-rich preparations or foams is recommended. Performing an appropriate test procedure if contact allergy is suspected should be considered. It is essential to prevent polypragmasia, to define a well-founded management concept and to communicate this to all suppliers.

REFERENCES

Atiyeh BS, Dibo SA, Hayek SN. Wound cleansing, topical antiseptics and wound-healing. Int Wound J 2009; 6: 420–430.

Hachem JP, Crumrine D, Fluhr J, Brown BE, Feingold KR, Elias PM. pH directly regulates epidermal permeability barrier homeostasis, and stratum corneum integrity/cohesion. J Invest Dermatol 2003; 121: 345–353.

Jungersted JM, Hogh JK, Hellgren LI, Jemec GB, Agner T. Skin barrier response to occlusion of healthy and irritated skin: differences in trans-epidermal water loss, erythema and stratum corneum lipids. Contact Dermatitis 2010; 63: 313–319.

Wohlrab J, Klauck D, Savtcheva E. [Regulatory requirements for topical preparations]. Hautarzt 2014; 65: 175–179.

Wohlrab J. [Basics of topical therapiy]. Hautarzt 2014; 65: 169–174.

39

Cornelia Erfurt-Berge
Allergy

─────── **Key notes** ───────

- Patients with chronic wounds have an increased risk of contact sensitisation and the occurrence of contact dermatitis.
- A skin patch test is carried out to clarify the allergic reaction. The patient's wound therapy

products should be examined in addition to carrying out the standard patch tests.
- Patients with chronic wounds should avoid the use of external agents with a high allergenic potential, such as those containing fragrances or preservatives.

39.1 Introduction

In the context of wound assessment, eczematous skin changes such as redness, flaking or erosion are often noticeable in the periwound skin. These not only influence the choice of wound care but also require the identification of its aetiology. Inadequate exudate management is the most common cause of irritative contact dermatitis. However, contact sensitisation and subsequently allergic contact dermatitis are increasingly found in patients with chronic venous insufficiency (CVI) or venous leg ulcers.

39.2 Contact sensitisation in patients with chronic wounds

Several studies have consistently described contact sensitisation rates of around 60% for patients with CVI and/or venous leg ulcers, with polysensitisations found in many cases. General risk factors for contact sensitisation include genetic predisposition, female gender and pre-existing skin barrier disorders. Patients with chronic wounds are exposed to multiple potential contact allergens in their periwound skin, due to the prolonged use of wound products, topical antibiotics, wound irrigation solutions containing preservatives, and wound treatments. Current data for Germany from the Informationsverbund Dermatologischer Kliniken (IVDK) show that the allergen spectrum of this patient group differs significantly from that of the general population (➤ Table 39.1).

The high contact sensitisation rates in the German-speaking countries were generally shown as declining in a comparison of data between 1994–2003 and 2004–2013, although they remain relevant in practice. Topical antibiotics were recognised as having a high contact sensitisation potential – their decline in use resulted in a reduction of the documented sensitisation rate.

Table 39.1 Frequent contact allergens in patients with chronic venous insufficiency or venous leg ulcers and their occurrence in wound treatment

Peru Balsam/fragrance mix	Fragrances in creams, ointments, cosmetics
Wool wax alcohol derivatives (lanolin alcohol/ amerchol L-101), cetylstearyl alcohol	Emulsifiers in creams, ointments, cosmetics
Tertiary butylhydroquinone, propylene glycol	Preservative in creams, ointments, cosmetics, hydrogels, fatty gauzes
Colophony	Adhesive dressing materials, hydrocolloids (also derivatives), plasters

39.3 Procedure in case of suspected contact dermatitis

Compared to atopic eczema, contact dermatitis presents with a nonspecific clinical presentation of skin changes, i. e. presence of itching, skin lesions in the surrounding area, and a delayed occurrence of skin changes a few days after allergen contact, due to the T-cell-mediated type IV immune response (delayed reaction). A skin patch test can detect possible sensitisation to a suspected contact allergen. Prior to the planning of a skin patch test, a detailed assessment of the patient's medical history is necessary, in which all externally applied substances, e.g. self-treatment with possible 'home remedies', application of possible herbal substances with high allergenic potential (i. e. arnica, tea tree oil or marigold) need to be queried. Furthermore, assessment should include current wound therapy and previously known contact sensitisations or the presence of an allergy history. Using the anamnestic data, a test panel of commercially available test substances is available to select from [sets from the German Contact Allergy Group (DKG)]. The substances used in the patient's self-treatment, including wound therapeutics, can also be tested in the patch testing. The substances are applied in a fixed concentration in a carrier substance to the patient's back and left there for 24–48 hours (➤ Fig. 39.1). Skin reaction will be observed and evaluated at a fixed time (48 h, 72 h, or a late reading after seven days, if necessary), on the basis of a presentation of erythema, infiltration, papules, and blisters. The skin reaction is expected to increase over a period of time, from 48 to 72 hours (so-called crescendo).

A positive reaction in a skin test is the first evaluation of proven contact sensitisation. A relevant contact allergy can only be assumed when looking at the patient's anamnesis in conjunction with the temporal relationship between the application of the positively tested allergen and the occurrence of typical skin changes at the application site.

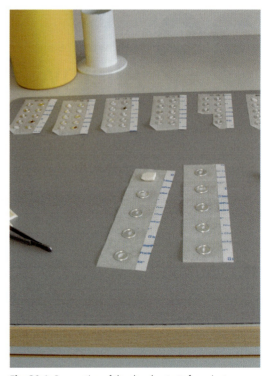

Fig. 39.1 Preparation of the chamber tests for epicutaneous testing. [T1061]

39.4 Contact allergies to modern wound dressings

The data available on the sensitisation rate to advanced wound care products is currently still inadequate and in some cases, very divergent. While French colleagues were able to demonstrate sensitisation in almost 20% of patients tested with wound dressings, the results in other test groups were significantly lower. Wound care products should be included in the epicutaneous testing. However, relevant assessment in conjunction with the patient's anamnesis is important.

39.5 Conclusion

The specific and increased sensitisation potential of patients with chronic wounds, in particular ulcus cruris venosum, must be taken into account. External agents used on the patient should be as free of fragrances and preservatives as possible. An epicutaneous test, which includes the patient's own external applications and the most recently used wound dressings, should be carried out if there is any clinical suspicion of contact sensitisation. In the event of a positive reaction to a wound dressing, it is advisable to contact the manufacturer to determine the individual components of the wound dressing and, if possible, to test them separately.

REFERENCES

Erfurt-Berge C, Geier J, Mahler V. The current spectrum of contact sensitization in patients with chronic leg ulcers or stasis dermatitis – new data from the Information Network of Departments of Dermatology (IVDK). Contact Dermatitis 2017; 77: 151–158.

Erfurt-Berge C, Mahler V. Contact sensitization in patients with lower leg dermatitis, chronic venous insufficiency, and/or chronic leg ulcer: Assessment of the clinical relevance of contact allergens. J Investig Allergol Clin Immunol 2017; 27: 378–380.

Mahler V. [Contact allergies in the elderly]. Hautarzt 2015; 66: 665–673.

Schnuch A, Aberer W, Agathos M, et al. Performing patch testing with contact allergens. Guideline of the Deutsche Dermatologische Gesellschaft (DDG) and Deutsche Gesellschaft für Allergie und klinische Immunologie (DGAKI). J Dtsch Dermatol Ges 2008; 6: 770–775.

Thyssen JP, Linneberg A, Menne T, Johansen JD. The epidemiology of contact allergy in the general population-prevalence and main findings. Contact Dermatitis 2007; 57: 287–299.

Valois A, Waton J, Avenel-Audran M, et al. Contact sensitization to modern dressings: a multicentre study on 354 patients with chronic leg ulcers. Contact Dermatitis 2015; 72: 90–96.

40

Anja Stoffel
Podiatry in patients with foot diseases

Key notes

- Podiatry is a profession which provides non-medical healthcare therapies for the foot.
- Pressure points on the foot show signs of unphysiological pressure conditions, such as friction and overloading, representing an early warning symptom for possible damage to the foot.
- With pathological corns and calluses, the layers which affect the elasticity of the skin are removed. However, a thin keratinised layer is left behind to protect the nonkeratinised tissue, which is too thin and can be painful or injured when walking under stress.
- Orthonyxia treatment is a treatment to help the nail grow wider in a transverse cross-section and to relieve discomfort caused by pressure, friction and irritation of the nail fold around the nail edges.
- Orthoses are individual, customised device aids to correct and protect against pressure and friction for malaligned toes.

40.1 Introduction

Podiatry is a profession which provides foot therapies which don't need a physician. Podiatrists treat pathological changes to the skin and nails as well as secondary diseases, such as diabetic foot syndrome, following a preventive and curative procedure within a multidisciplinary approach.

40.2 Taking care of one's own feet

Advising on the health and self-care of the feet is a crucial component of the podological consultation. The four main approaches are:

- **'The (medical) correct way to cut the nails'** always leaves a part of the free (white) front edge to avoid injuries to the tissue under the free edge, the hyponychium – a common entry point for onychomycosis infections. The nail corners should be filed fairly straight to spade-shaped; on no account should the nails be cut into the nail folds if there is no medical indication (acutely inflamed ingrown nails). The sulci or folds and the nail edges should be left as they are until their joint anatomical completion. Shortening the length of ingrown and deformed nails at home should only be done by using a nail file, because conventional instruments (nail clippers) tend to leave remaining splinters in the corners as well as jagged edges, which can penetrate the soft tissue and cause infections.
- The patient can self-treat their calluses or hyperkeratosis using a fine-grained file. Rotating grinding instruments (which cause heat!) or rough graters, not to mention planers, lead to more keratinisation due to the roughened surface and, in worst case scenarios, to injuries. If a file is used, it should be dry and not softened, to make the surface as smooth as possible and to not provoke new keratinisation.
- Skincare should make the skin supple, and maintain and strengthen its barrier. An intact acid mantle offers no entry points for microorganisms and infections. It reduces corneal formation, keeps existing calluses elastic, does not form rhagades and reduces pressure points forming on the soft tissue. Skincare should be executed according to the condition of the skin, i.e. cream must be applied several times a day if necessary,

to avoid secondary diseases such as rhagades and pressure points. To prevent transepidermal water loss, it is advisable to use skincare products which leave a slightly occlusive layer behind after absorption, retaining the moisture in the skin. Products containing irritants such as fragrances and essential oils should be avoided. Products with a high proportion of urea help to macerate hard calluses but are not suitable for permanent or extensive use. A reversal of the positive effect is possible with long-term use (a few weeks) or if unkeratinised skin is moisturised intensively with cream containing urea: the skin peels, and the acid mantle and barrier are disturbed.

- Podological treatment as a whole includes controlling the inside of the currently worn shoes as part of the therapy. Patients are trained to monitor their shoes daily before they wear them.

40.3 Treatment of nail changes

Nail changes are common as the keratin of the nail adapts to stress exposure, which leads to life-long physiological changes in shape, curvature and colour. In contrast, pathological changes are caused by infections, traumas, drug side effects, systemic diseases and malignant processes. The most common nail changes, their causes and treatments are listed in ➤ Table 40.1.

Table 40.1 Nail changes

Clinical picture	Causes	Therapy
Shape change in the sagittal or longitudinal growth direction	• Biomechanical incorrect loading (hallux valgus, pronounced foot mal-positions) • Conditional (congenital axial deviation) • Poor condition of care (onychogrypho-sis), systemic diseases	• Removal of the nail to achieve the best possible shape • For severe deformities, nail prosthetics for cosmetic correction
Infections Onychomycosis	• Acquired through microtrauma • Favoured by systemic disease or dis-position	• If a mycosis is confirmed by differential di-agnosis, the procedure which supports the indicated local or systemic treatment is the removal of the affected nail material • Disadvantage: often, mechanical growth disturbances remain due to damage to the nail bed during long periods of infec-tion and therapy • The prognosis worsens when the nail growth, the blood circulation and the overall condition of the patient is weak
Thickened nails, onychauxis	• Circulatory disorder, nail matrix supply disorder • Pressure exposure, trauma, com-pression load, safety shoes • Apex (end) of toe bulges after loss of nail plate • Drug side effects	• Grinding down to normal thickness with-out fracture grooves to avoid tearing • Nail is cut only after grinding it down thinly to prevent splintering • Avoid trauma to the nail due to inap-propriate footwear if possible
• Thin nails • Splintering and tearing of the nail plate (onychoschisis) • Irritations due to sharp nail edges in the nail fold	• Genetic disposition • Toddlers and adolescents	• Reinforcement and sealing of the nail plate with varnish or prosthetic material • In the case of problems with the fold of the nail, nail correction clips are indicated to shift and relieve the friction point between the nail and the fold

Table 40.1 Nail changes *(cont'd)*

Clinical picture	Causes	Therapy
Transversally ingrown nails, unguis convolutus	• Genetic disposition • Foot and toe malpositions • Tight shoes	• Nails must not be cut too short and should only be shortened by filing: the nail fold serves as an indication for the end point • If nail care is poor, nail slivers will remain in the fold, or a nail that is cut too short will push into the sensitive fold as it grows longer
Colour changes, dyschromias	**Yellow colouration:** thickening of the horny substance, a growth disorder, medication, discolouration due to nail polish and iodine	If possible, avoid triggering factors
	White spots, leukonychia: many microlesions of the cuticle, manipulation and nail-biting	• Avoid triggers • Skincare
	Brownish-yellow discolouration: with changes in nail plate transparency, structural changes and differently affected and stained areas: mycosis and psoriasis	• Psoriasis: grinding down to standard thickness; sealing possible • Mycosis: complete removal of the infection, external or systemic therapy
	Dark, almost black areas: haematoma, infection, necrotic foci or melanoma	If patient is not aware of any direct trauma, immediate assessment of its causal factor is necessary
	Pigmentation disorders such as melasma and **hyperpigmented lines** also appear symptom-free on the nails.	No therapy known
Onycholysis	Long-lasting exposure to pressure (footwear, sport) leading to reduced supply of the nail bed.	• Gentle cleaning out under nails • Keeping the nail at a standard length as protection and spacer for the fold • For large hollow spaces, underpinning with nail bed cushions/tamponades is possible

40

40.4 Prevention of pressure points

Pressure points are a sign of non-physiological pressure conditions, friction and overloading and represent an early warning symptom for possible damage to the foot. The relief of the compressed area is essential and should be checked and adjusted regularly to prevent subsequent problems. The prevention of pressure points is a consistent biomechanical off-loading, challenging in practice and requiring a high degree of adherence from all parties involved. Concrete measures are:

• Checking shoes and socks for friction points, seams and rough surfaces. The smoother and more friction-free shoes and socks are, the better.
• The size of the footwear must conform to the stressed shape of the foot. A visual representation of the width of the forefoot with an outline drawing can help. In lymphoedema/CVI, the shoe and sock material must be elastic to allow room for the increase in volume.
• There are countless protection measures to relieve the pressure points: made up of various skin-friendly materials, personalised by the podiatrist using dressings and relief materials, individually customised as an orthosis.

- It is advisable to follow professional shoe care recommendations from an early age.
- Skin with cornification disorders requires consistent care to retain its elasticity. Drier skin is more prone to cornification. There is more significant pressure damage to the deeper tissue layers when callosity is firmer and thicker.

40.5 Treatment of cornifications

The roles of a podiatrist include mechanical ablation, preventive counselling and treatment to relieve cornifications. Corneas are formed to serve the epidermis as a physiological protective factor in case of pressure and friction exposure. Elastic callosity physiologically protects against pressure and friction and does not provoke any discomfort in the soft tissue. The therapist has to weigh up in advance how much pressure can be applied to the tissue layers supplied with blood without causing damage, when polyneuropathy is also present. It is advisable not to remove physiological cornifications completely as this provokes a renewed, rapid stimulation of callosity and, in the long run, an increased formation of corns. The cornification is pathological if:

- There is no elasticity, and cracks/rhagades appear.
- The horn material is solid and hardened, and presses into the underlying tissue like a stone in the shoe, thus leading to an undersupply all the way to the ulceration/malum perforans.
- The corn tissue is exaggerated and grows excessively fast and thick. A doctor must clarify the causes.
- The surface is rough, fissured and excessively flaky. Here a mycosis infestation (mocassin mycosis), as well as chronic dermatosis, should be investigated. In practice, cornifications due to mycosis infestation prove to be resistant to treatment, which is why diagnosis and therapy are essential for skin restoration.

The distinction between hyperkeratosis and callosity is based on the clinical presentation and is helpful in the choice of therapy.

Callosity is a clearly defined, usually elastic, glassy, yellowish callus. Callositas acts like a layer of candle wax.

Hyperkeratosis on the other hand is not clearly defined, whitish-greyish, scaly, rough hornification which can affect the entire skin area of the foot. Patients have skin flakes getting stuck in their socks, and a smooth surface is difficult to achieve.

A unique form of punctual hyperkeratosis is the **clavus**, the corn. It appears on the skin surface close to the bone, the eye-shaped core pressing into deep tissue layers and it can cause severe pain. Consistent pressure relief leads to complete 'healing' of the clavus; many different clavi are to be differentiated in podiatry.

The cornification can be removed with a scalpel; cutting with a blade is preferable to scraping as there is less of a mechanical stimulus exerted on the skin. Rotating instruments and grinders are only used for smoothing and finishing off, as heat generation can also lead to increased formation of the callus.

All layers that impair the elasticity of the skin should be removed, until there is a slightly firmer surface compared to the non-keratinised tissue. Skin that is too thin and rosy will hurt when stressed with running. In exceptional cases, this procedure is repeated frequently – every two to three weeks. Additional skincare is essential to:

- Maintain the elasticity and suppleness of the skin,
- Avoid rhagades and injuries caused by cracks,
- Reduce increased horn formation due to rough surfaces,
- Regenerate the lipid and acid protective mantle.
- Reduce itching and prevent entry ports due to wounds from scratching,
- Make keratinised areas elastic to avoid pressure ulcerations and recurrences of malum perforans.

40.6 Nail correction clips

The nail correction brace or orthonyxia treatment is a measure to help the nail grow wider in a transverse cross-section and to relieve discomfort caused by pressure, friction and irritation of the nail fold through the nail edges (➤ Fig. 40.1). A variety of brace models is available, which enable therapy of any nail shape

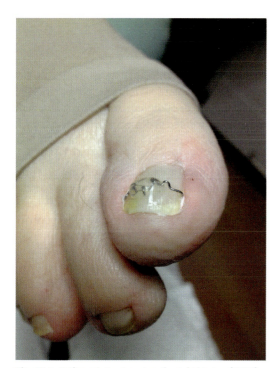

Fig. 40.1 Orthonyxia treatment on the right big toe. [P609]

and at any single stage of the disease. The indication is guided by the patient's complaints and not by the radius of the nail curvature.

Fields of treatment are:

- Chronic complaints in the nail fold, pressure pain, cornifications, clavi
- Long-term incorrect nailcare: condition after cutting a nail too short, atrophy of the nail folds, growing in of the lateral nail edges due to atrophy of the folds as a direction indicator
- Irritation of the sulcus due to sharp nail edges
- Ingrown nails, Unguis convolutus
- Inflammation due to ingrown nails left untreated
- Acute inflammatory ingrown nail
- Hypergranulation as a sign of massive mechanical irritation in the nail fold
- For nail growth disorders after traumatic nail plate loss, mycosis therapy
- With a genetic disposition to ingrown nails
- Malpositioning of the toes and the feet bio-mechanically promote ingrown toenails. Correction of the malpositioning avoids recurrences, in addition to the brace therapy

- Wedge resection/Emmert's procedure for persistent complaints can relieve orthonyxia treatment and reduce pain.

The ingrown nail parts are lifted dorsally by the tensile and/or restoring forces of wire applied to the nail or hooked in under the free lateral nail edges. As the nail grows, the transverse diameter widens. The tension must be adjusted accordingly as a delicate, thin nail plate is prone to tearing, whereas a robust and firm nail material requires more substantial pressure to achieve a result.

Absolute contraindications are not known. An experienced therapist can perform nail correction even in patients with pronounced neuropathy, circulatory disorders or nickel allergy. Relative contraindications are

- Defunct nail growth.
- Nail plate mycosis infestation. The structural strength of the nail is at risk if the nail plate is infected (usually via $1/5$ of the surface), and the nail may split and tear. Additionally, orthonyxia treatment impedes local treatment of mycosis, which explains the necessity of careful assessment and weighing up of treatments.
- Structural damage to the nail plate (such as Beau-Reil transverse furrows or strongly psoriatic nails) that cannot be exposed to tensile stress.
- Onycholysis.
- Nail edges are so traumatised that insertion of the wire hook is impossible.

Many different products are available on the market, all working on the same principle. Depending on the indication, the therapist chooses between adhesive clips and wire buckles.

Adhesive clips are not inserted into the nail fold, but are glued to the nail plate and develop a light to medium retraction force. They are the method of choice:

- For mild complaints or presumed short duration of therapy
- Severe inflammations, which prevents the insertion of the hooks into the folds
- For babies and toddlers up to primary school age
- For severe allergies to nickel and metal alloys
- In patients with anxiety who cannot tolerate braces
- For thin nails, which require only minimal tension

Corrrection braces always consist of the following parts: tiny hooks, the wire adjusted to the nail bulge, and an 'omega' as middle part, a little concave recess to buffer too much tension.

The lateral ends are hooked under the free side edges of the nail to fix down the sides. These tiny hooks are short and wafer-thin, fitting snugly until they are not noticed by the patient at all. Under no circumstances must a hook prick or press unpleasantly into the nail fold. The side wires, which lie in a perfect fit on the nail plate, exert an elastic restoring force dorsally on the nail plate. Correct adjustment of this force is essential for an effective result in guiding nail growth without traumatising the nail bed.

On the nail plate, a small recess formed like the greek letter 'omega' in the side wire construction offers a buffer function to prevent excessive tightening of the braces and to allow a minimal adjustment. A nail brace is always the preferred choice if it requires an effective outcome or a long period of therapy. When a nail is only ingrown on one side, lifting only one side of the nail plate is necessary, and a combination of products which have a more substantial pulling effect on just one side is required.

Wearing instructions

Patients are instructed to return immediately if the nail fold is pricked, or if there is redness or other complaints. In most cases, the patients do not feel the nail correction clips or braces at all, but only have a feeling of relief in the nail fold, which occurs immediately when the tension is adjusted. All everyday activities, including sports and swimming, may be carried out during this treatment.

The **duration of therapy** is between half a year and a year (with exceptions). The nail must have sufficient growth time to be able to broaden sustainably. Short treatments are prone to premature recurrences. A nail correction clip or buckle can be used on any size of nail, even on the little toe and fingernails.

The nail carries on growing wider after the treatment, unless the foot and toe position, or shoes worn too tightly despite a consultation, or when there is a genetic disposition of Unguis convolutus (coiling of nails), cause a recurrence of the ingrown nail. Repeated therapy is possible.

40.7 Orthoses

Orthoses are individual, custom-made aids for correction and protection from pressure and friction. Condensation- or addition-curing two-component materials with different degrees of hardness are used, depending on the desired function and durability. Soft materials give a more elastic, softer and cushioning effect to protect prominent friction and pressure points. Tougher orthosis materials have a corrective effect and can be used to underlay more delicate materials as a substructure, to increase the longevity of the orthosis.

Contraindications are allergy to silicone, open wounds and infections of the affected skin areas, footwear that is too tight and lack of compliance, and contracted joints that would have been placed under too much stress by orthosis (passive mobility test). In the case of pronounced neuropathy, circulatory and lymphatic drainage disorders, care should only be provided by an experienced therapist with clear information given to the patient on the maintenance and warning signs, to avoid consequential damage.

In Germany, more extensive and more complex orthoses are made by the orthopaedic shoemakers. Podiatric orthosis care is common in Germany, especially in the forefoot and toe area; however, there is no clear division or assignment of certain orthosis forms or sizes in the profession.

A relief of pressure is always given when the surrounding area around the pressure point is more prominently constructed than the pressure point itself, to redistribute and reduce stress directly at the pressure point. Hereby the pressure shift in the direction of movement during walking, i.e. from proximal to distal, must be taken into account. A compromise between the required thickness and the pressure exerted by the footwear is essential. If the patient is not compliant with the wearing of suitable footwear, an orthosis is an alternative prescription.

Various shapes are available:
- Toe wedge for relief of interdigital clavi
- Morton neuroma/neuralgia (toes 2–4 are placed together in a comb-shaped underlay. The material between the toes of the affected metatarsal spaces should be thicker to reduce the pain-inducing compression.)

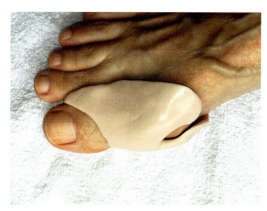

Fig. 40.2 A modified splint is shown as friction protection for hallux valgus on the right foot. [P609]

- Pads under the toes for apex relief in cornification/malum perforans in digitus flexus or digitus malleolus
- Pads over the toes at clavi on the DIP/PIP
- Spacers between D1 and D2, for relief in Unguis incarnatus (ingrown toenails) lateral U1

Orthoses serve as friction protection when friction causes pain and/or callosity:

- Splints for hallux valgus (➤ Fig. 40.2) or digitus quintus varus
- Splints for individual toes with clavus formation

Use of corrective orthoses when joint mobility is maintained:

- Ingrown toenail correction
- Hammer- and clawtoe correction
- Toe separator D1 for lateral deviation

The orthosis should be worn when the foot is under stress and removed when it is stressfree. After removing the orthosis, the skin should be meticulously examined daily for redness or pressure points. Wearing it should be interrupted immediately if any abnormali

ties are noticed, and a check-up appointment should be arranged. For cleaning, rinse under clear running wate – washing with soap is optional – then air dry. The orthosis must be dry before wearing it again.

Orthoses can help over a long period to relieve individual pressure problems and foot deformities that cannot be treated adequately with ready-made products.

REFERENCES

Di Chiacchio N, Kadunc BV, Trindade de Almeida AR, Madeira CL. Treatment of transverse overcurvature of the nail with a plastic device: measurement of response. J Am Acad Dermatol 2006; 55: 1081–1084.

Erdogan FG. A quantitative method for measuring forces applied by nail braces. J Am Podiatr Med Assoc 2011; 101: 247–251.

Erdogan FG, Erdogan G. Long-term results of nail brace application in diabetic patients with ingrown nails. Dermatol Surg 2008; 34: 84–86.

Grünewald K. Theorie der medizinischen Fußbehandlung; Angewandte Techniken. Band 2. München: Verlag Neuer Merkur; 2001.

Haneke E. Controversies in the treatment of ingrown nails. Dermatol Res Pract 2012; 2012: 783924.

Harrer J, Schöffl V, Hohenberger W, Schneider I. Treatment of ingrown toenails using a new conservative method: a prospective study comparing brace treatment with Emmert's procedure. J Am Podiatr Med Assoc 2005; 95: 542–549.

Liu CW, Huang YC. Efficacy of a new nail brace for the treatment of ingrown toenails. J Dtsch Dermatol Ges 2018; 16: 417–423.

Navarro-Flores E, Gijón-Noguerón G, Cervera-Marín JA, Labajos-Manzanares MT. Assessment of foot self-care in patients with diabetes: retrospective assessment (2008–2014). Foot Ankle Spec 2015; 8: 406–412.

Ruck H. Handbuch für die medizinische Fußpflege. Stuttgart: Hippokrates; 2005.

Scholz N. Lehrbuch und Bildatlas für die Podologie. München: Verlag Neuer Merkur; 2007.

40

41

Jan-Jakob Meyer, Knut Kröger, Joachim Dissemond

Pain therapy

Key notes

- Pain can occur in patients with chronic wounds due to the underlying disease, complications or therapeutic measures.
- Pain therapy for chronic wounds should always be a combination of causal and symptomatic treatment.
- Adequate wound therapy helps to reduce or avoid therapy-related pain.

- Medicinal pain therapy should be introduced and increased according to the WHO stage scheme.
- The use of analgesic combinations and medication on demand reduces pain and thereby pain chronification.
- The use of regional anaesthesia procedures or topical local anaesthesia should be considered in the therapy concept.

41.1 Introduction

According to the definition of the International Association for the Study of Pain (IASP), pain is defined as '… pain is that experience we associate with actual or potential tissue damage … always unpleasant and therefore also an emotional experience'.

Pain impairs the quality of life, has an unfavourable effect on the compliance of patients and, as an independent risk factor, delays the healing of wounds. Pain is a common problem in patients with chronic wounds. Pain therapy includes all the therapeutic measures that lead to a reduction of pain. Since the treatment of chronic pain, in particular, requires an interdisciplinary and individualised approach, the term 'pain management' is often used for this purpose.

In addition to the treatment of the causative factors of chronic wounds, the approach of multimodal pain therapy also includes treatment by physiotherapists, psychotherapists and pain therapists as well as other medical and non-physical disciplines, according to an individualised and standardised treatment plan.

41.2 Causes of pain

In providing pain therapy to people with chronic wounds, it must be differentiated whether:

- The pain is primarily attributable to the underlying disease, e. g. ischaemia in arterial circulatory disorders or vasculitic ulceration,
- it is specific complications of the wound, e. g. bacterial infectious diseases, that cause the pain, or
- it is the therapeutic measures of wound treatment, e. g. dressing changes or debridement, which are associated with the pain.

Vascular diseases are always associated with the risk of impaired tissue perfusion and accompanying tissue destruction. Effective pain therapy must not promote possible tissue destruction and should, therefore, only be used when clearly indicated. Besides the crucial signs from ischaemia pain, pain can be differentiated on the basis of whether it is caused by an infectious disease, a trauma, an edematous swelling or cooling. The transitions between the various causes of pain are fluid. Regular clinical checks are therefore necessary. Increasing the pain therapy for an undetected infectious disease can have fatal consequences.

The lack of pain perception in patients with advanced diabetic polyneuropathy is an excellent example of how vital pain is as a warning sign for the patient and the practitioner. Such patients usually come to the therapist quite late, and the extent of the tissue lesion is often underestimated.

The intensity and occurrence of pain can be differentially and diagnostically helpful. Skin changes caused by pyoderma gangrenosum, thrombangiitis obliterans or cutaneous vasculitis are usually many times more painful than skin changes of the same magnitude caused by PAD or CVI. If the subjective pain intensity is disproportionate to the physical appearance, such clinical pictures should also be considered. Therefore, standardised pain evaluation at the first contact and in the treatment course should be given to all patients with chronic wounds. The type of survey, documentation and re-evaluation should be clearly defined in the institution's internal standards. For example, if pain needs to be recorded daily, then the patient can be asked about the level of pain experienced over the last 24 hours.

41.3 Detection of pain

Various scales have been established for the objective assessment of pain intensity in everyday clinical life. In addition to the widespread visual analogue scale (VAS), a numerical rating scale (NRS) or a verbal rating scale (VRS), describing words, can be used. For a better evaluation of the subjective pain sensation, patients should be allowed to describe the pain in their own words using adjectives. Besides, the patient is often aware of what the worsening influences are on the pain, and these should be taken into account. Patients with chronic pain should also keep a pain diary. The primary evaluation of the different pain characteristics and qualities is essential, and the basis of the subsequent individual therapy. The

progress of pain during therapy should be recorded and documented at regular intervals.

41.4 Acute pain – chronic pain

Patients with chronic wounds often also have chronic pain. In the context of chronic wounds, patients without a long history of pain are an exception. The associated problems are manifold and include pathophysiological, pharmacological, social and psychological aspects. The changes associated with this long history of pain lead to a chronification of pain.

Acute pain has a warning function and protects the body from injury. Permanently occurring pain loses this warning function and leads to the development of pain memory. The pain persists even if the cause is cured and must be considered in the therapy of chronic pain. If pain lasts longer than 3–6 months, it fulfils the definition of chronic pain. ➤ Table 41.1 summarises the characteristics of acute and chronic pain.

The chronification of pain has pathophysiological, psychological and social aspects. A holistic therapy concept includes all aspects of therapy planning.

Permanent pain stimuli from the periphery lead to increased activity of neurons in the posterior horn of the spinal cord. These nerve cells, known as Wide-Dynamic-Range (WDR) neurons, change their excitability through repeated pain stimuli. Gene expression of IEG (immediate early genes) occurs. These processes

Table 41.1 Characteristics of acute and chronic pain

	Acute pain	Chronic pain
Function	Warning of acute damage	Pain, even without damage
Duration	Hours to days	Weeks to years
Aim of the therapy	Fast effect, no pain	Long-lasting effect, pain tolerance
Therapy duration	Hours to days	Months to years
Type of therapy	Mono- or combination therapy	Combination therapy
Application path	p.o., s.c., i.v., epidural	p.o., transdermal
Dosage	Titration, as required	According to time of day, consistent level
Duration of effect	Short-acting substances, combination with long-acting substances	Long-acting substances
Therapy control	Hourly, daily	Daily, weekly
Concomitant therapy	None or on-demand	Yes, medicinal, physiotherapeutic, psychotherapeutic

begin as early as 14 days after the onset of chronic pain. The alteration of these metabolic processes of the interneurons between the first and second neurons leads to independence of the pain process. The cross-linking of the altered interneurons also causes an increase in the peripheral receptive field. As a result, supra threshold stimulus responses can be triggered in a larger area than that of the chronic wound. The painful area is larger than the wound (widespread pain index). The change in intracellular metabolic processes cannot be reversed immediately with the onset of sufficient pain therapy. Even after the wound has healed, it can continue. This phenomenon, known as pain memory, means that pain therapy must be extended beyond wound-healing.

On the psychological level, chronic pain leads to an increased occurrence of depressive moods. Somatic pain results in a poor physical pain-relieving posture. The permanent occurrence of pain leads to withdrawal and inactivity, emotional instability and increased irritability, as well as fear of pain and associated avoidance behaviour, leading to a psychologically protective posture.

On the social level, performance reduction due to pain leads to a fear of loss of work or income. The decrease in mobility, possibly due to a reduction in driving ability, can lead to loneliness on the part of the patient. Sleep disturbances and restlessness also contribute to the exhaustion of psychological anti-chronification systems. The processing of mental and physical pain takes place in the same area of the brain and thus reaches a mutual end destination. Psychological and physical pain is therefore experienced in a similar way.

The consideration of a holistic therapy approach leads to better pain reduction, can prevent or reverse chronification processes and thereby increases patient satisfaction.

41.5 Pain therapy

When planning a pain therapy, the cause of the pain must be considered. The best pain therapy is therefore the causal treatment of the underlying disease, specifically for:

- PAD – revascularisation
- CVI – decongestion
- Lymphatic diseases – decongestion
- Pressure injury – pressure relief
- Infectious diseases – incision (e. g. abscess) or antibiotics (e. g. erysipelas)
- Autoimmunological diseases – immune suppression
- Vasculopathies – rheological therapy

In terms of differential diagnosis, the first question to be clarified is whether the pain is nociceptor-mediated or neuropathic. Nociceptor-mediated pain is a reaction to mechanical, chemical or thermal stimuli. It can be subdivided into somatic or visceral pain. Patients describe somatic pain caused by damage to the skin, muscles, bones or joints as sharp, stabbing, pressing, piercing and easily locatable. Visceral pain is described as dull, colicky and poorly characterised. Neuropathic pain, i. e. pain resulting from damage to the peripheral or central nervous system, is associated with paraesthesia, shooting or burning pain. Knowledge of the cause is essential for successful treatment. Burning pain is treated differently than stabbing pain. In the treatment of pain in chronic wounds, this sharp line between nociceptive and neuropathic pain is often blurred.

The initial pain assessment and the planning of the resulting pain therapy should be structured, ideally using standardised questionnaires. These include questions about the duration of the pain, first occurrence, localisation, radiating of the pain, patient's experiences regarding relief and pain intensification, the occurrence of sensory disturbances, paraesthesias, or a reduction in strength, the pain characteristic as well as the intensity. This information is highly relevant for a differential diagnosis as well as for therapy. Also, the structured procedure facilitates therapy control over more extended periods.

When dealing with opioids of WHO level 3, extensive patient eduction is required, to reduce any fear of this therapy on the one hand, and to use the drugs as they are indicated and required on the other hand. The following rules apply to therapy with opioids:
- Pain is a physiological antagonist of the dreaded respiratory depression; as long as the analgesic dose is titrated along with the pain intensity, there is no danger of clinically relevant respiratory depression (start low – go slow).

41

- Psychological dependence is rarely clinically relevant to pain patients.
- Always prescribe medication on demand for phases of higher pain intensity at the same time. Rule: ⅙ of the total daily dose of an opioid in the same group.
- Choose starting dose carefully; especially in opioid patients.
- Drug intake, according to a fixed schedule.
- Drug application as non-invasive as possible (p. o. or transdermal).

The concept of on-demand medication involves the patient closely in the therapy and represents an essential mainstay of pain therapy for patients with chronic wounds. Drug therapy includes not only retarded analgesics, usually of WHO group 2 or 3, supplemented by co-analgesics, but also the prescription of short-acting opioids of the same group. These allow the patient to exert influence in phases of higher pain intensity. Even the possibility of self-determination is pain-relieving. As a rule, ⅙ of the daily dose of the retarded opioid is prescribed in an unretarded form. The patient is free to choose the time and, within limits, the frequency of taking the opioid. A goal of this concept is it to intercept pain peaks and to thereby work against a chronification of pain. For example, if the patient receives 2 × 10 mg oxycodone, this corresponds to an equivalent dose of 60 mg oral morphine. In this case, 10 mg of unretarded morphine is prescribed as on-demand medication.

Also, a temporary accompanying systemic pain therapy may be necessary, following the WHO stage scheme in ➤ Table 41.2. This three-stage scheme originates from oncology, but has become widespread and can be used in patients with chronic wounds.

The following substances can be used as co-analgesics:

- Antidepressants (TCA > SNRI > SSRI) for burning pain, for example, amitriptyline, duloxetine, fluoxetine,
- Anticonvulsants with an effect on neuronal sodium channels against stabbing pain, e. g. carbamazepine, oxcarbazepine,
- Anticonvulsants with an effect on neuronal calcium channels against stabbing, shooting pain, e. g. gabapentin, pregabalin.

Adjuvants include laxatives, antiemetics, myotonolytics and bisphosphonates.

There is no internationally uniform recommendation for long-term therapy with opioid analgesics. The use of opioid analgesics with a therapy duration > 3 months is defined as long-term use according to the current guidelines. For all non-tumour-related chronic pain, therapy with opioid-containing analgesics should be regarded as an individual therapy due to insufficient data. In the guideline mentioned above, the possible indications for short-term (4–12 weeks) and long-term (> 26 weeks) therapy with opioid-containing analgesics are clearly stated:

- Chronic limb pain in ischaemic and inflammatory artery diseases (ICD 10 I70–I79)
- Chronic pain in stage 3 and 4 pressure ulcers (ICD 10 L 89.2 and L89.3)

According to the guideline, the analgesic effect of opioids (investigated substances: tramadol, codeine, morphine, oxycodone, fentanyl), based among other things on a meta-analysis of 60 RCTs, is clearly below the clinically relevant effect in chronic non-tumour-induced pain with a dosage in the lower to medium dose range (e. g. oxycodone maximum 60 mg per day, morphine maximum 120 mg per day) according to the VAS. Long-term use of the opioid analgesics investigated for up to three months showed weak but statistically significant pain relief. Even taking other literature into account, there was no difference

Table 41.2 WHO-level scheme

Level	Medication
Level 1	Non-opioid analgesic, e. g. non-steroidal anti-inflammatory drugs (NSAIDs), metamizole and paracetamol, possibly in combination with co-analgesics and adjuvants.
Level 2	Weak opioids, e. g. tramadol and tilidine, possibly in combination with a non-opioid analgesic, or co-analgesics and adjuvants.
Level 3	Strong opioids, e. g. morphine, hydromorphone, oxycodone, fentanyl, buprenorphine, tapentadol and methadone, possibly in combination with non-opioid analgesics or co-analgesics and adjuvants.

in the strength of action between opiates and level 2 analgesics (opioids) and level 1 analgesics (NSAIDs) in the clinical pictures for osteoarthrosis, neuralgia after herpes zoster, diabetic polyneuropathy, non-specific back pain and fibromyalgia investigated in the studies. Due to the limited pain-relieving effect of opioid analgesics in non-tumour-induced pain, a trial application of opioid analgesics should therefore only be carried out when additional measures are taken and after taking into consideration the possible side effects of stage 1 analgesics.

It is important to note that a combination of strong and weak opioids is not useful for combined therapies, as weak opioids have an antagonistic or partially antagonistic effect on strong opioids and thus cancel the impact of strong opioids.

41.6 Special features of patients with chronic wounds

Patients with chronic wounds usually have a long history of pain; chronification processes have already begun. This circumstance must be taken into account in the acute therapy of patients with chronic wounds. Due to the independence of the pain process, successful wound-healing often leads to a reduction in pain, but not to freedom from pain. A pain therapy that has already begun must therefore be adapted to the treatment plan. In this context, sudden discontinuation of long-term opioids leads to an increase in side effects and is therefore counterproductive.

In pain therapy for chronic wounds, local or regional anaesthesia procedures represent a sensible and essential addition and extension of the therapy spectrum. A distinction must be made between topical methods through the use of pain-relieving creams and invasive regional anaesthesia with catheter procedures. Neuraxial anaesthesia procedures such as peridural or spinal anaesthesia, spinal cord stimulation (SCS) or ganglion blockades do not play a significant role in the treatment of chronic wounds outside of multimodal pain therapy.

Local anaesthetics are used in the acute pain therapy of chronic wounds as topical or regional anaesthesia, usually only within a limited time frame. Local anaesthetics such as lidocaine, mepivacaine, bupivacaine or ropivacaine inhibit the transmission of an electrical impulse. Depending on the isolation of the nerves, with increasing concentration of the local anaesthetic, first the vegetative, then the sensitive and finally the motor nerves are blocked. Local anaesthesia in the area of chronic wounds must take into account the risk of bacterial spread and necrosis of infected ischaemic tissue.

A unique option for local pain relief in superficial chronic wounds, such as lower leg vascular ulcers, is the use of local anaesthetics and morphine in cream or gel form. EMLA® is a cream containing 25 mg lidocaine and 25 mg prilocaine per 1 g each. According to technical information, it is applied after mechanical cleaning in a layer of approx. 1–2 g/10 cm2 up to a total of 10 g and preferably covered with a sterile occlusive dressing (➤ Fig. 41.1). EMLA® cream has been used in studies for the treatment of leg ulcers up to 15 times within 1–2 months without any loss of efficacy or

41

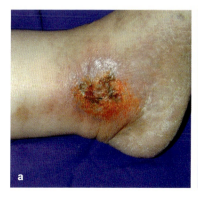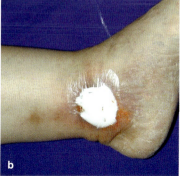

Fig. 41.1 Application of FMLA® cream to reduce pain before surgical debridement of a venous leg ulcer. EMLA® cream is applied, covered with an occlusive dressing and left for at least 30 minutes, preferably 1–2 hours. [O1089]

Table 41.3 Recipe for a morphine hydrochloride gel 0.1% for wound treatment, following a recipe from the University Hospital Essen, according to Dissemond and Geisheimer

Morphine hydrochloride trihydrate	0.1 g
Sodium edetate	0.1 g
Hydroxyethylcellulose 250 G	4.5 g
Polihexanide concentrate 20%	0.2 g
Aqua dest.	ad 100 g

increased local response. The maximum plasma concentration at application rates greater than 10 g cream for the treatment of lower leg ulcers was not tested. The application time should be at least 30 minutes. An extension of the application time up to several hours can further improve the anaesthesia. The intervention should begin immediately after re-moval of the cream. Occasional casuistic reports on the occurrence of contact sensitisations were made.

There is a polyurethane foam dressing with 0.5 mg ibuprofen incorporated per cm² of foam. The ibuprofen should be released continuously in a moist environment. It can be left on wounds for up to seven days depending on the amount of exudate, according

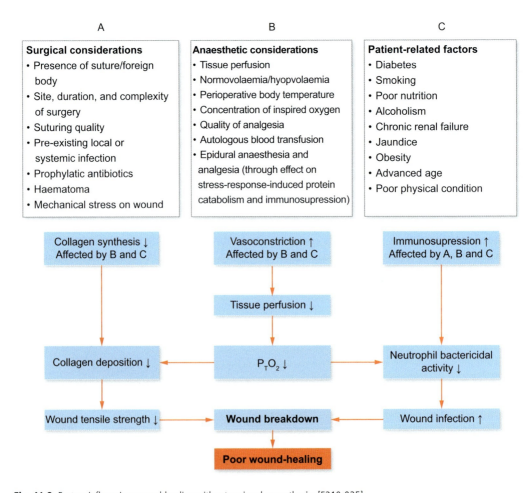

Fig. 41.2 Factors influencing wound-healing without regional anaesthesia. [F210-025]

to the manufacturer's instructions. There are several clinical studies on this subject. However, the topical application of ibuprofen also entails the risk of contact sensitisation.

There are several extemporaneous formulations for the production of a hydrogel for wound treatment that incorporates morphine for local pain therapy. At Essen University Hospital in Germany, a formulation to which polihexanide was added as a preservative has been developed and tested in studies for patients with painful wounds (➤ Table 41.3). It is covered, for example, with sterile fatty gauze. The morphine wound gel should be applied to the wound every 24 hours. Systemic resorption is to be expected for large wounds.

A significantly higher effort and expense characterises invasive procedures such as regional anaesthesiological blocking of peripheral nerves, compared to oral or topical application. Still, in addition to the actual pain-relieving effect, there are also some positive aspects supporting wound-healing. The main focus of regional anaesthesia procedures is on those that block the nerves of the lower extremities. Venous leg ulcers usually develop in the area of innervation of the ischiatic nerve, but can also affect parts of the femoral nerve in cranial expansion. The blockades are typically performed as catheter procedures with the aid of a medication pump. On the one hand, this offers the possibility of extending this procedure beyond the duration of a single-shot blockade, and on the other hand the option of better adapting the therapy to the patient's real needs through patient-controlled analgesia.

Regional anaesthesia methods block vegetative nerves. This sympathetic lysis leads to vasodilatation in the innervation area of the anaesthetised nerve. In addition to improving tissue oxygenation and the immune system, this results in a sympatho-adrenergic shielding of the wound (➤ Fig. 41.2), which results in a reduced washout of mediators and, as a result, less tissue and psychological stress. Less catecholamine washout leads to less vasoconstriction. The reduction of mediators results in lower tissue oedema and thus in better oxygen supply. These effects cannot be achieved with oral or topical pain therapy.

The use of regional anesthesiological procedures leads to decisive changes in nutrition and the oxygen supply of the affected wound. Sympathetic lysis, as a result of regional anaesthesia, leads to a reduction in vasoconstriction, after which tissue perfusion is improved and this, in turn, increases tissue oxygen partial pressure. Structural changes such as collagen incorporation and wound stability as well as improvements in the immune system lead to an improvement in wound-healing (➤ Fig. 41.3).

Through the use of regional anaesthesia procedures, a therapeutic approach can be pursued on several levels. In addition to relieving pain, these procedures also lead to an improvement in wound-healing. By letting the patient control the anaesthesia (Patient

41

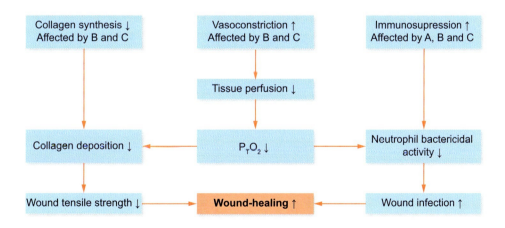

Fig. 41.3 Influence of regional anaesthesia on wound-healing. [F210-025]

Controlled Regional Anaesthesia, PCRA), the anaesthesia procedures can be better oriented to the actual needs of the patient. Negative effects of high-dose oral pain therapy such as sedation, fatigue or immobilisation can thus be reduced. Last but not least, the fact that dressing changes can be performed much more painlessly in this way represents a positive effect for the patient that should not be underestimated.

41.7 Conclusion

The treatment of pain in patients with chronic wounds is an essential part of therapy and a prerequisite for successful wound-healing. Whenever possible, pain should be reduced by prompt treatment of the underlying disease. For wound therapy, external agents can be used to avoid pain or for direct pain therapy. If this is not sufficient, systemic medicamentous pain therapy should be initiated, which should follow the WHO scheme. This drug therapy can be given in individual cases as an individual treatment attempt over several months. Regional anaesthetic procedures can also lead to an improvement in wound-healing in the initial phase of wound therapy in addition to a reduction in pain.

REFERENCES
Buggy D. Can anaesthetic management influence surgical-wound-healing? Lancet 2000; 356: 355–357.
Deutsche Schmerzgesellschaft e.V. S3-Leitlinie, Langzeitanwendung von Opioiden bei nicht tumorbedingten Schmerzen (LONTS), AWMF-Leitlinien-Register Nr. 041/003. www.awmf.org/uploads/tx_szleitlinien/145-003l_S3_LONTS_2015-01.pdf (last accessed 12 October 2020).
Kommission Leitlinien der Deutschen Gesellschaft für Neurologie. S1-Leitlinie Pharmakologisch nicht interventionelle Therapie chronisch neuropathischer Schmerzen, AWMF-Registernummer 030/114. www.awmf.org/uploads/tx_szleitlinien/030-114l_S1_Neuropathischer_Schmerzen_Therapie_2014-abgelaufen.pdf (last accessed 12 October 2020).
Von Korff M, Saunders K, Thomas Ray G, et al. De facto long-term opioid therapy for noncancer pain. Clin J Pain 2008; 24: 521–527.

42

Finja Reinboldt-Jockenhöfer, Anna Lena Kahl, Manfred Schedlowski

Placebo

Key notes

- Mechanisms that control placebo response should be used to optimise the effectiveness of pharmacological interventions and medical treatments in general for the benefit of the patient.
- There are currently no clinical studies that support the theory of a placebo-induced positive influence on wound-healing concerning the ob-

jective parameters. However, there is evidence that subjective parameters, such as quality of life, can be influenced by expectation-induced placebo effects.
- In the future, these aspects should be increasingly taken into account in education and training in the medical professions, but also the effective treatment of patients with wounds.

42.1 Introduction

The word placebo comes from Latin and means 'I shall be pleasing' in the original sense. In the modern medical context, however, a placebo is defined as a sham treatment or a sham drug without a pharmacologically active substance. The so-called placebo effect caused by the use of a placebo, i.e. the positive physiological and psychological changes, is composed of various factors, such as the natural course of the disease and the fluctuation of symptoms, or statistical phenomena, such as regression to the mean. The individual placebo response, which constitutes a significant part of the placebo effect and consists of the following three interdependent components: the patient's expectations regarding a possible therapeutic effect, associative learning processes such as classical conditioning, and the quality and quantity of doctor-patient interaction.

42.2 Placebo effect

The placebo effect only became the focus of medical research in the 1950s with the introduction of controlled randomised trials. In this context, the placebo effect is often seen as a disruptive factor that makes

it difficult to assess the efficacy of pharmacological and non-pharmacological treatments. In pharmaceutical clinical trials, placebos are an indispensable component. They are used to treat a control group for comparison purposes with the premise that either no drug effects or otherwise specific therapeutic effects are produced. Nevertheless, these control groups regularly show effects that are normally only achieved by a specific drug. Assuming that a placebo is a non-pharmacologically active substance, it remains to be explained how a placebo administration produces these effects.

To date, there are far more studies in which placebo groups are used as comparison groups than there are studies on the effect itself. Nevertheless, the scientific and clinical relevance of the placebo response is becoming increasingly important in many areas of medicine. Recent scientific research has shown that a better understanding of the neurobiological and neuropsychological mechanisms of the placebo effect is of enormous importance and has significant implications for clinical practice. These mechanisms underlying the placebo effect have already been studied in healthy subjects as well as in the context of various diseases such as chronic pain and neurological, psychiatric and gastrointestinal diseases.

The research results of these studies document that placebo effects are mainly controlled by cognitive processes such as expectations and associative learning. Thus it could be documented that the clear expectation of a person taking part in the test to receive or not to receive a strong pain medication significantly increased or eliminated the pain-relieving effect of the administered opiate. Conditioned pharmacological reactions, which can also develop without a directed expectation of the patient, were proven in different physical systems, e. g. the pain system, the motor system, the immune system or the autonomous nervous system.

Neuroscientific investigations over the past three decades have impressively demonstrated that these neuropsychological phenomena can substantially influence the overall success of a therapy. In various clinical studies, the administration of placebos documented the reduction of the symptoms of an existing disease and positively impacted the healing process. For example, even the open administration of a placebo, i. e. the pure expectation, substantially reduced the severity of the symptoms in patients with irritable bowel syndrome compared to an untreated control group. Furthermore, in Parkinson's patients, simply the expectation of receiving an effective drug led to an improvement in motor symptoms and additionally to a dopamine release in the striatum. Kidney transplant patients showed increased immunosuppression after implementation of a conditioned placebo response in the existing medication.

However, the significance of expectations and associative learning processes for placebo effects in connection with different physiological systems is still unclear. The neuroscientifically best-investigated placebo response is placebo analgesia. Various studies using imaging techniques of the central nervous system have shown that reduced pain perception is accompanied by activation of the descending pain-inhibiting system and thus reduced activity in the classical pain-processing areas of the brain. Activation of areas such as the pain inhibiting system has been demonstrated to produce placebo responses associated with emotions. The common and different contributions of different brain areas regarding placebo responses affecting other physiological systems are still unclear.

There is also a sizeable interindividual variance in the development of a placebo effect, which manifests itself in varying degrees. While some patients or people taking part in clinical trials respond well to placebo interventions and thus show pronounced placebo responses (responders), others do not respond at all to these interventions (non-responders). In this context, intensive research is currently being conducted into so-called predictor variables, i. e. psychological, neuroendocrine and genetic factors that are associated with a placebo response and have a corresponding predictive value. Thus, psychological variables on the part of patients or subjects, such as anxiety, depression or optimism, seem to explain part of the variance in placebo response. A genetic component could also play a role here. The individual brain anatomy also appears to influence the ability of placebo responses.

42.3 Placebo in wound-healing

There are older studies which show that psychological factors, especially stress and pain, influence wound-healing processes. However, systematic reviews on the significance of expectation-induced placebo effects on wound-healing are scarce.

One study investigated whether the mere expectation of receiving a drug for wound-healing also accelerates it. These were artificial wounds induced by an ablative laser, i. e. acute wounds in 22 healthy men. Wounds were inflicted on both thighs; the verum group received a supposedly innovative wound gel on one side and a neutral, inactive gel on the other. The control group received the latter on both sides. In reality, both groups received an identical, neutral, inactive wound gel. The wound size reduction was determined by planimetry on days 1, 4 and 7 after the trauma and clinically assessed from day nine during the daily dressing changes with the application of the hydrogel. Overall, no significant intra- or inter-individual differences in duration or wound-healing was found in this examination. Thus, this cohort observed no expectation-induced placebo effects regarding wound-healing of acute wounds.

Against the background of these findings, an RCT investigated expectation-induced placebo effects in patients with chronic leg ulcers (duration > eight weeks). It was observed over 12 weeks whether the wound-healing processes, as well as physiological factors, including quality of life, could be influenced by the mediation of an expectation of receiving a new, particularly effective preparation. A total of 20 patients with chronic leg ulcers were recruited and evaluated. Here, too, there were two experimental conditions (each n = 10). The verum group was informed that the applied product was a special new gel preparation that could have a positive effect on wound-healing and any pain; the control group received a particularly closely monitored and detailed documented treatment with the same gel, but with the information that it was a conventional wound gel. The preliminary results document that the objective parameters such as wound surface reduction and pain do not differ in either group. Still, the quality of life of the patients in the verum group, measured by the Wound Qol (quality of life questionnaire), seems to have improved significantly.

42.4 Conclusion

Overall, the experimental and clinical findings to date on placebo response in the various physiological systems and end organ functions document that the mechanisms that control placebo response (effective communication with the patient that influences patient expectations as well as associative learning processes) should be used; specifically, to optimise the effectiveness of pharmacological interventions and medical treatments in general for the patient's benefit. There are currently no clinical studies that support the thesis of a placebo-induced positive influence on wound-healing concerning the objective parameters. However, the studies mentioned above provide first indications that subjective parameters such as quality of life can be influenced by expectation-induced placebo effects.

In the future, these results should be increasingly taken into account in education and training in medical professions, but also for the effective treatment of patients with wounds.

REFERENCES

Bingel U, Wanigasekera V, Wiech K, et al. The effect of treatment expectation on drug efficacy: imaging the analgesic benefit of the opioid remifentanil. Sci Transl Med 2011; 3: 70ra14.

Enck P, Bingel U, Schedlowski M, Rief W. The placebo response in medicine: minimize, maximize or personalize? Nat Rev Drug Discov 2013; 12: 191–204.

Jockenhöfer F, Knust C, Benson S, Schedlowski M, Dissemond J. Influence of placebo effects on quality of life and wound-healing in patients with chronic venous leg ulcers. J Dtsch Dermatol Ges 2020; 18: 103–109.

Schedlowski M, Enck P, Rief W, Bingel U. Neuro-bio-behavioral mechanisms of placebo and nocebo responses: Implications for clinical trials and clinical practice. Pharmacol Rev 2015; 67: 697–730.

Vits S, Dissemond J, Schadendorf D, et al. Expectation-induced placebo responses fail to accelerate wound-healing in healthy volunteers: results from a prospective controlled experimental trial. Int Wound J 2015; 12: 664–668.

Walburn J, Vedhara K, Hankins M, Rixon L, Weinman J. Psychological stress and wound-healing in humans: a systematic review and meta-analysis. J Psychosom Res 2009; 67: 253–271.

42

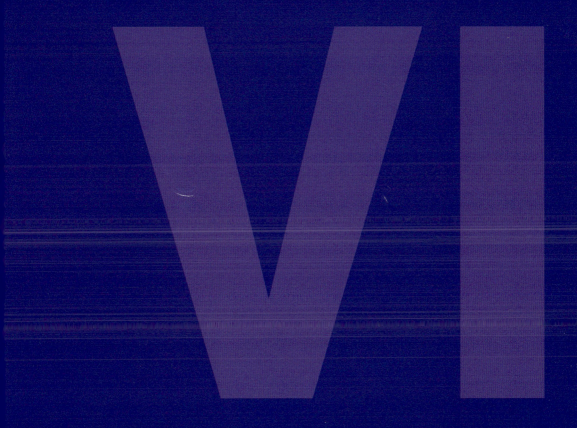

VI Living with a wound

43

Alexander Risse
Body perception

Key notes

- 'Body perception' is a post-platonic, anthropological-dualistic construct.
- The 'subjective body' and 'embodied experience' actually constitute human experience (subjectivity).
- The subjective body is an assemblage of surfaceless spaces, perceived body parts, with a real, specific dynamic in the area of the physical body.
- Asomatognosia is the loss of perception of body parts caused by polyneuropathy and is the only necessary and at the same time sufficient condition of diabetic foot syndrome.
- Subjective facts are stronger than objective facts.

43.1 Introduction

The term body perception presupposes that something (a body) is perceived by something. The thing which is doing the perception is called something else: consciousness, psyche, spirit, mind, reason, and so on. In recent times, the brain is also more frequently presented in this way. With the prevailing Babylonian confusion of language, all authors have an ancient, unquestioned anthropological concept in common: the division of the human being into a body and a soul (consciousness etc.). This concept is called 'anthropological dualism' and was constructed about 3,000 years ago by the philosophers Plato and Aristotle – with far-reaching consequences for human self-understanding. The mind was seen as the primary and essential part that has the task of keeping the inferior body with its impulses and drives under control. The Christian doctrine has reinforced this position and further morally charged it with hostility towards sex and anorexic dietary restrictions. One of the medical specialities holds the Platonic concept in the title: psychosomatic (psycho = self, soma = body).

43.2 The perceived body

A considerable subjective area between body and mind has been forgotten: the perceived body. *'The perceived body* ['Leib' in German] *is defined as that which one feels in the area of one's own body, directly from oneself.'* In our world today, both patients and health care professionals are first and foremost physical; intellectual interpretations are subordinated to physical events. While the academic tradition places too much emphasis on the intellectual dimension and thus overlooks the bodily dimension, the members of professions who deal with the body (wound managers, nursing) are in close contact with this phenomenon, which is often lacking in well defined concepts. Further approaches to the bodily dimension follow below.

43.3 Chronic wounds and their health care professionals

In the problematic horizon of chronic wounds, their treatment and the care of affected patients, the interpretative concept of anthropological dualism reaches its limits, especially in the case of the diabetic foot syndrome. With the usual style of thinking in therapeutic practice, the body is the primary place of action, and the psyche of the patient comes predominantly under scrutiny as a disturbing factor under the concept of 'poor compliance'.

Health care professionals aim for objective results ('objective reality'); patients live in a world of subjective truths. Health care professionals and patients thus consistently meet on entirely different anthropological levels. The significance of this fundamental anthropological conflict for patients and relatives is that they are permanently misunderstood. The significance for health care professionals consists of bewilderment about the patients' behaviour, often with aggressive blaming and shaming as 'poor compliance'. Why do patients not wear their compression stockings? Why do patients walk around on their diabetic foot lesions? How can compliance be improved? Many questions remain unsolved despite enormous technical progress.

In all chronic wounds, the injured physical integrity plays an essential role. The changed body dynamic, i. e. the deep anthropological layer, also determines the course of the disease before any psychological processing.

43.4 Classical psychological interpretations of body perception by the psyche

Psychologists and psychotherapists have also investigated particularities in the behaviour of patients with DFS. In the psychosomatic thinking style of these professional groups, there is also the underlying assumption of the dichotomy of the human being as a psyche and a physical body, with the psyche visualising the adherent physical body. The concepts of 'body image' and 'body image disorders' arise. With this perspective in DFS, there is a disturbed connection between the foot and the brain. Here, deep and differentiated insights into the problem of polyneuropathy are already surfacing: being pain free is bewildering under threatening conditions. The absence of this otherwise reliable symptom of inflammation or vascular problems creates a contradiction between one's own experience and the information conveyed by the doctor: a foot that looks normal and does not hurt is supposed to be severely threatened?

A further approach is attempted with the neurological and psychological conceptualisation of neglect: *'Parts of the body are no longer visualised by the brain, so that they virtually cease to exist.'* Neglect, however, is not appropriate for interpreting patient behaviour, because the outer representation is preserved: patients

can talk about their feet. Further, psychologically comprehensible consequences such as occupational hazard, change of social role, loss of independence, and loss of sexual identity are described. Depressive symptoms are often mentioned.

All these considerations from the usual objectification viewpoint of psychological-reductionist-introjectionist anthropology are helpful but do not offer any clues for understanding the fundamental dynamics.

43.5 Physical body and perceived body

For medical theory and therapeutic practice, therefore, it makes sense to extend anthropological dualism and its concept of 'body perception' through the dimension of the 'perceived body'. To follow the trail of this perceived body, you should try to turn inwards with your eyes closed. You will notice immediately that this does not work continuously as we can touch ourselves. What we encounter here is a loose succession of parts in the area of our physical body: perceived body parts. Constantly present are the perceived body parts of the mouth (oral zone), a genital and anal part and always also the two perceived body parts which are the feet. In some people, a perceived body part that has gone unnoticed for a time becomes very noticeable around noon: the gastral perceived body part (hunger). Accordingly, the consciousness shrinks to only include the immediate present (concentration disorders). The cursory description above can be read in more detail in the extensive literature.

After World War I, perceived body parts as a concept was researched in patients who had to suffer amputations due to war injuries and suffered from 'phantom pain'. Surprisingly, many patients had similar complaints in the area of the amputated, missing limbs. Despite missing that part of the body, the physical sensation persisted: phantom limbs are therefore a perceived body part without being part of a physical body. These psychiatric research results are old and have consequently been forgotten in diabetology and medicine as a whole.

If you follow the concept of perceived body parts and the phenomenon of the perceived body at all, for example in diabetic polyneuropathy – in contrast to the phantom limb experiences (perceived body without physical body) – we now find the 'physical body without the perceived body': one can see the legs, but perceiving them as body parts has disappeared due to polyneuropathy. The body part is no longer viewed with any subjectivity. One could also speak of an 'internal amputation'. This is a condition known as asomatognosia.

Spontaneously, i. e. without thinking, people (patients as well as health care professionals) live in a world of sensations and perceived body parts: the world of subjectivity (subjective reality). It is this world of subjectivity that drives us and urges us to take action: no patient goes to the doctor, for example, with the complaint: *'Doctor, help me, my nerve conduction velocity has decreased, and my lipoprotein lipase is working too slowly!'*

The underlying drama of diabetic (and other) polyneuropathies is that the loss of sensation also leads to a loss of subjectivity in perceiving the body parts which are the feet: people with polyneuropathy treat their feet as if they were environmental components. Not only the warning function of pain is lost, but also the spontaneous concern for the feet. So it is not only a loss of perception – asomatognosia changes the whole person from the ground up.

Polyneuropathy has further consequences. Those affected have the feeling that they no longer have both feet 'on the ground' – when buying shoes, people often choose shoes that are several sizes too small. The reason: the surface sensation is lost; one has the sensation of not wearing a shoe. If the shoes are chosen more tightly, the dull, protopathic pressure that then arises gives you the feeling of security that you are wearing shoes again (subjective reality). In this case, it is not helpful to draw around the feet and compare this with the outline of the shoes (objective reality). The patient's behaviour will not change because it is not the perception that is disturbed, but physical caution. Lost subjectivity and a lack of pain sensation will then also explain why patients no longer wear the prescribed ugly, wide, flat shoes or the annoying orthoses and thus repeatedly end up with injuries by applying pressure. In the hospital, patients stand up shortly after a small amputation – *'Just going to the toilet!'* – and tear open the fresh surgical sutures, etc.

43.6 Consequences for the doctor-patient relationship

Incorrect signal transmission to the therapist due to lost subjectivity of the patient's feet is seen as 'poor patient compliance' from the therapist's point of view. Not only the perception of the patient seems to have changed, but their change in physical caution also seems to change the habitual perception of the doctor. The lost subjectivity of the feet results in completely incorrect signals being transmitted to the treating therapist. Despite sometimes grotesque injuries, the patients are relaxed and give the doctor the indication that everything is fine, there is nothing to worry about. This could explain why even health care professionals often do not act fast enough. Conversely, as long as the health care professionals have the body and mind (psyche) as the starting point, they cannot understand the patient whose subjectivity has been altered by polyneuropathy. They call this behaviour 'bad compliance' and become either aggressive, cynical or resigned. This is especially true when the previous frequently taught training content is repeatedly forgotten at a cognitive level. A deeper, anthropologically correct viewpoint could help here to improve mutual understanding: diabetic polyneuropathy not only leads to a loss of perception but also to the condition of asomatognosia, which changes the whole person. It remains a lifelong threat to the feet of people with diabetes, even after the defective function of that body part has been corrected. It is not a simple problem of nerve conduction, but interferes with the person's subjectivity. Training and other educational measures are therefore not enough.

43.7 HSAN and BID

Patients with hereditary sensory and autonomic neuropathy (HSAN) show similar phenomena as in DFS. In essence, children who are born without feeling pain suffer multiple injuries and mutilations at an early age and have an extremely shortened life expectancy.

Even stronger indications are shown by people who, in a healthy state, do everything possible to get rid of

43

a body part because their underlying perception does not include it. The clinical picture of Body Integrity Disorder (BID; previously called apotemnophilia, 'love to cut off') causes the same lack of understanding in an anthropological-dualistic interpretation as with DFS. In the context of the body, this becomes immediately understandable.

43.8 Conclusion

Radical changes in physical caution and thus in the human being and their living environment in its entirety, such as encountered in polyneuropathy or BID, do not cause a disorder in body perception, i. e. a loss of the perception of the physical body by the psyche. It is instead a disorder caused by asomatognosia which causes a radical change in physical caution

and thus affects the entirety of the person and their living environment.

If patients trigger the counter-transference of incomprehension, bewilderment or even aggression in health care professionals, this is an indication of physical phenomena that go beyond pure body perception disorders.

The concept of body perception has to be investigated in the wider context of the body.

REFERENCES
Brand P, Yancey P. Pain: The gift nobody wants. Zondervan: HarperCollins; 1993.
Risse A. Der etwas andere Zugang zum diabetischen Fuß-Syndrom, angewendete Neue Phänomenologie. In: Uschok A (ed.): Körperbild und Körperbildstörungen. Bern: Hogrefe 2016; 153–165.
Schmitz H. System der Philosophie. Bd. II, Teil 1: Der Leib. Bonn: Bouvier; 1965.
Schöning D. Krankheitserleben bei diabetischem Fußsyndrom und Ulkusrezidiv. Diabetologe 2012; 8: 207–212.
Woods S, Clever HU. Psychologische Aspekte des diabetischen Fußsyndroms.;1; Diabetologe 2006; 2: 18–26.

44

Christine Blome, Matthias Augustin

Health-related quality of life

Key notes

- Chronic wounds have a significant impact on health-related quality of life; it is therefore recommended to have a regular measurement of quality of life.
- Among several standardised questionnaires, the Wound-QoL is the recommended tool for

measurement of the quality of life of patients with chronic wounds.
- Based on the data collected, treatment can be planned and adjusted during the course of treatment when necessary.

44.1 What is health-related quality of life?

While the global quality of life refers to all areas of life, **health-related quality of life** only looks at the aspects that are influenced by health and illness. It analyses a multidimensional construct which represents a patient's well-being and functionality from their own perspective. The dimensions considered may differ depending on the definition and tool used; for example, the impact on an individual's body, emotions, social life, and functional capacity are often included.

There is a distinction between general or generic disease, and a specific disease, in measuring a patient's quality of life. On the one hand, tools that measure the generic quality of life allow a comparison between patients with different diseases, as well as between them and the general population. On the other hand, a disease-specific tool can measure more exactly how the patient's quality of life has been affected by the disease. It enables the clinician to formulate a treatment plan that meets their requirements.

44.2 Why is it important in wound care to measure quality of life?

Chronic wounds have a severe impact on the patient's quality of life, i. e. physically, psychologically and

socially. Examples of physical impairments are pain, reduced mobility, odour, exudate, and sleep problems. Mental stress often arises from perceived dependence, body image changes or the impact on their social life. Besides, there are often occupational stresses and strains caused by the treatment.

Measuring these impairments of the quality of life of patients with chronic wounds is essential and helpful for various reasons. One is that this information allows a more differentiated assessment of the treatment that is needed. For example, depending on the focus of the current limitations, treatment can be adapted, or supportive measures can be adopted. Repeating this measurement of the quality of life during treatment provides information on the success as well as quality control of the current therapy. The subjective feedback from the patients is an essential assessment, in addition to objective measurements by the practitioner. An example is the wound size: from the patient's perspective, the improvement in the quality of life is ultimately decisive for the success of the treatment but it is often only partly correlated to objective measurements. Thus, a patient's subjective benefit of the therapy should not solely be based on the clinical improvement or deterioration of the wound.

Additionally, the assessment of the quality of life in wound care provides a basis for discussion with patients about the stresses and strains they are facing. Practitioner-patient communication can influence patient satisfaction, which allows patient compliance towards therapy. Patient compliance towards treatment plays an important role, for example, in patients with diabetic foot syndrome, because the requirements to be compliant with their diabetes treatment are high and include dietary restriction, smoking cessation, physical activity, medication, and blood glucose monitoring, as well as preventive measures to avoid aggravating existing wounds.

44.3 How can quality of life in wound care be measured?

Usually, the time available for the care of the individual patient is limited. It is therefore recommended to use a simple and time-saving tool to measure their quality of life. The questionnaires should be easy to understand and require little interpretation for both patient and practitioner. Various tools are available for the standardised measurement of quality of life, developed partly for diseases in general, partly for specific indications such as pressure ulcers or diabetic foot ulcers (DFU).

44.3.1 Measuring tools for chronic wounds in general

The short questionnaire 'Wound-QoL', supplemented by the practical tool 'Wound-Act', was developed based on three other, more comprehensive surveys. These are the 'Freiburg Quality of Life Assessment for Wounds' (FLQA-w), the 'Cardiff Wound Impact Schedule' (CWIS) and the 'Würzburg Wound Score' (WWS). These tools are described in more detail below.

The **FLQA-w** measures the wound-specific quality of life with 24 questions, each with five possible answers. It comprises the following dimensions: physical complaints (5 items), everyday life (5 items), social life (3 items), psyche (4 items), therapeutic burden (4 items) and satisfaction (3 items) as well as three 10-step scales on health status and overall quality of life. Apart from the total values for each of these dimensions separately, calculation of an overall value for the quality of life as a whole is possible. Investigations of the measuring accuracy of the FLQA-w showed a sufficient internal consistency with a Cronbach's alpha > 0.85. The results of a repeated measurement

within four weeks ('test-retest reliability') also attest to excellent measuring accuracy. Depending on the comparison tool, convergent validity, i. e. agreement with other questionnaires on related constructs, was also given.

The **CWIS** consists of three scales (dimensions): well-being (7 items), social life (14 items) and physical symptoms and daily living (24 items); five response options are available for each. Two additional items assess the overall quality of life using a ten-step scale. The CWIS refers in particular to the quality of life of people with leg wounds. The original English language version of the CWIS showed convergent validity concerning the generic quality of life tool SF-36, and measurement accuracy indicated that a repeat test of the CWIS after 5–7 days correlated strongly with the first survey (r = 0.86 to 0.93). The CWIS also proved to be valid and reliable for example in the German-language translation: the internal consistency was at Cronbach's alpha = 0.76 to 0.88; the instrument correlated with the SF-36 at medium to high levels and differentiated between subjects with open and healed wounds. However, the people being tested described the tool as challenging to understand.

The **WWS** comprises 17 individual questions and covers the areas of pain, emotions and psychological mood, sleep, finances, everyday life, mobility, holidays, social isolation, feelings of illness or disability, convidence in being healed, fear of amputation, and assessment of reduced life expectancy due to the wound (five-step answers given in each case). There is however only a calculation on the overall value for the quality of life as a whole, no dimension-specific values. There are additional questions about the use of mobility aids or support shoes and the time required for wound care. The convergent validity of the WWS was confirmed for patients with leg wounds by correlating with questionnaires on generic quality of life (Nottingham Health Profile and SF-36). The WWS was also able to map clinical changes more sensitively than the two generic surveys mentioned.

The tools mentioned are either quite extensive with a length of up to seven pages or, in the case of the WWS, do not map different dimensions of quality of life. Thus it prompted the authors of these tools to develop the Wound-QoL jointly. For this purpose, the three questionnaires described above were first answered in the course of routine care of 154 test patients with leg wounds. Based on these data, those items were selected from a total of 92 items that were not redundant in content, covered the most important areas of quality of life, and had good psychometric or measurement theory characteristics. A team of experts optimised and standardised the formulations, possible answers and instructions and derived subscales for individual dimensions using factor analyses.

The thus developed **Wound-QoL** (➤ Fig. 44.1) is composed of 17 questions in three subscales. Question 1–5 refer to physical impairments, e. g. 'In the last seven days my wound hurt', question 6–10 refer to the psyche, e. g. ' … the wound has made me unhappy', and question 11–16 refer to everyday life, e. g. ' … the wound has limited my leisure activities'. Question 17 also records the patient's financial burden due to the wound but was not assigned to any subscale. Five possible answers are available for each question (not at all, a little, moderately, quite a lot, very much).

If a self-assessment of the patient is not possible (e. g. due to cognitive impairment), a related person can assess the patient's quality of life using the Wound QoL. Here it is important to note that representatives tend to evaluate the quality of life somewhat worse than the patients themselves, as initial studies show.

The overall Wound-QoL value is the average value of all items. Subscales can also be calculated and can be useful if a patient assesses his quality of life as very different in the different areas. It allows adjustment of the treatment accordingly. For practical use of the Wound-QoL, the Wound-Act is also available, an additional form developed by wound experts and comprising one page. For each item of the Wound-QoL in which the patient indicates a significant impairment, the Wound-Act can be used to document the corresponding supporting measure taken. The Wound-Act contains various suggestions for these measures.

In the meantime, several validation studies have been investigating the measurement properties of the Wound-QoL. Good internal consistency in all subscales and on the global scale was shown and also the retest reliability, convergent validity and sensitivity to change were confirmed. The instrument can therefore be considered reliable, i. e. accurate in measurement, and valid, i. e. giving the quality of life as a snapshot and mapping it well over time.

44.3.2 Measuring tools for certain types of chronic wounds

The 'Pressure Ulcer Quality of Life Questionnaire' (PU-QOL) is a tool that was developed specifically for assessing the quality of life of people with pressure ulcers. This tool is currently only available in English. However, given the substantial pieces of information for future translation provided by the developers of this questionnaire, it may be assumed that additional language versions will soon be available. The survey is aimed at adult patients suffering from a pressure ulcer of any localisation and severity. It comprises a total of ten subscales (pain, exudate, odour, sleep, vitality, mobility, everyday activities, well-being, self-perception and appearance, as well as social participation) with a total of 81 questions with three possible answers each. The PU-QOL was extensively validated in 400 patients in England – also using modern psychometric methods (Rasch analysis). With an average processing time of 40 minutes, it is possibly less practicable in practice; however, it is possible to collect individual scales of interest separately.

The 'Diabetic Foot Ulcer Scale' (**DFS**) is available specifically for people with diabetic foot ulcers. It maps the dimensions of leisure, physical health, everyday activities, emotions, non-compliance, family, friends, treatment, treatment satisfaction, positive attitude, and finances. Since the original tool is quite extensive with 58 items, the short version **DFS-SF** (Diabetic Foot Ulcer Scale – Short Form) was developed, with 29 items. In the validation studies for both tools, it proved to be internally consistent, reliable, valid and sensitive to change.

Conclusion

A number of easy-to-use and validated questionnaires are now available to measure the health-related quality of life of wound patients. There is a choice between tools for chronic wounds in general and specific tools for DFU or pressure ulcers. The results recorded with these questionnaires can help healthcare professionals to understand patients' needs as well as being better able to evaluate the effectiveness of previous therapy, and to adjust treatment plans accordingly.

44

Wound-QoL questionnaire on quality of life with chronic wounds

The following questions are designed to find out how your chronic wound(s) affect(s) your quality of life.

Please check one box per line!

In the <u>last seven days</u>…

		not at all	a little	mod erately	quite a lot	very much
1	…my wound hurt	O	O	O	O	O
2	…my wound had a bad smell	O	O	O	O	O
3	…the discharge from the wound has upset me	O	O	O	O	O
4	…the wound has affected my sleep	O	O	O	O	O
5	…the treatment of the wound has been a burden to me	O	O	O	O	O
6	…the wound has made me unhappy	O	O	O	O	O
7	…I have felt frustrated because the wound is taking so long to heal	O	O	O	O	O
8	…I have worried about my wound	O	O	O	O	O
9	…I have been afraid of the wound getting worse or of getting new wounds	O	O	O	O	O
10	…I have been afraid of hitting the wound against something	O	O	O	O	O
11	…I have had trouble moving around because of the wound	O	O	O	O	O
12	…climbing stairs has been difficult because of the wound	O	O	O	O	O
13	…I have had trouble with everyday activities because of the wound	O	O	O	O	O
14	…the wound has limited my recreational activities	O	O	O	O	O
15	..the wound has forced me to limit my contact with other people	O	O	O	O	O
16	…I have felt dependent on help from others because of the wound	O	O	O	O	O
17	…the wound has been a financial burden to me	O	O	O	O	O

"Wound-QoL" questionnaire on Health-related Quality of Life in Chronic Wounds | Version English (U.S.), Augustin et al. 2017, Blome et al. 2014

Fig. 44.1 The 'U.S. English Wound-QoL' questionnaire for recording the quality of life in people with chronic wounds. [F1025-001]

REFERENCES

Augustin M, Conde Montero E, Zander N, et al. Validity and feasibility of the wound-QoL questionnaire on health-related quality of life in chronic wounds. Wound Repair Regen 2017; 25: 852–857.

Augustin M, Herberger K, Rustenbach SJ, Schäfer I, Zschocke I, Blome C. Quality of life evaluation in wounds: validation of the Freiburg Life Quality Assessment-wound module, a disease-specific instrument. Int Wound J 2010; 7: 493–501.

Blome C, Baade K, Debus ES, Price P, Augustin M. The "Wound-QoL": a short questionnaire measuring quality of life in patients with chronic wounds based on three established disease-specific instruments. Wound Repair Regen 2014; 22: 504–514.

Gorecki C, Brown JM, Cano S, et al. Development and validation of a new patient-reported outcome measure for patients with pressure ulcers: The PU-QOL instrument. Health Qual Life Outcomes 2013; 11: 95.

Sommer R, von Stülpnagel CC, Fife CE, et al. Development and psychometric evaluation of the U.S. English Wound-QoL questionnaire to assess health-related quality of life in people with chronic wounds. Wound Repair Regen 2020; 28: 609–616.

ACKNOWLEDGEMENT

We would like to thank Ms. Alina Bruhns for her support in the preparation of the manuscript.

45

Alexander Risse

Secondary illness gain

Key notes

- The term Munchhausen syndrome is used too often and senselessly by health care professionals.
- Primary or secondary illness gain is nothing to be ashamed of but needs to be acknowledged.
- Properly treated wounds which are not healing are indicative of self-abuse.
- Artefacts cannot be treated with wound therapy.

45.1 Introduction

When dealing with secondary illness gain in the context of chronic wounds, there is an implication that the patient is resistant to the healing of his wound. Through the further assumption that the patient is deliberately undermining the efforts of the therapist out of personal interest, a strong pejorative or derogatory connotation is formed. Furthermore, it is significant that the term Munchhausen syndrome is generally used by physicians where patient-induced self-injury or another illness seems to be present and it initially presents as an artefact syndrome. Since the healing process of chronic wounds is often complicated and the delusions mentioned above arise occasionally, it is worth taking a closer look at the subject area of illness gain.

45.2 Definitions

Illness gain The benefits which an ill person derives from the circumstance and nature of his illness. Within European culture, someone who is ill can usually count on care and compassion. The distinction between primary and secondary illness gain goes back to Sigmund Freud. He writes: *'Under average conditions, we recognise that the ego gains a certain amount of inner disease through the avoidance of neurosis. In some life situations, this is accompanied by a tangible external advantage, which in reality can be more or less appreciated.'* The interpretations and attempts at explanation thus relate mainly to the treatment of intrapsychic processes relative to mental illness and are therefore far removed from the question of secondary illness gain in the treatment of chronic wounds. Here, the mental health of the patient should always be the first consideration.

Primary illness gain Inner benefits that a patient can draw from his neurotic symptoms and a retreat into the illness; e. g. he can avoid situations that are perceived as painful. Although the symptom itself is unpleasant, it allows him to avoid unpleasant conflict situations or worse.

Secondary illness gain External benefits that a sick person can draw on retrospectively from pre-existing neurotic symptoms, e. g. a disability pension. These are often so blatant that the benefit gained by the illness is mistakenly thought to be the sole cause of the symptoms. In the case of the primary illness gain, the development of the disease symptoms is closely related to the resulting benefit, but with secondary illness gain the symptoms occur initially by chance, e. g. as a result of an accident. However, it is not always possible to draw a sharp line between primary and secondary illness gain. With chronic wounds, it is primarily a physical illness without it being an inter-psychic conflict accompanied by neurotic symptoms, as with a primary illness gain. Even without a neurotic base, the secondary gain from the illness could here come from the fact that socially isolated patients are ensured regular contact with a caregiver because of the chronic nature of their wound treatment. Prof. Siebolds speaks here of the patient's delay in recovery.

Table 45.1 Phenomenology of self-harming illness

1.	Feigned/self-induced symptoms from all medical fields
2.	Striking medical knowledge
3.	High percentage from medical professions
4.	Complicated medical history
5.	Start often after real illness, after trauma, in a life crisis
6.	Socially adapted patients
7.	Significant predominance of the female sex
8.	Addictive need for repeated hospital stays and invasive diagnostic and therapeutic procedures
9.	Noticeable willingness to submit to these measures
10.	Initially an apparent lack of motivation with regard to personal circumstances
11.	Pathological doctor-patient relationship

Wound management in this instance therefore does not need deep psychological considerations to clarify the socio-economic context or the offer of a secure space in which wound treatment can take place without the possibility of any accompanying issues.

Tertiary illness gain   Benefits not achieved by the ill person in question, but by a third party, such as relatives, psychotherapists or healthcare workers. Example: the feeling of being needed. As a rule, all healthcare professions benefit from tertiary illness gain. Related to the topic: in the context of this disorder, patients inflict wounds on themselves, artificially induce symptoms of illness or interfere in a highly negative way with ongoing therapy, e. g. in preventing the healing process of an injury by introducing infectious material into the wound. Although these manipulations take place in a destructive self-dialogue between the patient and his body, they only acquire their interactive significance when doctors become involved. In the context of psychosomatic collusion, secondary and tertiary illness gain, i. e. the interaction between patient and therapist, can lead to a mutually satisfactory chronification of the wound and its treatment, without therapeutic progress having to be achieved or even being sought.

45.2.1 Self-harming illnesses, self-harm, artefacts

These disorders are characterised by the fact that the affected patients feign, aggravate or produce disease symptoms, mainly physical, but also psychiatric. The motivation initially remains unclear. The aim is not to gain certain direct advantages, as is the case with simulation. The behaviour is used to assume the role of the patient, to receive medical treatment and a hospital admission, as well as invasive medical procedures. The leading phenomena shows ➤ Table 45.1.

45.2.2 Factitious disorder

A factitious disorder presents itself when a patient, in social distress or due to an inherent personality disposition, pretends to be ill to escape from distress, or assumes the role of a sick person, in order to achieves defined external benefits. This behaviour usually serves as a form of self-protection and not in conflict with it, although a possible dissocial component must not be overlooked.

45.2.3 Munchhausen and other syndromes

These syndromes are reserved for that particular group of patients with chronic factitious disorders. In addition to secret self-harming with often bizarre physical symptoms, the syndrome is characterised by features of pseudologia phantastica, signs of social uprooting with numerous failed relationships, frequent dissocial developments with delinquency and drug addiction, and extensive wandering from hospital to hospital as the dominant lifestyle. For information on further rare and psychiatric entities (addictive self-harming; deliberate self-harming; Munchhausen-by-proxy; self-harming in the context of psychotic disorders, skin-picking syndrome), please refer to the relevant literature.

45.2.4 Transitions: conscious, unconscious

The transitions from conscious action (delusion) to unconscious neurotic or psychotic processes are fluent. From unconscious to conscious in ascending order are: psychosomatic > hypochondria > self-harming illnesses > eating disorders > conscious > factitious. Artefact syndromes therefore also contain unconscious active components that are difficult to differentiate in an actual medical setting.

45.3 Epidemiology of artefact syndromes

Self-harming illnesses aimed at secondary gain appear to be rare overall, although reports from wound care therapists tend to indicate a greater frequency. The availability of data is patchy, so the number of unreported cases is probably high. The one-year prevalence of artificial disorders is reported to be 1.3–1.8%. In most cases, the diagnosis is made only after months or even years of progression of the illness or not at all. Munchhausen syndrome, 5–10% of the total group of artificial disorders, is extremely rare. American authors estimate the prevalence of artificial disorders at 4% in the general population and 21% in a clinical context. Experts estimate the prevalence to be 0.05–0.4%, with 5–8 times higher prevalence in women. The DSM-5 describes the prevalence of artefacts as unknown, *'presumably because of the deliberate deception in this clinical picture'*, but estimates that about 1% of patients in hospitals show corresponding behaviour. Epidemiological data on self-induced disorders in chronic wounds are lacking.

45.4 Cutaneous artefacts

In scientific literature, the data on dissociative disorders are casuistic and contingent. Dissemond gives a synoptic interpretation of disorders in leg ulcers and other skin diseases.

He regards the following features as significant:
- Cutaneous artefacts describe mental disorders.
- They are autoaggressive actions.
- They occur more frequently in women between the ages of 20 and 40, especially in patients with medical knowledge.
- In some patients, these cutaneous artefacts manifest as a secondary illness gain.
- Use of chemical substances, needles, razor blades or constricting bands.
- Mechanical manipulation by scratching, rubbing or squeezing.
- Cutaneous artefacts are usually located in areas that are easily accessible by hand, circumscribed or striated, well separated from the surrounding skin.
- Often the patient's medical history is already indicative, with prevalence of the word 'overnight'.

Dissemond takes the characteristics mentioned from a European Society of Dermatology and Psychiatry position paper, which has also served as a citation source for many other authors. Again, information on the frequency of occurrence is missing. Most of the papers dealing with self-induced wound disorders refer to patients with defined psychiatric diseases and not to the presumably frequent connection between the delay in wound-healing to the securing of social contacts (wound care therapists, doctor's appointments, etc.), i. e., motivations which can be understood in normal psychological terms and which could easily be clarified with an empathetic discussion.

45.5 Secondary illness gain: a synopsis for wound care therapists

Intrapsychic conflicts and psychiatric illnesses can lead to self-harming illnesses that manifest themselves on the skin or even cause wounds with serious endangerment. Artefact syndromes are a result (rarely: Munchhausen syndrome), in which case a psychotherapist or psychiatrist should be involved therapeutically. To solve the problems with the means of wound care management is not advised. It is the task of the wound care therapist to be mindful if this is the case and, if necessary, to enlist appropriate professional competence. Practitioner reports suggest that even in mentally healthy patients, unconscious, preconscious or conscious actions may be taken to delay the wound-healing process, e. g. mechanical irritation with knitting needles, files, flushing of wound areas, the introduction of dog or cat excrement into the wounds, etc. The secondary gain from the disease then consists – easily understood from a normal psychological point of view – of an attempt to maintain contact with the wound care therapists. Here too, the wound care therapist's task is not to openly, possibly even aggressively, confront the patient's behaviour (harming!), but to deal with the problem in a cautious, empathetic and appreciative manner, possibly without addressing it openly and accepting a delayed healing process, which ensures the integrity and dignity of the patient. In this perspective, secondary illness gain is not a call for detective work, but a phenomenon to which patients are entitled.

REFERENCES

Eckhardt A. Das Münchhausen-Syndrom, Formen der selbstmanipulierten Krankheit. München: U&S; 1989.

Ferrara P, Vitelli O, Bottaro G. Factitious disorders and Munchausen syndrome: the tip of the iceberg. J Child Health Care 2012; 17: 366–374.

Freud S. Vorlesungen zur Einführung in die Psychoanalyse. Ges. Werke Bd. 11. Frankfurt: S. Fischer; 1944.

Kapfhammer HP. Artifizielle Störungen und Simulation. In: Möller HJ, Laux G, Kapfhammer HP (Hrsg.): Psychiatrie und Psychotherapie. Heidelberg: Springer 2003; 1456–1457.

Willi J. Die Zweierbeziehung. Reineck Hamburg: Rowohlt; 1990.

VII

Structures

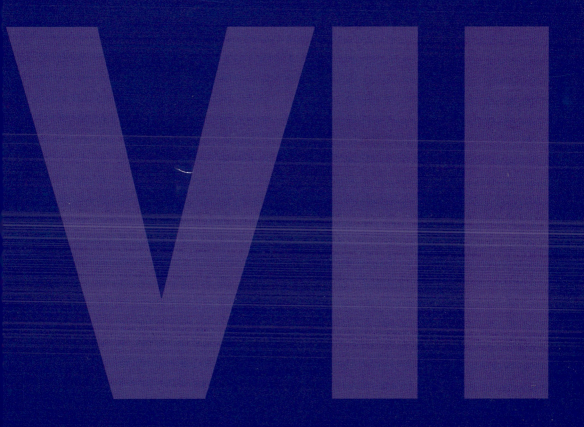

46

Kerstin Protz, Finja Reinboldt-Jockenhöfer

Wound documentation

46.1 Wound anamnesis and assessment

Key notes

- Well-executed and comprehensible wound documentation is an essential basis for communication among the relevant health care providers in the treatment process.
- Wound documentation is a communication tool that prevents breaks in therapy and supports patient care.
- Photographs support the written wound documentation, but are not an adequate substitute.

- Photographs enable a visual diagnosis of the wound, may be necessary for billing purposes, support telemedicine, can visualise the healing process and make it comprehensible as a series of images.
- Conventional photographs are not able to capture wounds three-dimensional, and depict pockets or fistulas.

46.1.1 Introduction

In many countries, the (model) professional code of conduct for physicians (and nurses) makes it mandatory to document the measures taken. It is a reminder for the practitioner and is in the patient's interest as a proper documentation of his therapy. Accordingly, this must be made available for inspection on request.

Wound documentation is the basis for coordinated therapy. It represents the type of measures carried out, guarantees the verifiability of the activities performed and is the basis for uniform wound treatment. In addition, it monitors the healing process and provides necessary facts for a prognosis assessment. Problems are quickly recorded and can be remedied. Adequate wound documentation makes the treatment process comprehensible for all professional groups involved in care, prevents interruptions in care and counteracts interface problems. In addition to its functions as a means of coordination and billing, it is also an essential component of quality assurance.

In the event of a legal dispute, complete documentation is considered as proof of the work done ('What is not documented is considered not done'). The work carried out personally and promptly must always be

recorded in the documentation, within 24 hours. This can neither be done in advance nor delegated to colleagues. If a hand sign legend is available, a hand sign is sufficient as signature. The hand sign legend must be updated annually, as the handwriting changes over time. New employees register immediately. If corrections have to be made, they must be marked accordingly. The use of correction fluid, oversticking, blackening or even the removal and rewriting of entire pages can be legally consideredas a forgery of documents. Facilities that fail to provide the necessary written documentation for the supply process can be threatened with recourse claims and termination of the treatment contract in the event of damage.

Wound documentation serves in many respects as a legal safeguard. For example, if the patient refuses care or aspects of it, the therapist also records this in the documentation. If the patient refuses, the risks of his decision must be presented to him in a comprehensible manner. This instruction must also be recorded in the documentation.

In addition to legal protection, wound documentation also facilitates the transfer of relevant information and helps with the organisation. Standardised wound documentation enables the presentation of the wound care performed in the care process and thus ensures the quality of treatment. This increases the safety in care. Even after long periods of absence of the treating physician, e. g. due to vacation or illness, the treatment is immediately apparent from the documentation. The practitioner may understand what has to be considered therapeutically and when and with which materials the wound care has to be carried out. Problems such as complications or allergic reactions are promptly recorded and treated. This increases the quality of care and ensures the continuity of therapy. Wound documentation is part of the whole documentation within the framework of the treatment and care contract. It includes the initial assessment, the healing process and the course of therapy.

46.1.2 Preconditions

Specialised knowledge is required to meet the preconditions of wound documentation, such as wound assessment, presentation of the healing process and identification of problems. It includes comprehensive knowledge of the anatomy and physiology of the skin, development of wounds, phases and stages of wound healing, knowledge of the current state of science and proper documentation. Only a fundamental knowledge about these aspects enables adequate recording of the facts to be included in the wound documentation.

Wound documentation forms the basis of the therapeutic and nursing care of people with chronic wounds. The external form of the wound documentation sheet prevents any problems that may arise when filling it out. Simple wound documentation sheets help to record progression, simply, clearly and promptly. The data should be entered predominantly by ticking the appropriate box. Free text fields bear the danger of 'writing novels', which makes it difficult to understand progressions quickly or at all. The pre-formulated, generally understandable definitions of a checkbox avoid subjective assessments such as 'wound stains', 'looks good', 'seems okay' etc. Conspicuous features that are not defined by the pre-formulated descriptions on the sheet should be entered, for example, under the field 'other' or recorded in the general documentation sheet. Such wound documentation sheets prevent possible comprehension problems caused by language, typeface and printout. A further advantage is that changes can be recognised promptly at first glance. Therefore, only one wound per sheet should be documented.

Currently there are no generally valid, standardised wound documentation sheets in most countries. Each institution and practice often works out and implements its own documentation sheets, tailored to individual priorities, within the framework of a working group.

46.1.3 Medical and nursing wound anamnesis

The facts recorded in the wound anamnesis form the basis for adequate wound documentation. It includes information about the social environment, the clinical picture, psychosocial aspects and factors that trigger wounds and have a negative influence on healing. Exemplary contents are:

Patient/relatives knowledge about:
- Cause of wound(s)
- Importance of special measures, e. g. compression therapy, exercise, pressure distribution
- Symptoms, e. g. wound moisture, odour, itching
- Wound-healing and estimated time for recovery

Wound- and therapy-related limitations, e. g.:
- Pain, e. g. strength using a visual analogue scale or by external assessment, quality, localisation, duration, frequency, previous experience with pain relief measures, situation-related occurrence
- Mobility/activity restrictions, e. g. climbing stairs, going shopping
- Unpleasant odours, exudate quantities, itching, oedema
- Difficulties with personal hygiene
- Dependence on other/external help
- Psychosocial aspects, e. g. frustration, grief, depression, social isolation, fears, worries
- Restrictions on the choice of clothes and shoes
- Sleep disorders

Pre-existing wound-related aids:
- Donning devices, medical compression stockings, orthotic shoe care, pressure-relieving mattresses, seat cushions and positioning aids

Self-management skills of patients/relatives for:
- Dealing with restrictions caused by wounds and therapy (see above)

- Dressing changes
- Nutrition
- Blood glucose adjustment
- Smoking cessation
- Vascular sports
- Skin protection and care
- Decongestive measures, such as activation of the muscle pumps, raising the legs above heart level
- Maintaining mobility and everyday activities, e. g. walks, hobbies, shopping
- Disease-specific measures, e. g. foot care and in-spection, movement exercises, compression therapy

In addition, the following information should be taken into account:

- Age
- Medication
- Allergies
- Social environment, e. g. how and with whom does the patient live (ground floor, staircase without elevator, relatives, etc.). Are they self-employed, or do they need help? Who has cared for the patient up to now (medical, domestic, nursing)?
- Immune status, tumours
- Concomitant and metabolic diseases, surgical in-terventions
- Recording of the mental and spiritual state
- Living habits, e. g. smoking, alcohol, sport
- Information about the clinical picture and atti-tude towards it
- Continence situation

46.1.4 Wound assessment: criteria of wound documentation

Wound documentation illustrates both the previous treatment process and the healing process or current condition of the wound. Exemplary contents for a wound assessment or a wound evaluation are:

- **Medical wound diagnosis:** underlying disease, wound type/classification and severity of the wound or underlying disease.
- **Examples of wound classification:** e. g. venous leg ulcer/arterial/mixed, diabetic foot ulcer, pres-sure ulcer, burn, postoperative wound-healing disorder.
- **Examples of severity classification:** pressure ulcer classification, e. g. according to European

Pressure Ulcer Advisory Panel (EPUAP), classifi-cation of diabetic foot ulcer according to Wagner/Armstrong, classification of chronic venous in-sufficiency (CVI) according to Widmer or CEAP, classification of peripheral arterial desease (PAD) according to Fontaine or Rutherford.

- Previous diagnostic and therapeutic measures for wound care and the underlying disease.
- **Wound location:** formulated in writing and also via a diagram; photograph taken if necessary.
- **Wound duration:** necessary to estimate stress, treatment times and healing time for the patient.
- **Recurrences:** recording of number and recur-rence-free time; allows indications of possible problems in prevention.
- **Wound size:** gauging by using the perpendicular method, e. g. 'six o'clock' or 'twelve o'clock', i. e. the greatest length and width (at 90° to the length) in cm, depth in cm, recording of pockets/under-mining/fistulas using clock terms.
- **Wound margin/surrounding area:** e. g. under-mined, vital, macerated, livid, necrotic, edema-tous, bulging, reddened, itching, dry, cracked.
- **Wound base/tissue type:** e. g. necrosis, fibrin coating, granulation tissue, bone, tendon.
- **Wound odour:** yes/no.
- **Exudation:** quantity, texture, colour.
- **Signs of infection:** redness, swelling, overheat-ing, impaired function, pain.
- **Wound pain:**
  - Intensity based on, e. g. visual analogue scale, smiley scale, numerical ranking scale, verbal rating scale or by external assessment.
  - Situations associated with pain and those that lead to improvement.
  - Quality: e. g. throbbing, burning, piercing.

It should also contain information about the medi-cation, such as full product name and given quantity (e. g. required for repeat order), date and signature of the person performing the treatment.

Wound documentation should include each dressing change and the noticeable differences to the previous condition. A complete wound assessment that includes wound measurement, is performed at chronic wounds at the latest after two to four weeks and additionally after wound-related interventions or acute changes, e.g. surgical debridement, infec-tion. In acute wounds, weekly wound assessment

46

with wound measurement is required. Additionally, there should be a routine review and documentation on the effectiveness of all measures at intervals of no more than four weeks. Any necessary changes should also be included in the plan of action and the wound documentation.

Individual assessment criteria are included in more detail below.

Size of the wound

The change in wound size is regarded as an essential factor in assessing the healing process. Description of the wound size should not include statements which are no exact specifications such as 'palm-sized', 'tomato sized', 'pinhead' or 'pound coin-sized'. Statements such as 'wound looks good', 'wound without findings', do not belong in wound documentation, due to lack of meaningfulness.

Wound measurement is usually measured with a disposable paper ruler (➤ Fig. 46.1). However, this method cannot depict the shape of a wound. Multiple possible measuring instruments such as stoma calipers, riveted plastic rulers and templates cannot be disinfected properly or only with great effort and expense, thus encouraging the spread of germs. Therefore these instruments should not be used.

As an alternative to the above-mentioned perpendicular method of **measurement**, the most significant distance between the wound edges is calculated vertically (length → foot-head-axis) and horizontally (width). The length and width axes are at a 90° angle to each other when measuring. The corresponding part of the body is both written out and illustrated with a stylised drawing. For this purpose, many wound documentation sheets/systems schematically depict a human body on which the exact localisation can be indicated. The team must agree on the measurement points and must not take measurements at other points at every wound inspection.

One method that is not using the body axes but the orientation of the wound is the **clock method.** Regardless of the position of the wound, the longest extension is measured here. To do this, the alignment of the clock should be defined as clearly as possible within the team. The orientation is the face of the clock, i. e. twelve o'clock points towards the head, six o'clock towards the foot.

Tracing the outline of the wound as accurately as possible helps to give a more precise idea of the wound, for which a sterile double-sided film can be used. The film is applied to the wound and a waterproof pencil is used to trace its contours without exerting too much pressure (pain trigger!). When using a double-sided sterile film, the upper, non-contaminated part can be filed in the wound documentation. The contaminated adhesive side remaining on the wound will be disposed after use. In addition, the preparation date and the location of the wound should also be included. The use of a film with a grid can also provide information on the wound area by recording the number of boxes (➤ Fig. 46.2). One box corresponds to a size unit of 1 cm². Every box of which more than half has

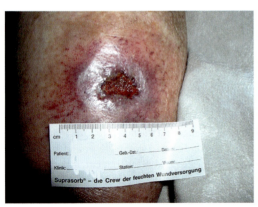

Fig. 46.1 Measurement of the wound with disposable paper ruler. [M291]

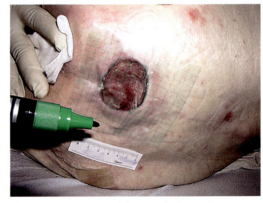

Fig. 46.2 Measurement of the wound using tracing or planimetry. [M291]

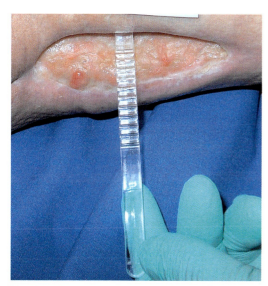

Fig. 46.3 Measurement of the wound depth with sterile tweezers. [M291]

been marked is considered counted. This procedure is called **tracing** or **planimetry**. This method can also be carried out by computer. In addition, various computer programs for wound documentation are available, which independently calculate the wound area after a punctiform recording of the wound margin (by defining a size scale, e.g. disposable paper ruler).

Wound depth

There are various possibilities for determining the depth of the wound, such as sterile tweezers (➤ Fig. 46.3), sterile scaled probes, sterile button cannulas or sterile irrigation catheters. If the wound is undermined, the deepest wound location is measured in each case.

Caution: the use of sterile cotton swabs is not recommended as they may leave residues in the wound.

With **undermined wounds,** it is advisable to use the clock face as a guide when specifying the location of each wound pocket. On the feet or hands, toes and fingertips are defined as 'twelve o'clock', with heel and wrist defined as 'six o'clock'.

The so-called **calibration method** determines the volume of the wound in millilitres. The wound is firstly covered with a sterile transparent film; then warmed Ringer's/or physiological saline solution is injected into the wound using a syringe and cannula. The volume of the wound in millilitres can be read off the syringe scale.

Caution: this elaborate method is cost-intensive, as it requires a great deal of time and material. It also has the potential to injure the patient and is often perceived as unpleasant. If the patient lies in a different position to when the method was previously done, the result can be different.

Wound exudate

Wound exudate varies according to the wound condition, size, phase, stage and clinical picture of the wound. The amount of exudate is a relative quantity and cannot be described objectively. Terms such as amount, medium, moderate, low or less describe only subjective perceptions. The treatment team should agree on the respective meaning. An indication of the amount of exudate can be given by the frequency of dressing changes, the number of soaked dressings and the choice of material, with regard to its absorbency, absorption capacity and retention. A corresponding definition of the in-house standard facilitates the assessment. The exudate should also be assessed for colour ➤ Table 46.1) and consistency (➤ Table 46.2).

Wound margin

The appearance of the wound margin allows conclusions to be drawn about the healing process and, in some cases, about the aetiology. Here, for example, bleeding, hyperkeratosis or necrosis occurs. Wound documentation includes wound margin conditions, which can, for instance, appear livid, hyperkeratotic, undermined, edematous, reddened or macerated.

Periwound skin

The assessment of the wound environment also allows conclusions to be drawn about the healing process and, in some cases, about the aetiology. Here there are indications, e. g. of infection, skin

46

Table 46.1 Exudate colours and their possible meaning*

Transparent, clear, amber	Cloudy, milky or cream	Red, pink
Normal, serous appearance or, e. g. due to lymphatic/urinary tract fistula	Fibrin threads due to inflammation, infection	Blood cells in exudate, e. g. from injury
Yellow, brown	**Green**	**Grey, blue**
Intestinal/urethral fistula, residues from wound dressings, e. g. hydrocolloid dressing, scab components	Infection by *Pseudomonas aeruginosa*	Residues of wound dressings containing silver

* Photos: [M291], at the bottom right: [O1014]

Table 46.2 Possible causes of different exudate viscosities

Thick, sticky or high viscosity	Thin, weeping or low viscosity
• High protein content due to an inflammatory process • Residues of dressing material, e.g. hydrocolloid dressing or topical preparations • Necroses in autolysis • Secretion from intestinal fistula	• Low protein content, e.g. due to malnutrition, venous disease or decompensated cardiac disease • Secretion from lymphatic fistula, joint fistula or urinary tract fistula

care status, exudate management, inadequate pressure distribution or skin lesions due to insufficient compression therapy. Wound documentation should include periwound skin, which can, for example, appear dry, scaly, overheated, hyperpigmented, eczematised or macerated.

Wound bed

The wound bed allows conclusions to be drawn about the healing process. The type of tissue is determined, e.g. necrosis, sclerosis, fibrin, granulation and the extent of the affected tissue layers, e.g. epidermis, dermis, subcutis, exposed structures such as bone, tendon or muscle. Colour models should not be used as they are too imprecise. For example, the colour black indicates necrosis. In a softened state, however, it can also be yellow. However, tendon and bone structures or fibrin coatings are also yellow.

Wound odour

Among other things, the wound odour allows conclusions about the microbiological status of a wound. It also has serious effects on the patient's quality of life. An atypical wound odour should be documented with 'yes/no'. Specifications such as sweet, sour, putrid, septic, stinking or faecal refer to subjective impressions and are not precise. A statement about wound odour should therefore be limited to whether or not it is present.

46.2 Wound photograph(y)

46.2.1 Introduction

In addition to the written wound assessment, the documentation with digital photographs serves to illustrate the care provided.. A frequently expressed reservation about digital photo documentation is the possibility of manipulation. Nevertheless, digital photographs are valid in court, as alteration can happen in any type of documentation.

A prerequisite for wound photography is following the legal aspects. Photographic documentation has the advantage of monitoring the healing processes visually in an understandable way and a non-contact manner. There are limitations in recording the three-dimensionality of a wound because the full extent of ducts, fistulas, wound pockets/cavities and colours cannot be shown adequately. Photographs do not replace written documentation; they can only be supplementary. They are also the basis for wound assessment in the context of telemedicine. This is becoming increasingly important, particularly in rural areas with few specialists, in areas where hardly any specialists are available due to structural requirements, and in inpatient care for the elderly.

Photo documentation must meet specific criteria. It serves to visualise the current state of the wound and illustrates the healing process, whereby the sequence of images can be considered as a follow-up. It applies particularly to discharge or transfer reports.

A photo of a wound is taken **after** wound cleansing, unless certain conspicuous features, e. g. in the dressing material, are to be recorded in advance. The size of the wound should also be apparent. It can be ensured, for example, by including a disposable paper ruler when taking a photograph. The disposable paper ruler should not be white, because the scales, numbering and notes will not be visible in the photograph, especially when using a flash. For this reason, the disposable paper ruler should have a slight colouring, e. g. yellow, grey, etc. A patient code or the patient's name, first name and date of birth, the date of the photograph and the wound location must be written on the ruler for each photo, to ensure that it can correctly be assigned to the relevant patient. In the clinic, patient labels with all the data are available for this purpose.

46

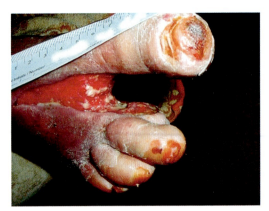

Fig. 46.4 Shadowing. [M291]

The photo documentation must also be comprehensible. Using a macro function with an identical incidence of light (flash if necessary), the same resolution and distance, and taken from the same angle, should be consistent when taking wound photography. The photographer must make sure that the incidence of light and the perspective do not cast any disturbing shadows on the subject (➤ Fig. 46.4), which may be misinterpreted afterwards as necrosis, pockets or similar. The patient should always lie or sit in the same position. The use of a neutral, calm background, e. g. by using surgical towels or other unicolored towels (➤ Fig. 46.5a), strengthens the significance of the photo. The surface/background should be uniform, but not white (➤ Fig. 46.5b), to prevent white balance problems while using the flash.

The fundamental prerequisite for photo documentation is the consent of the patient or, if applicable, his relatives or caregivers. The patient should be adequately informed about the reason for the execution of the photographs as well as where they are kept. The patient can revoke his consent at any time, and it must be recorded in writing in the patient's file and enclosed with the documentation. Photo documentation should also be carried out at least every four weeks in the case of chronic wounds, as well as in the case of severe changes in the wound situation. It is advisable to draw up an internal standard within the institution regarding the requirements for the respective criteria for taking photographs.

46.2.2 Preconditions and procedure

- Educate and inform the patient about the photo and where it will be kept.
- Obtain the consent of the patient or the legal guardian and record it in writing in the file; the consent can be revoked at any time.
- Retroactive consent should be established in exceptional cases, e. g. to collect evidence in case of relocation, or photos taken before obtaining consent. If the patient refused, discard the photographs accordingly.
- Always use the same camera.
- Always take photos under the same conditions in order to make them meaningful.

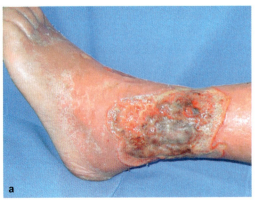

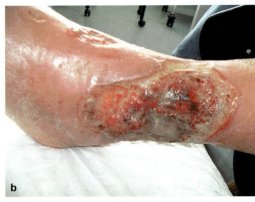

Fig. 46.5 a Wound situation is clearly recognisable against a neutral, calm background; **b** wound against a white, restless background. [M291]

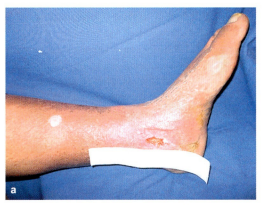
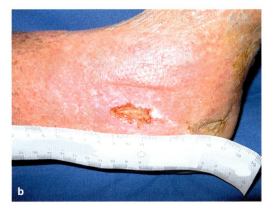

Fig. 46.6 a Creation of an overview image; **b** Creation of a close-up. [M291]

- The photo must be assignable to the relevant patient: note the patient code, patient label, or name and date of birth next to the date of creation.
- Use a disposable measuring paper ruler or graduated photo card to indicate the size and course of the wound; if necessary, indicate the body area/side; always place the measuring paper ruler in the same place.
- To avoid measuring errors, mark points of the wound measurement on the photo if necessary.
- Take one close-up and one overview photo (➤ Fig. 46.6).
- Always take the photo after wound-cleansing (➤ Fig. 46.7). Exception: recording of certain conspicuous features in advance.
- Use a neutral, calm background, e. g. use a monochrome cloth (not white because of problems with the white balance; ➤ Fig. 46.5a).
- Ensure sufficient image sharpness, both at the wound and the surrounding area; use macro or automatic focus and image stabiliser.
- Avoid creating shadows.
- Ensure that lighting conditions are the same as for previous shots, with realistic colour reproduction and high resolution.
- Ensure that the distance, angle (parallel to the point of exposure) and position of the patient are the same as in previous exposures; after initial exposure, note these details in the documentation.
- The decision of taking a close-up or overview image without (➤ Fig. 46.8) or with flash (➤ Fig. 46.9) depends on the lighting conditions;

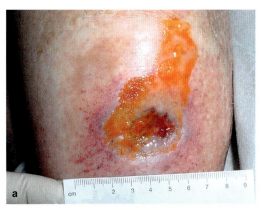
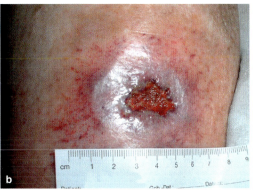

Fig. 46.7 a Photo documentation before wound-cleansing; **b** Photo documentation after wound-cleansing. [M291]

subsequent shots should stick to this decision. Always take wound photographs at the same time of day and under the same lighting conditions; avoid reflections/mirroring by the flash; if necessary, provide supporting lateral lighting.

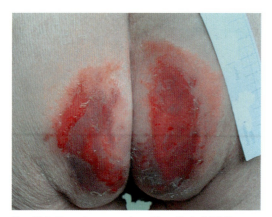

Fig. 46.8 Photo documentation without flash. [M291]

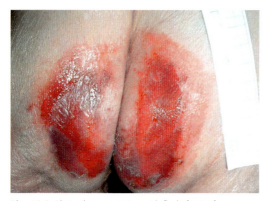

Fig. 46.9 Photo documentation with flash. [M291]

- The wound should take up at least one-third of the photo.
- Finally, ensure the photo is assigned correctly to the corresponding patient file.

46.2.3 Technical preconditions

A digital camera should have the following functions and features:
- Flash and macro function; a ring flash would be ideal (weigh up within the institution for cost-effectiveness).
- Large LCD (at least 2 inches, i.e. 5.1 cm diagonal), so that it is possible to check the suitability of the image immediately.
- The standard resolution for taking photographs should be at least 1,984 × 1,488 pixels (3 MB).
- Automatic recording of date and time.

- Image stabiliser.
- Sufficiently large external memory card.
- Computer criteria include archiving software with search function, camera connection options such as USB, colour printer and photo paper.
- To trace subsequent changes, the archiving software must be able to control changes and make them visible in the system.

Photos should be downloaded from the memory card and saved daily if possible on an external medium.

> **Tip**
>
> The printed image may vary depending on the processing software, printer and paper used. There are limits to the photo documentation for specialised wound courses, such as undermining or fistula tract. Such wound conditions can be clarified by adding sterile tweezers (➤ Fig. 46.3) or transparent film laid over the wound area with drawn-in markings.

Three-dimensional wound photography

Three-dimensional (3D) wound photography is a method in image documentation in which three planes are photographed, recording the following parameters:
- Length
- Width
- Depth

Calculation of the scope and volume is possible with this information. Over time, it is then possible to display statements, such as area reduction, average depth or maximum size.

With the two-dimensional (2D) surveying techniques used so far, usually only length and width are recorded. These methods are highly variable, particularly in their interrater-reliability, i.e. the extent to which the results match those of different performers, so that new combined systems for more precise wound observation, evaluation and documentation were required and are now available with 3D wound photography.

One of these 3D systems will be presented below as an example. The Silhouette system (ARANZ Medical, Christchurch, New Zealand) consists of a 3D camera that connects to a computer which has had special software installed (➤ Fig. 46.10). The system enables 3D wound photography with measurements on

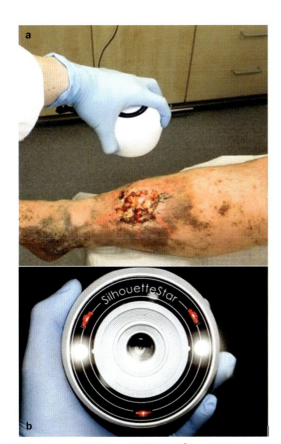

Fig. 46.10 a ARANZ Medical Silhouette® Application example; **b** Camera underside with three lasers, two LED flashes and the 3D camera. [T1060]

all three planes and a documentation system with its patient database. Due to its small size (100 × 67 mm) and weight (240 g), and its spherical structure, the camera can be operated with one hand. A five-megapixel camera sits in the middle of the casing, which has automatic exposure with two LED flashes (10,000 Lux each) and a fixed focus for the fastest possible (1.2 seconds release time) and uncomplicated photo documentation. Accordingly, the maximum working distance (distance camera – wound) is specified by the system. Three lasers are arranged at equal distances around the camera and meet at the optimum working distance of 235 mm (max. 285 mm) at a point where the most significant possible measuring accuracy and image quality are achieved. On the side of the casing, there is a button for one-handed use of the camera. The photo that is taken is immediately transferred to the PC and stored in the system.

Obtaining a 3D photo of a wound uses the same procedure as for a 2D photo. It means that every 2D photo created with the system contains the data required for a 3D measurement.

The system specifies photo-taking parameters in terms of distance, autofocus, exposure and resolution. The system can measure a wound by using the computer mouse to define the wound margin, or a special pen for a touch screen, to record the above parameters. The creation of a 3D photo, including the measurement, takes about one minute, depending on the size of the wound. The minimum wound size is two × 2 mm, and the maximum wound size is 250 × 180 mm, because the camera lens in combination with the fixed lasers has a defined field of view. The user creates a patient record for each patient, which can contain any amount of patient information.

Documenting a new wound in this system will require the anatomical location of the wound so that the system can automatically assign it correctly and provide reports with as much wound information as possible. After creating a 3D wound photo, the wound is defined manually on the computer by moving the mouse around the wound margin. The system calculates the above measurement data, which is then entered into the patient's medical record, and compares it with previous measurements so that changes in size are calculated simultaneously as a percentage by the system. Furthermore, this data can be presented as graphs for a more accurate display. If an overview report is required, the program creates a clear PDF report with all available patient/wound data, photos and graphs (➤ Fig. 46.11).

46.3 Electronic Data Processing (EDP)-supported wound documentation

For the requirements of timely data transfer, especially in the case of patient discharge and transfer, computer-assisted wound documentation is a helpful organisational tool. Such systems are of great importance for interdisciplinary and interprofessional cooperation and networking of the persons involved in wound care. They guarantee the prompt, transparent

46

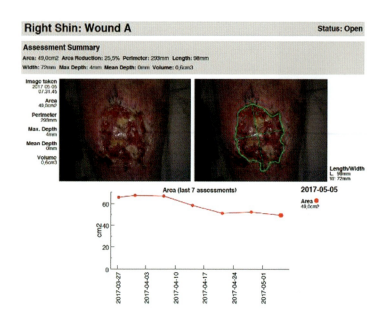

Fig. 46.11 Documentation system with created PDF report of an example wound (patient data was removed for data protection reasons). [T1060]

and comprehensive exchange of relevant data, enable continuous therapy and prevent interface problems. The patient's declaration of consent is a prerequisite for the transfer of their data to third parties. After querying the primary wound data, some such programs offer a selection of the wound care products and calculate the respective costs once selected. The working time required for wound care is one of the accounting factors. The data can also be used for statistical analysis. The results and progressions of the Electronic Data Processing (EDP)-supported documentation are easily retrievable, uncomplicated to process, send and duplicate, for example, the discharge/treatment and transfer reports. It is superior to handwritten documentation if the system is established within a network, as the entries are sent by remote data transmission. Secure connections are a prerequisite for this. Also, different access rights for various professional groups/providers are possible.

Usually, digital wound images can be included in the EDP-supported documentation. The size scale is defined, individual points at the margin of the wound

are marked on the digital photo by a mouse and the distance and position of these points are used to determine the **size of the wound area**. This procedure allows more precise results than measuring or copying by hand.

REFERENCES

Chiang N, Rodda OA, Kang A, Sleigh J, Vasudevan T. Clinical evaluation of portable wound volumetric measurement devices. Adv Skin Wound Care 2018; 31: 374–380.

Dissemond J, Bültemann A, Gerber V, Jäger B, Kröger K, Münter C. Diagnosis and treatment of chronic wounds: current standards of Germany's Initiative for Chronic Wounds e.V. J Wound Care 2017; 26: 727–732.

Kieser DC, Hammond C. Leading wound care technology: The ARANZ medical silhouette. Adv Skin Wound Care 2011; 24: 68–70.

Protz K. Moderne Wundversorgung. 9. A. München: Elsevier; 2019.

Röhlig HW, Nusser B. Rechtliche und praktische Aspekte der Wundbehandlung und -dokumentation. WundForum 2010; 2: 9–19.

Wundzentrum Hamburg e.V., Standards. www. wundzentrum-hamburg.de/standards.

47

Veronika Gerber

Requirements in wound management

47.1 Requirements for a wound team

Key notes

- People with chronic wounds need tailored care, structured around their complex requirements and tasks.
- Caring for people with chronic wounds requires an interprofessional and cross-facility team, which can only function if all players are well trained.

- The greater the number of people who are involved in the treatment of a patient with a wound, the more important it is to clarify everybody's responsibilities. Documentation plays an essential role in communication and securing of information.
- The structure of the wound management depends on the institution.

47.1.1 Introduction

People with chronic wounds need tailored care, structured around their complex requirements and tasks. A mere look at the wound will only clarify some of the requirements. A careful analysis of the causes, treatment for the causes (local as well as accompanying therapy) and patient eduction are required to achieve sustainable success. It also involves putting together an interprofessional and interdisciplinary wound team, operating across all facilities. In addition, hospitals need internal regulations to govern the various responsibilities in the diagnosis and treatment of chronic wounds. Here, the establishment of an in-house wound management system with freelance nursing wound experts and an assigned specialist has proved to be a success. This chapter focuses on the presentation of an internal clinic wound team. The presented case study below demonstrates the complexity of the subject. ➤ Chap. 47.2 will show the approaches for channeling cooperation across institutions.

47.1.2 The case-related team

Caring for people with chronic wounds requires many practitioners. As an example, a patient with a diabetic foot ulcer illustrates the complexity of the team

involved: Mrs. X, 64 years old, comes to the intensive care unit with sepsis caused by a previously undiscovered foot ulcer (➤ Fig. 47.1). She is almost blind due to diabetes, which has been poorly controlled for decades and her polyneuropathy is severe. The **internal medicine specialist** treats the sepsis; the **diabetologist** adjusts the completely derailed blood sugar level; and the **trauma surgeon** is consulted on the first day to plan any amputation that may be necessary. The **nursing ward team** takes over the intensive care measures, and the **wound care specialist** of the clinic works together with the diabetologist on the wound care. In this case, negative pressure therapy is applied after wound debridement.

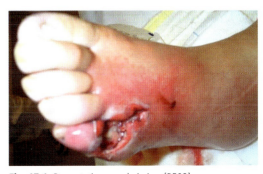

Fig. 47.1 Presentation on admission. [P592]

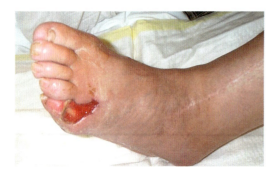

Fig. 47.2 Discharge condition, 14 days after admission to hospital. [P592]

The patient is transferred to the internal ward after seven days, where the diabetologist is involved. The wound expert continues to carry out the dressing changes with a PU foam dressing which is sufficient, as the infection has completely subsided. Amputation was not necessary. The patient's involvement starts now: the **dietary assistant** provides a diabetes consultation. The wound expert includes advice on shoe care, and discusses dressing changes at home with the patient and her caregiver who will support her with everyday tasks (➤ Chap. 48). The patient is discharged to her home on day 14 (➤ Fig. 47.2).

A home **nursing service** which assesses the wound and carries out dressing changes as well as providing instructions for skincare, is activated. The **general practitioner** monitors the state of health. The **resident diabetologist** will monitor the patient's diabetic control and take care of the insulin dosage; reports are linked to the clinic. The **wound care centre** prescribes the dressings and adjusts local wound care. A **podologist** takes over the complex podological treatment and checks the feet for lesions or other abnormalities in the long term. The patient is instructed by the wound expert to shake out her shoes before putting them on and to feel whether the little toe is in the correct position, as there is damage to the toe lifter tendon. The composition of the case-related wound team depends on:
- The location of the patients, e.g. clinic, rehabilitation clinic, home environment, nursing home
- The clinical aspect, e.g. vascular disease, diabetes, dermatological disease
- The type of wound treatment, e.g. the surgical team for negative pressure therapy

- Regional conditions, e.g. city/country, availability of experts
- The mobility and financial position of patients

Eleven different professions and institutions were involved in this particular case. It is possible to have more than 20 people involved in the same case. There should be at least three different people included in nursing services alone, due to holidays and illness; the wound care centre should have doctors and nursing wound experts at the very least; the ward team will involve a higher number of staff members. Excellent coordination, a standardised procedure and clear and complete documentation are required.

47.1.3 Structures

The structure of wound management depends on the institution. At least two nursing wound experts should be assigned to the hospital wards which usually treat people with chronic wounds. Their roles involve discussion of the local wound care with the attending physicians, carrying out dressing changes, assessing and documenting the progress, patient education and the regulation of post-operative care.

The establishment of central wound management and central wound treatment rooms (outpatient wound departments) has proven to be effective. The advantages are:
- Pooling of time and personnel resources
- Specially trained team develops routine
- Interdisciplinary use is possible
- All necessary materials are nearby
- Equipment for diagnostics and special therapies can be provided and thereby used economically, such as ultrasound-assisted debridement, cold plasma therapy, laser technology
- Wound cleansing facilities provided
- Treatment table facilitates the work
- Camera for wound photography and other equipment available
- Digital wound documentation with an interface to external treatment providers
- Quiet working area offers a suitable place for discussion of anamnesis and education
- Nursing wound experts on the staff can also provide a 'consultation service' for those areas which do not have nursing wound experts and only

rarely treat people with chronic wounds (ENT department, paediatric clinic, …). It is ideal if a senior physician is responsible for the consultation service and, if necessary, arranges for a diagnostic test and determines the therapy. An additional qualification in the field of wound diagnostics and treatment will be required.

Personnel occupation

The number of staff members required in central wound management depends on the number of patients and the medical orientation of the clinic. As there is a need for continuation of care in the event of staff members being ill or on holiday, it is advisable to have a nursing position and to recruit smaller hospitals (up to 500 beds) with part-time staff members. On top of a fundamental qualification in healthcare and nursing, nurses should have completed a basic and advanced course in wound management, in order to function as a nursing expert according to expert standards. For assigned physicians, there is a recommendation to obtain a wound-related qualification in addition to their specialist training.

It is recommended to have a wound treatment room staffed by wound care experts in rehabilitation clinics with a high number of wound patients. A consultation service should be available for immobile patients. Medical care for the chronic wound is more difficult in specific rehabilitation clinics with a fixed speciality (for example, internal medicine, neurology or oncology), as the treating physicians rarely encounter patients with chronic wounds during their training. In this case, the physician should thus have an additional qualification in the field of wound diagnostics and treatment.

For hospitals and rehabilitation clinics, there are interfaces to the internal departments of wards, outpatient clinics, discharge management, operating theatre, physiotherapy, hygiene management, kitchen, laboratory, central purchasing, pharmacy and administration as well as to specialists in private practice, general practitioners, nursing services, nursing facilities and homecare companies. The establishment of a database aids the network partners with additional information for clinicians to assess and communicate a treatment plan for the patient.

Qualification

The care of people with chronic wounds requires a well trained interprofessional and cross-facility team to function. Current situations show a gap in the continuation of care provided for the same patient when they transfer from one institution to another: therapies which had been started are not continued on an outpatient basis, or the local treatment is qualitatively unacceptable. The progress of the wound is not assessed correctly and documented, leading to a gap in timely interventions.

All professions involved deem the topic of 'chronic wounds' as taking a subordinate role in vocational training and studies. Offering further professional development is therefore urgently needed. There are specialised courses for this in the respective professional societies which should be certified and externally reviewed. A continuous update of knowledge can be acquired through sitting in on lectures in recognised wound centres to acquire training points, since practical application contributes to quality. A common theoretical basis is an ideal prerequisite for a wound team. Quality can be improved continuously in internal training courses and case discussions.

47.1.4 Process organisation

The more people are involved in the treatment of a patient with a wound, the more important it is to clarify everybody's responsibilities. Without a consultation, there is always an overlap in content which leads to duplicate or incorrect information. It begins with the medical anamnesis which focuses on diseases, diagnostics and therapy. The nursing wound anamnesis should contain the following parameters:
- Wound diagnostics:
  - Comorbidities
  - Previous diagnostic and therapeutic measures
- Wound localisation: graphic and written
- Wound duration, severity
- Recurrence rate
- Influencing factors
- Mobility and other limitations, pain, nutritional status, mental health
- Knowledge of the patient/resident and his/her relatives about the causes and healing of the wound

47

- Self-management skills

There will be duplicate entries with the medical anamnesis obtained. In both doctor and nursing documentation, they require the recording of some data which is essential for treatment planning. For example, the Wound-QoL questionnaire, which the patients fill out themselves, is suitable for recording the quality-of-life. The following step in the process will be an agreement with the patient on their treatment objective. Wound assessment should also be carried during the visit, as should the planning of local treatment. An internally defined assessment grid helps to ensure that the assessor does not overlook anything.

Example of a grid for wound assessment:

- Wound size: length, width, depth, cm^2
- Wound condition: tissue type, coatings, pockets
- Exudate: quantity and quality
- Wound odour: yes/no
- Wound margin: shape, colour, condition
- Wound environment: skin condition
- Signs of infection, allergies
- Wound pain

The more detailed the communication between physician, patient and nursing wound expert during the initial presentation, the smoother the rest of the treatment course will be. The physician can delegate data entry to the nursing wound expert during the visit. If unexpected events occur, a discussion must resume immediately. Experience and trust are a great advantage to the team.

The assignment of tasks between the wound care centre and the wound experts on the wards must be carefully defined. Depending on the workload, discharge management can be assigned to the Centre or to the wards. Without a consultation with the patient, everybody relies on the information provided by the others, i.e. recording of wound assessment on admission and discharge, wound anamnesis, patient education and target review.

Regular meetings of working groups (wound care circles) should involve 'wound care specialists' to ensure everybody in the team is kept in the loop on the patient's progress, so that everybody will be able to adapt to new circumstances promptly when they happen. Discussions in these meetings include the selection and use of wound materials (with the involvement of the central purchasing department and/or pharmacists) concerning the wound condition.

A regular evaluation of the treatment results provides information about the effectiveness of the initiated therapy, improves the quality, motivates those involved by talking about successful treatments and leads to objective analyses of their actions. Hospital management should support these wound care circles and the decisions made there should be binding for the hospital. In this way, the entire hospital can ensure an economical and high-quality process in wound management.

47.1.5 Communication structures

Documentation plays an essential role in the sharing of information. It pays off to utilise a well-structured documentation system which provides a quick overview of diagnostics already initiated, agreed targets, therapies commenced and the wound-healing progress, as well as the institutions and practitioners involved. Taking wound photos at every dressing change allows the attending physician to obtain information on the wound condition at any time without removing the dressing. It prevents unnecessary removal of wound dressings which interrupt the healing process and maximises the time and resources of the doctors and nursing staff when there is a shortage of nursing staff in clinics.

The recommendation to use a digital system for recording and documenting the wound progress helps to facilitate the transfer of information across institutions, and for quality assurance. Some hospital information systems include rudimentary wound documentation; however, these systems do not allow an interface with the outpatient sector due to data protection and safety. Therefore, an isolated web-based application for the wound outpatient department may be a possibility in this case.

Advantages:

- Central collection of all wound parameters
- Possibility of statistical analysis and thus quality control
- Control over material consumption
- Detection of problems, e.g. increase in multi-resistant pathogens
- Communication with the network: transfer documents created automatically
- Requirements for telemedicine

- Treatment plans can be printed out and given to the wards
- Contact information for network partners can be stored

47.1.6 Conclusion

A wound team can be seen as a department within the institution, consisting of the responsible physicians and nursing wound experts. Interface functions to all areas of the institution are created and described in the best possible way by clarifying the information pathways and responsibilities. Nursing wound experts should have a proper job description. For the medical sector, clarification of duties is necessary on an inter-disciplinary basis. If 'wound specialists' are appointed by the board of directors, they usually have a multi-disciplinary role. In other institutions, respective specialists are responsible. At least one suitable treatment room and appropriate wound documentation software are required. Progress depends on the competence of the clinician, the implementation of the concept and suitable communication structures.

REFERENCES
Bauer P, Otto U (eds.). Mit Netzwerken professionell zu-sammenarbeiten. Band II: Institutionelle Netzwerke in Steuerungs- und Kooperationsperspektive. Tübingen: dgvt-Verlag; 2005.
Deutsches Netzwerk für Qualitätsentwicklung in der Pflege (DNQP). Expertenstandard Pflege von Menschen mit chronischen Wunden. www.dnqp.de/fileadmin/HSOS/ Homepages/DNQP/Dateien/Expertenstandards/Pflege_ von_Menschen_mit_chronischen_Wunden/ChronWu_ Akt_Auszug.pdf (last acessed 12 October 2020).
Initiative Chronische Wunden e.V. (eds.). Lernbegleitbuch ICW. 3. ed. Eigenverlag; 2017.
London F. Informieren, Schulen, Beraten. Praxishandbuch zur Patientenedukation. 2. ed. Bern: Hans Huber; 2010.
Panfil EM, Schröder G (eds.), Pflege von Menschen mit chro-nischen Wunden. 3. ed. Bern: Hans Huber; 2015.
Schicker G. Praxisnetze im Gesundheitswesen. In: Schubert H (ed.): Netzwerkmanagement. Koordination von professionellen Vernetzungen. Wiesbaden: VS-Verlag für Sozialwissenschaften 2008; 146–166.
Voigt W (ed.). Kommunikation und Transparenz im Gesund-heitswesen. Marburger Schriftenreihe. Baden-Baden: Nomos; 2015.
Wimmer A, Wimmer J, Buchacher W, Kamp G. Das Bera-tungsgespräch. Skills und Tools für die Fachberatung. Wien: Linde; 2012.

47.2 Requirements for discharge management and structured outpatient wound care

---

Key notes

- The patient's discharge from the clinic must be well prepared.
- There should be communication between the various facilities.
- A functioning network facilitates intersectoral cooperation.

47.2.1 Discharge management

To be able to continue the treatment process initiated in the clinic on an outpatient basis, a structured transition is required. A letter of discharge to the family doctor is not sufficient, as other practitioners usually have to be involved. Depending on the clinical picture and the patient's self-care possibilities, the composition of the people and institutions to be informed varies. The work of transitional care therefore includes a needs analysis, identification of the outpatient practitioners, the need for aids, the required materials and services. Every patient with post-surgical care and support needs should receive individualised discharge management to ensure continuous and needs-based care. The prerequisite is the written consent of the patient. The patient has an unlimited right of choice in the selection of outpatient service providers. Prepared transfer protocols facilitate structured documentation provided to the patient. If necessary, the clinician can prescribe wound dressings and medication for the first seven days after discharge to avoid interruptions in care.

47

47.2.2 Requirements in the out-patient wound care sector

Information and coordination are even more challenging for the clinician in the outpatient setting than in the hospital, as there is no universal documentation basis and no clear assignment of tasks.

Example: A patient with a venous leg ulcer is cared for by his family doctor, the vascular surgeon, the physiotherapist and the nursing service. Who prescribes the compression therapy? Who trains the patient in health-promoting behaviour? Who checks the outcome of compression therapy? An explicit agreement between the parties involved is a good prerequisite for successful co-management. Role assignment should take into consideration the cost-effectiveness and legal requirements.

Based on the above example, there is a suggestion of how the process could be in Germany, for example. Internationally, the professional groups involved can be very different: the general practitioner recognises the necessity of the treatment and refers the patient to the vascular surgeon. The vascular surgeon carries out the diagnosis and treats the causal factors. He prescribes manual lymph therapy as well as the wound dressings and a multi-layer system for compression therapy, and calls in a nursing service for wound care and compression equipment. The medical assistant with an additional qualification for wound treatment will measure the calf circumference, apply the first dressing and compression bandage correctly and advise the patient on elevating the legs several times a day to support the therapy. When the patient is again presented to the vascular surgery practice, they will review the calf circumference measurement to assess the effectiveness of the treatment.

The tasks mentioned above can also be distributed differently depending on the clinician and the situation. Therefore, communication and documentation are indispensable in these processes.

47.2.3 Quality assurance

It is a significant challenge to ensure the universal quality of care for people with chronic wounds due to the difference in standards among institutions and the partners involved. Professions should implement the specified therapy plan, regularly monitoring the effectiveness of the therapy and changes should be recognised and reported back. It requires a good selection of the partners involved, with the establishment of suitable communication structures.

Case study example: Mrs. Z, a patient with a mixed leg ulcer, was diagnosed with a multi-resistant *Pseudomonas aeruginosa* wound infection by her family doctor. There is a need for immediate interventions as follows: the need for implementing local wound care, notifying a nursing service, providing the vascular surgeon and care team with the relevant information, and instructing patient and relatives on the cleansing protocol.

Suitable instruments are therefore required to measure and ensure quality across institutions. In addition to documentation, communication is essential. Keeping a 'wound passport' and bringing it to each visit with the doctor may be beneficial for the patient. It can include diagnostic and therapeutic measures as well as the wound condition. Corresponding documents are already available, such as the ICW wound passport. It aims to avoid duplication of examinations, to assess the course of treatment and to check the effectiveness of the therapy.

Network establishment

The establishment of regional networks greatly facilitates cooperation. Within the framework of quality circles, communication structures can be agreed upon among the partners to prevent redundant discussion for each new case.

The formation of a regional network is regarded as best practice. Yet this is still a conclusively agreed preliminary draft for the definition of required quality:
- The network ensures interprofessional, interdisciplinary and trans-sectoral care in the field of chronic wounds and/or palliative wound treatment.
- In this network, care sectors and professional groups involved in care, work together transparently, continuously and with quality assurance.
- Those involved in the network first develop the necessary regional, structural and process criteria to then jointly define the tasks, responsibilities and pathways of communication. For self-organi-

sation, the system designates network coordination.

- The network develops standards for all necessary process steps.
- The network ensures that a guide is available for each wound patient. The task of the guide is to coordinate the network partners.
- Each network partner is responsible for their own work and undertakes to provide care following the guidelines and care, completeness, accuracy and time efficiency.
- The comprehensive documentation of all steps taken is obligatory.
- The network creates a common communication platform to enable a routine, low-threshold and structured exchange of information between the parties involved.
- The network holds regular network meetings, case conferences and quality circles.

47.2.4 Conclusion

The success of wound treatment is mainly dependent on the quality of the implementation of prescribed measures. A reliable network enables continuous development and facilitates the transfer of information. Unfortunately, the necessary expenditure is not counter-financed at present. Conduction of similar pilot projects should take place in the form of a study to demonstrate the benefits and form a basis for the transfer of case management to standard care.

REFERENCES

Bauer P, Ullrich O (eds.). Mit Netzwerken professionell zusammenarbeiten. Band II: Institutionelle Netzwerke in Steuerungs- und Kooperationsperspektive. Tübingen: dgvt-Verlag; 2005.

Deutsches Netzwerk für Qualitätsentwicklung in der Pflege (DNQP). Expertenstandard Entlassmanagement in der Pflege. 2009. www.dnqp.de/fileadmin/HSOS/Homepages/DNQP/Dateien/Expertenstandards/Entlassungsmanagement_in_der_Pflege/Entlassung_Akt_Auszug.pdf (last acessed 12 October 2020).

Schicker G. Praxisnetze im Gesundheitswesen. In: Schubert H (ed.): Netzwerkmanagement. Koordination von professionellen Vernetzungen. Wiesbaden: VS-Publisher for Sozialwissenschaften 2008; 146–166.

Voigt W (ed.). Kommunikation und Transparenz im Gesundheitswesen. Marburger Schriftenreihe. Baden-Baden: Nomos-Verlag; 2015.

48

Health economics and people-centred wound care

Matthias Augustin, Rachel Sommer

Key notes

- Chronic wounds have a considerable socio-economic meaning and require early and appropriate action due to the high level of patient suffering and frequent escalation of findings.
- From a health economics perspective, the prevention of wound deterioration through rapid identification and timely treatment of the causes with evidence-based treatment is essential.
- The benefits of health economics are:
  a. to ensure specific qualifications of the doctors and nurses providing standardised care,
  b. the use of guidelines and standards,
  c. working with networks,
  d. communication between caregivers about the individual patient, and
  e. the availability of relevant information on the spot.
- Digital technologies will contribute to an increase in economic efficiency in these areas.
- The determinants of costs as well as the possibilities of cost avoidance are well described and require continuous attention in practice.

48.1 Costs and care situation of chronic wounds

Chronic wounds are a global problem with a considerable socio-economic burden for the state and society as well as individuals and their relatives, i.e. a relevant loss in the quality of life. The main determinants of these direct and indirect costs are the prolonged course of the disease which can extend over years or even decades. There is considerable co-morbidity of the patients, and noticeable physical, psychological and social complaints as a result of the wounds. Due to its prolonged origination time and the preceding development of the underlying pathology (e. g. vascular diseases), there is a long-term demand for the continuity of care, which in many countries is often not adequately covered.

The economic significance of chronic wounds lies not only in the monetary costs incurred by the patient, their relatives, the health insurance companies and the taxpayer but also in the intangible costs, i.e. the burdens on those affected and their environment. For example, more than 90% of patients with leg ulcers show a considerable loss in their quality of life and a sustained impairment in their living conditions. The latter concept is known as 'Cumulative Life Course Impairment' (CLCI). It goes from the premise that failure to improve the wound situation at an early stage leads in some cases to irreversible damage for the patient ('missed opportunities'), even if the wound heals again.

Prolonged suffering over time is also an extra economic premium. Approximately 80% of those affected suffer from severe pain, of which about 50% suffer without any relevant improvement from previous pain therapy. Patients are affected by a large number of other stresses and demands from their therapy besides pain and treatment frequency. Based on the 22 items in the 'Patient Needs Questionnaire', it was shown that in addition to the primary goal of complete wound-healing, intermediate goals such as pain reduction, improvement of mobility, decrease in unpleasant odours and exudate management are also of great importance. Patient-related stresses such as 'fear of disease progression' or 'loss of autonomy' also play a significant role in the planning of patient-centred care.

These intangible costs are an essential argument for treating chronic wounds timely and consistently or – even better – to avoid them. The yardstick for economic action is most important for the United Nations (UN) in their 'sustainable goals' and for the World Health Organisation (WHO) for timely and sufficient access to appropriate 'people-centred health-care'.

According to the current findings of research in health services, the treatment of these wounds falls short of its potential. This chapter aims to characterise significant health economic findings on the care of patients with chronic wounds, based on study data and surveys. There is an emphasis that an economic approach and solidarity-based care are not contradictory, but rather are essential in the care of chronic wounds.

48.2 Methods

The following methods are used for processing:
1. Systematic literature analysis in the international medical databases (Pubmed), including supplementary manual searches
2. Multisource data analysis through own primary and secondary data sources

48.3 Results

48.3.1 Systematic literature research

Up to 2017, a total of 492 relevant studies were found in a survey of the health economics of chronic wounds, spread relatively evenly across leg ulcers, diabetic foot syndrome, pressure ulcers and wounds in general (➤ Fig. 48.1).

The most frequent topics of health economic analyses were costs in general (56%), followed by cost-effectiveness studies (22%), healthcare cost studies (13%) and modelling (7%; ➤ Fig. 48.2).

Work on general wound care (50%) dominated in publications on therapeutic measures followed by local therapies (20%) and compression therapy (15%). Surgical interventions were less frequently represented (7%; ➤ Fig. 48.3).

The health economic analyses derived from clinical studies (59%), followed by meta-analyses (18%), systematic reviews (13%) and epidemiological studies (10%; ➤ Fig. 48.4).

The findings from the published literature are summarised synoptically below.

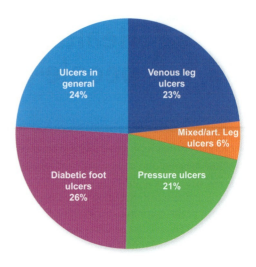

Fig. 48.1 Health economic analyses of chronic wounds: distribution of indications (n = 492 studies). [P593/L231]

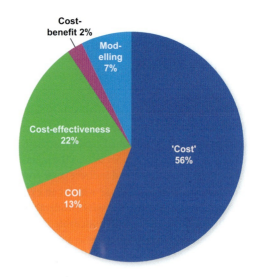

Fig. 48.2 Health economic analyses of chronic wounds: distribution of cost issues (COI = cost-of-illness studies). [P593/L231]

48.3.2 Findings from the published literature

Chronic wounds are frequently associated with high direct costs.

Due to demographic change, the diverse etiologies and the intrinsic risk diseases, such as peripheral vascular disease and diabetes mellitus, the

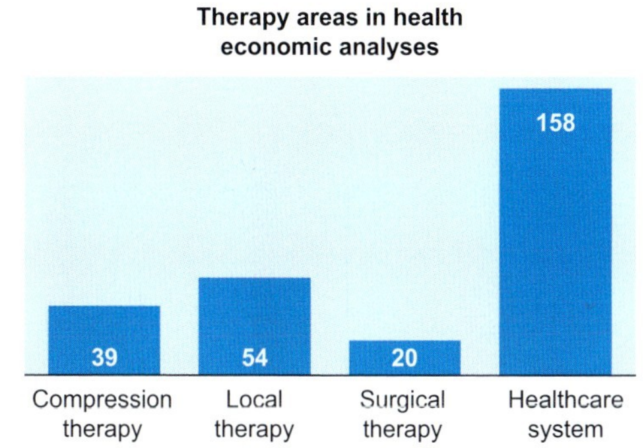

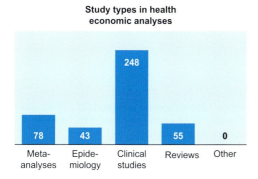

Fig. 48.3 Health economic analyses of chronic wounds: distribution of therapeutic areas. [P593/L231]

Fig. 48.4 Health economic analyses of chronic wounds: distribution of study types. [P593/L231]

about € 8,000 were found for a leg ulcer, with even more than € 10,000 per patient per year for arterial ulcers.

Chronic wounds are associated with considerable intangible costs (loss of quality of life) and a high burden of disease. These determine the goals of treatment.

Almost all patients (> 95%) are affected by quality of life problems in all areas, such as physical and psychological well-being, social contacts, work and leisure, and the therapy itself (➤ Fig. 48.5).

Identification on the loss of quality of life and the high disease burden of these patients' results have a significant impact and is essential to determine therapeutic goals ('patient needs') (➤ Table 48.2). The achievement of these objectives is considered a relevant economic benefit of the treatment. The most frequently mentioned therapeutic goals after complete healing are the reduction of pain, exudate and odour, but also general concerns such as less dependence on doctors and clinics and a return to everyday life (➤ Table 48.2).

The most substantial cost factors for chronic wounds are inpatient hospital treatment, followed by resource commitment for nursing staff and wound material.

Using the example of the leg ulcer, the major cost factors in the care of chronic wounds are inpatient treatment and outpatient care, followed by topical wound therapeutics (➤ Fig. 48.6).

Clinical predictors of medical costs include wound size, wound duration and the presence of arterial circulatory disorders.

In a comprehensive real-world study involving patients from all areas of care, the regression analysis revealed inpatient therapy and clinical differences as significant predictors (➤ Table 48.3, ➤ Table 48.4).

Low compliance and adherence are drivers of higher costs.

socio-economic significance of chronic wounds is also increasing. Several primary data studies have equally shown that the treatment of chronic wounds is of high relevance in terms of annual costs, particularly from the perspective of the funding agencies (➤ Table 48.1). For example in Germany the average yearly cost of leg ulcers was € 9,500 (corresponds approximately 11,700 USD $). Mean high annual costs of

Table 48.1 Prevalence and medical costs of venous leg ulcers in Germany based on direct costing

Wound type	Prevalence (approx.)	People (approx.)	Mean time to heal (month)	Direct costs per patient/year (euro)	Annual costs (in bn. euro)
Diabetic foot ulcer	0.31	254,200	48	10,000	2,54
Pressure ulcer	0.35	287,000	72	8,000	2,30
Leg ulcer	0.42	344,400	65	12,000	4,13
Total		**885,600**			**8,97**

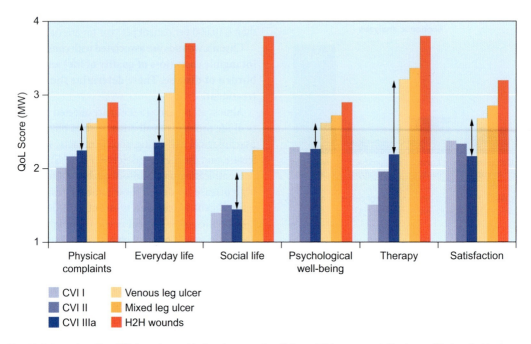

Fig. 48.5 Loss of quality of life in patients with chronic venous insufficiency (Widmer stages I–IIIa, in grey-blue) and with ulcers (in orange-red) In the different dimensions: poorly healing wounds (hard-to-heal [H2H] wounds of any aetiology) have the highest disease burden. The quality of life potentially gained by ulcer-healing is shown in blue. [P593/L231]

Table 48.2 The most frequently mentioned goals in the treatment of venous leg ulcers from the patient's perspective, measured on n = 290 patients with the Patient Benefit Index (PBI)

10 most frequent therapy targets for wounds	% of patients
Be healed from the wound(s)	100
Be free of pain	97
Be less dependent on doctor and clinical visits	96
Be able to lead a normal everyday life	94
Have confidence in the therapy	92
Have no discharge from the wound	92
Have no unpleasant smell from the wound	89
Have no fear that the disease will become worse	86
Find a clear diagnosis and therapy	85
Need less time for daily treatment	84

Conversely, in a study with venous leg ulcer patients, the improvement in adherence led to a doubling of healing rates. Recurrence rates were 2 to 20 times higher when patients did not become compliant with the use of compression stockings after ulcer-healing. The authors concluded that the non-adherence to compression therapy had a negative therapeutic outcome on ulcer care and that the patient adherence had to be improved to maximise the therapeutic result. In another study by Erickson, patients with strict compliance showed a shortened time to healing (p<0.02) and a longer time to relapse (p<0.004) compared to less compliant patients.

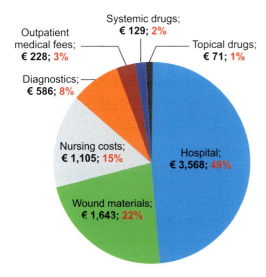

Fig. 48.6 Cost distribution in the care of chronic wounds by cost groups (n = 526 patients). [P593/L231]

The early initiation of appropriate care supports the avoidance of costs and the burden of disease, becoming one of the essential measures in terms of health economics.

Early, appropriate intervention and the introduction of consistent causal therapies can avoid the wound worsening and becoming chronic (➤ Fig. 48.7). It avoids not only higher costs but also the burden of disease for the patient.

Investment in early interventions and treating causal factors makes economic sense in the long term, even with higher initial costs.

Treatment of causal factors often requires an initial higher outlay in terms of care, which usually pays off again in the medium term through higher healing rates (➤ Fig. 48.8). Assessment of this principle is required for each therapy based on the cost-benefit data, but it is demonstrated for many therapies. It also applies to the prevention of wounds, especially in patients with venous insufficiency. The continuous material costs for compression systems were more than compensated economically by avoiding new wound formation (➤ Fig. 48.9). Conversely, the lack of causal therapy induces higher costs because the duration of the wound course is considerably prolonged.

Qualification and quality of the nursing staff and doctors providing care determine a higher level of efficiency.

These can be checked by using quality indicators based on the scientific guidelines (➤ Fig. 48.10). It is noteworthy that for example in Germany, care by qualified health care professionals and nursing staff has already led to a measurably better quality of care. The introduction of standards in care can also lead to higher economic efficiency. Against this background, the national consensus conference on chronic wounds has a high health-economic relevance.

The involvement of specialised doctors and nurses improves patient benefits and increases efficiency.

Based on the Patient Benefit Index (PBI), it shows what additional benefits patients with chronic wounds would have if admitted to a specialised wound care centre. The PBI records the needs and goals of patients from a list of 25 potential items and summarises these into a single benefit value by therapy. At the transition to specialised care, the distribution of these benefits was (➤ Fig. 48.11 right) significantly better.

In the outpatient and inpatient treatment of chronic wounds, the use of wound dressings that need less changing can improve cost-effectiveness.

Table 48.3 Correlation analysis and regression analysis (➤ Table 48.4) with the predictors or group differences of higher costs in the care of the leg ulcer

Parameters	Unit	Correlation with costs r =	p	n
Hospital stays	Numbers	.651	< 0.001	502
Wound size	cm^2	.472	< 0.001	502
Number of wounds	N	.437	< 0.001	502
Wound duration	Years	.321	< 0.001	502
Quality of life	FLQA score	.267	< 0.001	502
Quality of care	Quality index	.257	< 0.001	502

Table 48.4 Correlation analysis (➤ Table 48.3) and regression analysis with the predictors or group differences of higher costs in the care of the leg ulcer

Parameters	Subgroup	Average costs/year [€]	Test
Wound type	Venous leg ulcer	8,847	
	Arterial ulcer	13,060	
	Mixed ulcer	11,917	p<0.01, Chi-Square test
Treatment at	Wound centre	11,802	
	General practitioner	9,011	p<0.001, Chi-Square test
Nursing service	Yes	7,057	
	No	14,971	p<0.001, Mann-Whitney-U-test
Wound closure	Intermittent	8,606	
	No	10,894	p<0.001, Mann-Whitney-U-test
Living alone	Yes	11,063	
	No	9,366	p<0.01, Kruskal-Wallis-test

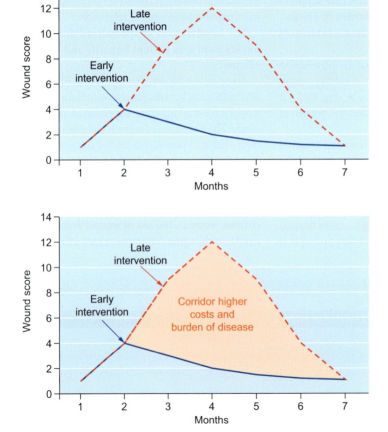

Fig. 48.7 Diagram of the benefits of early interventions by averting escalation with higher costs and disease. [P593/L231]

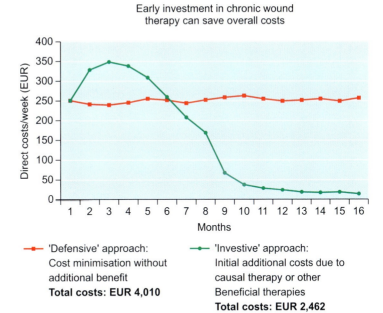

Fig. 48.8 Schematic representation of the cost-effectiveness
of the early use of higher-priced
treatment methods that are
associated with better causal
therapy or other higher benefits.
[P593/L231]

Early investment in chronic wound
therapy can save overall costs

━■━ 'Defensive' approach:
Cost minimisation without
additional benefit
Total costs: EUR 4,010

━●━ 'Investive' approach:
Initial additional costs due to
causal therapy or other
Beneficial therapies
Total costs: EUR 2,462

Korn 2002: J Vasc Surg 35: 950-7
'Why insurers should reimburse for
compression stockings in patients
with chronic venous stasis.'
Economical Markov model
for the United States

Life-time costs of venous leg ulcers

a) Whithout compression	$ 20.492
b) With compression	$ 14.588
Difference:	$ 5.904

Fig. 48.9 Greater cost-effectiveness of chronic venous
insufficiency care with lifelong use of compression systems.
Although the latter tie up higher material costs, the overall
benefit of avoiding ulceration is higher. [F1026-001]

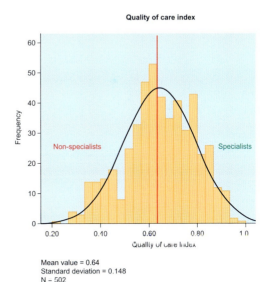

Mean value = 0.64
Standard deviation = 0.148
N – 502

Fig. 48.10 Distribution of the quality of care for patients
with leg ulcers in general care, measured by the degree to
which quality indicators have been achieved. A low index
means the low achievement of the indicators, a high index
high achievement (1.0 – 100% achieved indicators). In the
regression analysis, a high care index is associated with significantly more frequent involvement of wound specialists in
the medical and nursing profession. [P593/L231]

Qualified nursing staff are one of the most critical
resources, but also cost drivers of the wound therapy
(➤ Table 48.5). Nursing staff should assess and
control the use of materials in a way that mini-
mises frequent dressing changes as far as possible.
Material and personnel costs must always be seen in
conjunction with each other, and the benefit threshold
between personnel commitment and additional costs
for less frequent dressing changes must be determined
in each case.

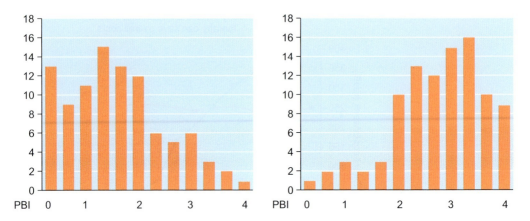

Fig. 48.11 Added value through the use of a specialised wound care centre, measured by the Patient Benefit Index (PBI) in primary care (left) and in specialised care (right). PBI = 0 means no patient-relevant benefit, PBI > 2 is a high benefit. The distributions of n = 100 patients are shown. [P593/L231]

Table 48.5 Comparison of the use of personnel and materials between conventional and hydroactive wound dressings in wound care (data from CWC Hamburg, Germany)

Day	Conventional Personnel	Hydroactive Personnel	Conventional Dressing	Hydroactive Dressing	Conventional Cumulative costs (€)	Hydroactive Cumulative costs (€)
1	9.45	9.45	5.52	15.89	14.97	25.34
2	9.45		5.52		29.94	25.34
3	9.45		5.52		44.91	25.34
4	9.45	9.45	5.52	15.89	59.88	50.68
5	9.45		5.52		74.85	50.68
6	9.45		5.52		89.82	50.68
7	9.45	9.45	5.52	15.89	104.79	76.02
8	9.45		5.52		119.76	76.02
9	9.45		5.52		134.73	76.02
10	9.45	9.45	5.52	15.89	149.70	101.36
11	9.45		5.52		164.67	101.36
12	9.45		5.52		179.64	101.36
13	9.45	9.45	5.52	15.89	194.61	126.70
14	9.45		5.52		209.58	126.70
15	9.45		5.52		224.55	126.70
16	9.45	9.45	5.52	15.89	239.52	152.04
17	9.45		5.52		254.49	152.04
18	9.45		5.52		269.46	152.04
	170.10	**56.70**	**99.36**	**95.34**	**269.46**	**152.04**

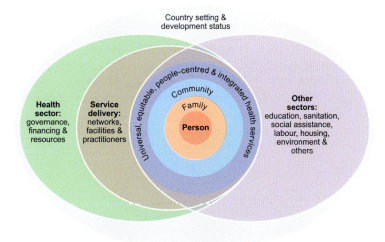

Fig. 48.12 'People-centred Health Care' as the basis of care and as a model for the improved care of chronic wounds. [P593/L231]

48.4 Conclusion

Economics of wounds in the context of ethical and social law

The treatment of chronic wounds is of considerable economic importance. As the most important predictors of costs, disease burden and possible solutions can be identified based on evidence and studies.

The measures of control and insufficient implementation of chronic wound care were identified as the more significant health economic hurdle.

It requires action, and the WHO has made a significant call for the concept of 'People-centred Health Care' (➤ Fig. 48.12). The central message is: *'Active consideration and inclusion of the needs and requirements of people with chronic diseases at all levels of participation and across sectors'*. It also applies to those countries, which despite a highly developed economic status are not sufficiently prepared to provide appropriate care for people with chronic wounds.

Economic decisions are essential here but require constant guidance by clinical necessity and the social and legal entitlement of patients in the respective countries.

REFERENCES

Augustin M, Brocatti LK, Rustenbach SJ, Schaefer I, Herberger K. Cost-of-illness of leg ulcers in the community. Int Wound J 2014; 11: 283–292.

Augustin M, Conde Montero E, Zander N, et al. Validity and feasibility of the Wound-QoL questionnaire on health-related quality of life in chronic wounds. Wound Repair Regen 2017; 25: 852–857.

Augustin M, Debus ES (eds.). Moderne Wundversorgung – im Spannungsfeld zwischen Qualitätsanspruch, Zuständigkeiten und Sparzwang. Bd. 2. Bonn: Beta Verlag; 2011.

Herberger K, Rustenbach SJ, Grams L, et al. Quality-of-Care for leg ulcers in the metropolitan area of Hamburg – a community-based study. J Eur Acad Dermatol Venereol 2012; 26: 495–502.

Heyer K, Herberger K, Protz K, et al. Epidemiology of chronic wounds in Germany: Analysis of statutory health insurance data. Wound Repair Regen 2016; 24: 434–442.

Purwins S, Herberger K, Debus ES, et al. Cost-of-illness of chronic leg ulcers in Germany. Int Wound J 2010; 7: 97–102.

Index